BIOCHEMISTRY
AND
THERAPEUTIC ATTRIBUTES
OF
CULINARY HERBS

BIOCHEMISTRY AND THERAPEUTIC ATTRIBUTES OF CULINARY HERBS

Authors

Dr. Bina Rani
Former Associate Professor
Department of Chemistry and Environmental Engineering
Poornima College of Engineering
Jaipur (Rajasthan)

Dr. Raaz K. Maheshwari
Former Professor
SBRM Govt. PG College, Nagaur
Rajasthan

Dr. Lalit Mohan
Assistant Professor
Department of Zoology
Dayalbagh Educational Institute
(Deemed to be University)
Agra, Uttar Pradesh

Co-Authors

Dr. Upma Singh
Head
Department of Applied Chemistry
University School of Vocational Studies and Applied Sciences
Gautam Buddha University
Greater Noida, Uttar Pradesh

Lakha Ram
Assistant Professor
Department of Chemistry
SBRM Govt. PG College
Nagaur, Rajasthan

Dr. Ravi Sharma
Jai NarainVyas University
Jodhpur, Rajasthan

Dr. Manish Maheshwari
Associate Professor
Department of Zoology
Dharam Samaj (PG) College, Aligarh
Uttar Pradesh

Dr. Jaswant Ray
President
Society for Environment Health, Awareness of Nutrition and Toxicology
(SEHAT-INDIA)
F-119, Pandav Nagar, Meerut-UP-250003

DPH

DISCOVERY PUBLISHING HOUSE
INDIA

Published by:

DISCOVERY PUBLISHING HOUSE
4383/4B, Ansari Road, Darya Ganj
New Delhi-110 002 (India)
Phone : +91-11-23279245; 23253475; 43596065
E-mail : discoverybooksindia@gmail.com
discoverypublishinghouse@gmail.com
namitwasan9@gmail.com
web : www.discoverypublishinggroup.com

***First Edition:* 2023**

ISBN: 978-93-94917-06-4

Biochemistry and Therapeutic Attributes of Culinary Herbs

CO-AUTHORS

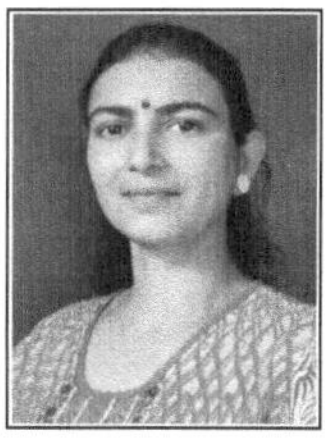

Dr. Upma Singh, is serving as Head, Department of Applied Chemistry, University School of Vocational Studies and Applied Sciences, Gautam Buddha University, Greater Noida. She did her Ph.D. in the field of metal complexes. She has published more than 50 research papers, review articles and book chapters encompassing the field of coordination compounds, natural products, bio-pesticides, environmental issues and dietary habits. She authored a book entitled, "Green Technologies for Environmental Security". She has participated and presented papers in number of Conferences/Seminars/Workshops, and chaired the sessions also. More than 15 students did their M.Sc. projects and awarded two Ph.D. degrees under her supervision. She is associated to various scientific and academic societies. She takes pride in being into the teaching profession and has been into teaching for nearly two decades.

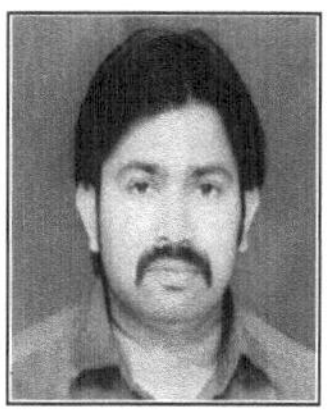

Dr. Ravi Sharma is a freelance researcher in the field of environmental Chemistry and presently working in Jai NarainVyas University Jodhpur, Rajasthan, as a research fellow in enviro-chemical lab. He pursued his Ph.D., in hydro-geo chemistry. He has been awarded by various societies. He served for 3 years as anresearch assistant in department of chemistry, JNV University Jodhpur. He has in his credit more than 30 review/research publications in Journals of International repute. He is founder of forum Enviro 9 focussing on environmental issues, multidisciplinary awareness programmes and environment literacy in India. He guided 20 DST- Inspire scholars at UG and PG level.

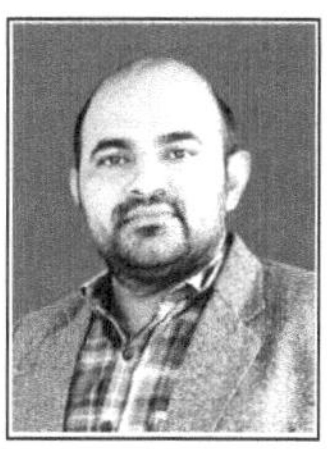

Mr. Lakha Ram, is working as Assistant Professor in the Department of Chemistry, SBRM Govt. PG College Nagaur, Rajasthan. He has guided 10 Inspire (Innovation in Science Pursuit for Inspired Research)-DST, Projects New Delhi of UG level. He is young research fellow member (SYRFM) of Scholar Academic and Scientific Society, Member of American Chemical Society, Member of Intellectuals Society for Socio-Techno Welfare, Life member of National Environmental Science Academy, New Delhi, Fellow of Koshambi Foundation, India (FKFI). He has published 3 book chapters, 17 review articles and 4 research papers in journals of national and international repute. His area of research is hydrochemistry, Nano-Technological approaches to purify of contaminated underground water, Green Chemistry. Mr. Lakha Ram has been awarded Best Innovative Researcher of the Year award 2021 by DHS Foundation, New Delhi, Young Environmentalist Award by Koshambi Foundation India, Agra, UP and Young Scientist of the Year award by National Environmental Science Academy, (NESA) New Delhi.

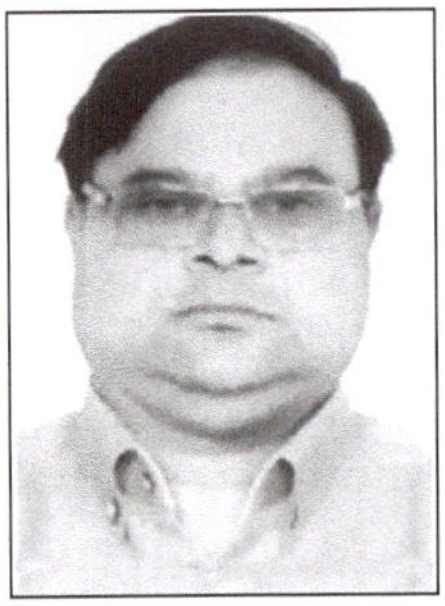

Dr. Manish Maheshwari has been serving in the field of Higher Education Science 2009. Currently, he is Associate Professor, Department of Zoology, DharamSamaj (PG) College, Aligarh, Affiliated to RMPSS University, Aligarh, previously Affiliated to Dr. BRA University, Agra from Aug. 2021 and previously work as Assistant Professor in NREC College, Khurja (Bulandshahar) Affiliated to CCS University, Meerut. Dr. Maheshwaridid his M.Phil and Ph.D., in Zoology from Dr. BRA University, Agra. He published more than 15 research article in various reputed journals and books. He has actively participated in more than 60 national/international seminars, conferences, workshops and Webinars. His area of specialization are Environmental Toxicology, Endocrinology and Fisheries Sciences.

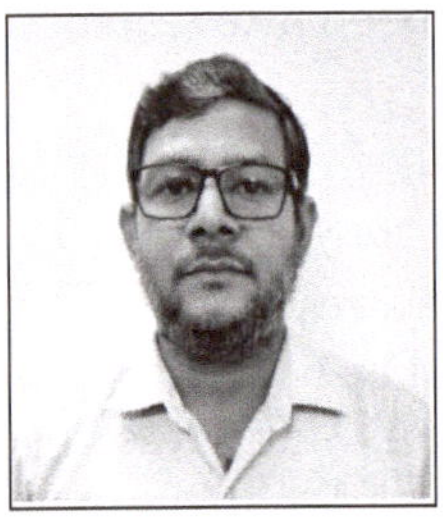

Dr. Jaswant Ray is working as a Manager (Research & Development) in AGSS Analytical and Research Lab (P) Ltd, Delhi; He has completed M.Sc. in Toxicology, B. Ed, UGC-NET, DPT, DYT, Auditor- ISO/IEC 17025, ISO 9001; 14001; 45001 and B.A.S.M (Alternative Medicine). His area of interest is Toxicology, Eco-Toxicology, Food Toxicology, Pesticides, Microbiology, Water and Environmental pollution, Alternative Medicine- Physical Therapy & Naturopathy. He is serving as President, *Society for Environment, Health, Awareness of Nutrition and Toxicology (SEHAT)* and social activist and consultant of Scientific laboratory/industries for Research & Development. He organized various health, environment, agriculture & farming awareness programs and organized National and International conferences, seminar. He published many paper, articles (+25) and books (+20). Membership of National and International Scientific Organization: He has membership of Society of Toxicology, India (STOX), which is the part of International Union of Toxicology (IUTOX); The Academy of Environmental Biology, India; Krishnamurthy Institute of Algology, India; British Toxicology Society (BTS); Member of International Society for Infectious Diseases (ISID).

**Dedicated to our Parents and
Specially dedicated to our beloved son
Late Mr. Aishwary Raaz**

(Dr. Bina Rani)

(Dr. Raaz K. Maheshwari)

Preface

India is the largest producer and consumer of some important common spices which are an important range of horticultural products. According to a report of International Organization for Standardization (ISO), 120 spices are grown in various regions of the world and more than 70 spices are grown in India. India has been recognized as the 'Land of Spices' from the dawn of time because India is the only country in the world with such a broad range of spice crops. India is one of the world's leading spice producers and exporters, accounting for around 25-30% of the global spice commercially. The scent, flavor and pungency of Indian spices are well-known. According to the tradition and research findings, spices have been recognized to serve more than only as flavorants. They have a lot of applications in ethno-medicine as the extracts and essential oils of spices are utilized in perfumery, insecticidal, cosmetic and pharmaceutical sectors. Moreover, they abundantly use in the manufacturing of Ayurvedic medicines and in the food industry as value added goods are in high demand. In addition, spices enhance shelf life of the food by preventing and delaying the spoilage and by preserving the sensory attributes of food products. Spices contain several important phytochemicals like aromatic compounds, essential oils, phenolics and pigments which impart characteristic flavor and aroma and gives a herbal appeal to the food and beverages and enhances their consumer acceptability. Spices are valuable plants that provide significant prospects for national economic security through agricultural output. Through local and international trade, this will create employment and offer a source of earning for the countries.

Spices derived from seeds are high in fat, protein and carbs. Spices are important sources of micro and macronutrients in the diet. Calcium, phosphorus, magnesium, and micronutrients like zinc are abundant in many spices. Spices are also high in phenolic compounds, which have antioxidant properties that influenced nutrition in a variety of ways. They react with a fat free radical or a surrogate radical to delay or hinder the commencement of the propagation stage. They may also stop a free radical chain reaction from continuing by providing hydrogen or electron to free radicals and converting them to stable compounds, i.e. they operate as hydrogen donors and free radical acceptors. Spices have antimicrobial effects that can be classified as bactericidal, bacteriostatic and fungicidal. Volatile components of Cardamom and Turmeric have an inhibiting impact on Gram-negative bacteria. The essential oil of Cinnamon, Clove, Oregano and Thyme stopped the mycelia of many species of fungi from growing. Nutmeg extracts were found to be effective against twenty-five different types of bacteria. The phytonutrients of spices explains the robust link between greater intakes, illness prevention in humans and plays a crucial pathogenic function such as cancer, arthrosclerosis, and arthritis. Lipid peroxidation is significantly linked to ageing and cancer development. Spice antioxidants in the diet may protect against peroxidative damage. Antioxidant capabilities have been documented. Spices are also used to treat diarrhea, gastro-intestinal problems, fever, post-partum discomfort, tapeworms, tonsil and throat irritation in a variety of traditional medicines. Clove oil is used as an antiseptic during surgery, Nutmeg to relieve coughs and Black pepper to speed up the healing of tiny wounds. Because of their carminative characteristics, several spices have been recognized to aid digestion, antipyretic and diuretic properties.

Furthermore, spices also have food preservation, repellent and insecticidal properties due to their volatile oils and oleoresins. Spices have the potential to be employed in pest control, and it has been proposed that the pungent odor of essential oils or oleoresin can provide insect protection. Nutmeg and Clove essential oils proved efficient against insects infesting maize in storage. Black pepper have insect repellent abilities and used to protect garments from moths. Under hermetic conditions, screened pepper fruits were shown to destroy all life stages of *Callotsobruchus maculatus* in preserved cowpea. Phytochemicals of spices are terpenes such as cineole, pinene, camphene, camphor and eugenol are linked to the insecticidal and repellent characteristics. Spices also contained alkaloids, glycoside, saponins, flavonoids, reducing compounds, polyphenol, phlobatannins and anthraquinones. The nutritional and medicinal qualities of the spices demonstrates that they have enormous health benefits. Overall, the spices are significant because of their numerous beneficial properties.

In addition the active components of these herbs and spices are endowed with tremendous functional properties and medicinal values providing several health benefits and immunity. The era of Covid-19 has seen spiked consumption of spices and herbs based health drinks and concoctions for providing these health benefits and immunity. The present book deals with the characteristics of some important Indian spices, their usages, active components present in them along with exploring their health benefits, functional and immunomodulant properties. The toxicological aspect and adverse effects of the spices are not covered in this book.

–Authors

Contents

CHAPTER

1

Contemplation towards Potentiality of various Pharmacognostic, Phytochemical and Pharmacological Profiles of Indigenous India Herb Ajwain (*Trachyspermum ammi* L.)

ABSTRACT

Ajwain fruit (seed) is claimed to be very important in the treatment of many ailments in humans. The plant, *Trachyspermum ammi* Linn., is a grassy, aromatic annual plant, which falls in the family Umbelliferae. This plant is grown in India, Iran, Pakistan, Egypt, etc. for its medicinal benefits. Tribals of India use it for the treatment of diarrhea, arthritis, colic and gastrointestinal problems. Ajwain seed analysis has revealed that it contains fibres, carbohydrates, tannins, glycosides, moisture, proteins, fats, saponins, flavones, nicotinic acid and mineral matters containing calcium, phosphorous and iron. The Ajwain fruits yields brownish essential oil, with thymol as the major constituent. Thenonthymol fraction (thymene) contains para-cymene, γ- terpenine, α- and β-pinenes, dipentene, α-terpinene and carvacrol. Minute amounts of camphene, myrcene and α-3-carene also have been found in the plant. Alcoholic extracts contain a highly hygroscopic saponin. From the fruits, a yellow, crystalline flavone and a steroid-like substance have been isolated and it also contains 6-O-β-glucopyranosyloxythymol, aglucoside and a yield of oleoresin containing volatile oil (thymol, γ- terpinene,para-cymene, and α- and β- pinene). The plant is used traditionally as a stimulant and carminative for flatulence and also for the treatment of atonic dyspepsia, diarrhoea, abdominal tumors, abdominal pains, piles, and bronchial problems, lack of appetite, galactogogue, asthma and amenorrhoea. It also possess various pharmacological activities like antifungal, antioxidant, antimicrobial, antinociceptive, cytotoxic, Hypolipidaemic, Antihypertensive, antispasmodic, Antilithiasis, diuretic, Abortifacient, Antitussive, Nematicidal, Anthelmintic and Antifilarial activity and broncho-dilating actions. The present review summarizes the information concerning the pharmacognostic, photochemistry and pharmacological studies of *Trachyspermum ammi*.

Keywords: Flavone, α- and β-pinenes, Saponin, 6-O-β-glucopyranosy-loxythymol, Carminative, Hypolipidaemic, Antihypertensive, Diuretic.

Introduction

Name for *Trachyspermum ammi* (ajwain) belongs to the family of Apiaceae (Umbelliferae), of the genus; *Trachyspermum*. The Umbellifers are the members of carrot or parsley family, which includes many herbs and spices such as dill, fennel, anise seed and caraway, is an annual herbal plant growing up to 3 feet in height bearing feathery leaves and red flowers. Some of the common names for the seeds are Bishop's Weed, Ajowan, carom, Caraway and thymol seeds etc. Carom seeds are ovoid and light brown in color. They have narrow green leaves and small delicate flowers. The fruits pods of these plants are often called seeds for their seed-like appearance. The Carom plants are believed to have originated from Egypt in Middle East. They are widely grown in India, Afghanistan and Iran [1-3]. In India, the major ajwain producing states are Rajasthan and Gujarat, where Rajasthan produces about 90% of India's total production. When the seeds are ripe, they are dried and threshed. In Ajwain, the major phenolic compound thymol has been reported to be an antispasmodic, germicide and antifungal agent [4-5]. In the essential oil of *T. ammi*, the principle active constituents are phenols, mainly thymol and some carvacrol. Both the phenols are responsible for the antiseptic, antitussive and expectorant properties. Carvacrol also possesses antifungal properties. It also prevents indigestion, abdominal pain and all other abdominal disorders. The plant is used traditionally as a stimulant and carminative for flatulence and also to treat diseases like atonic dyspepsia, diarrhoea, abdominal tumors, abdominal pains, piles, bronchial problems, lack of appetite, galactogogue, asthma and amenorrhoea. Medicinally, it has been proven to possess various pharmacological Activities like Antifungal, Antioxidant, Antimicrobial, Antinociceptive, Cytotoxic, Hypolipidaemic, Antihypertensive, Antispasmodic, Antilithiasis, Diuretic, Abortifacient, Antitussive, Nematicidal, Anthelmintic, Antifilarial activity and Broncho-Dilating Actions. The roots are diuretic in nature and the seeds possess excellent aphrodisiac properties. The seeds contain 2-4.4% brown coloured oil known as ajwain oil [6-7]. The main component of this oil is thymol, which is used to cure gastrointestinal ailments, lack of appetite and bronchial problems. The oil exhibits fungicidal, antimicrobial and anti-aggregatory effects on humans. The present review paper highlights the phytochemistry, pharmacological activities and traditional benefits of the plant.

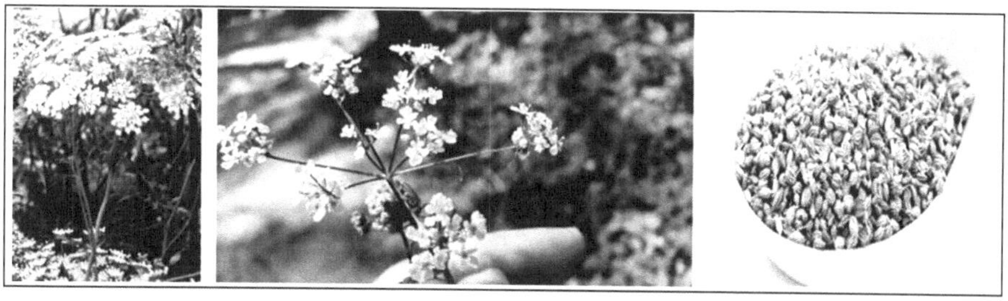

Trachyspermu ammni **Plant and fruits**

Phytochemistry and Pharmacological Profile

Traditional therapeutic uses of *Trachyspermum ammi* fruits include: galactogogue, stomachic, carminative, expectorant, antiseptic, amoebiasis, antimicrobial seeds fried in oil and used as a thin soup as a galactogogue, used in curing diarrhoea, Parasiticidal, and given in treatment of amenhorroea, Bronchitis, colic pain, Antipyretic and febrifugal. The seed of Ajwain is bitter, pungent and it acts as anthelmintic, carminative, laxative, and stomachic [8-9]. It also cures abdominal tumors, abdominal pains, and piles. Presence of terpenes, glycosides and sterols in plant has been found to exert active anti-inflammatory effects.

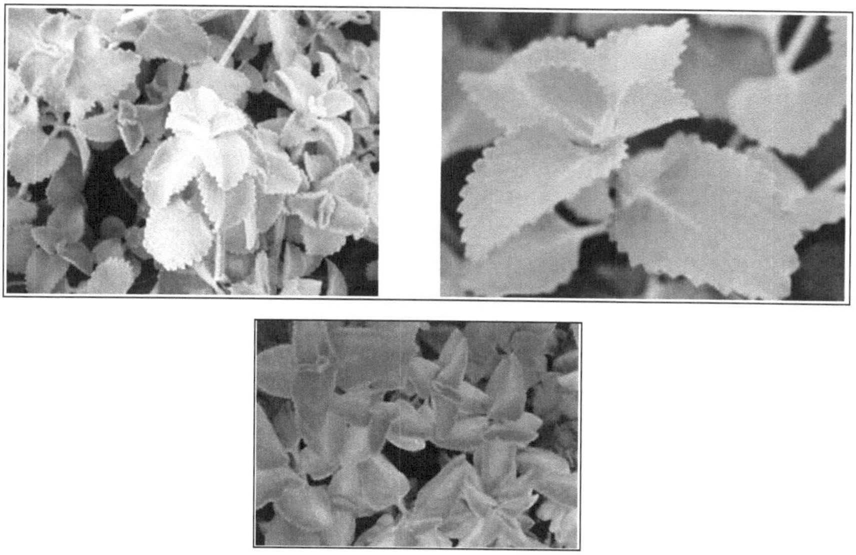

Trachyspermum ammi **(Ajwain leaves)**

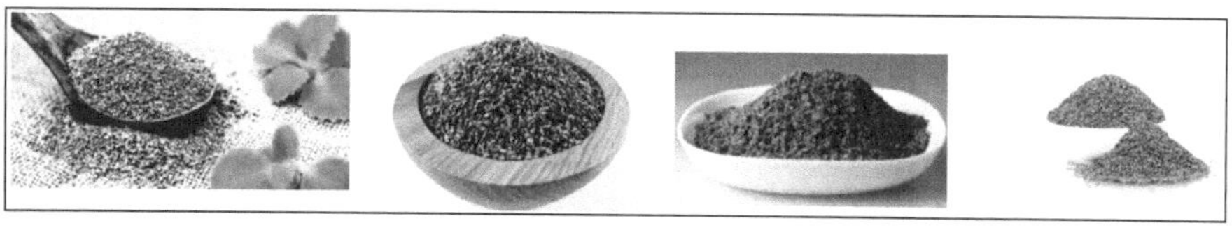

Ajwain seed is very valuable for its oil contents. It is a high value medicinally important seeds. Ajwain is most widely used for the treatment of many diseases in both animals and humans. Ajwain seeds are most commonly used as a household remedy for diarrhea, asthma, colic, and dyspepsia and they also have antifungal, antibacterial, antihelminthic, antioxidant properties. The active components of ajwain essential oils are phenolic carvacrol and mainly thymol. Both are responsible for antitussive and antiseptic properties. The phenolic compound thymol, is germicide, antifungal, and an antispasmodic agent. Ajwain essential oil showed the presence of 26 identified components which account for 96.3% of the total amount [1-13]. Thymol (39.1%) was found as a major component along with p-cymene (30.8%), γ-terpinene (23.2%), γ-pinene (1.7%), terpinene-4-ol (0.8%) whereas acetone extract of ajwain showed the presence of 18 identified components which account for 68.8% of the total amount. The major component was thymol (39.1%) followed by oleic acid (10.4%), linoleic acid (9.6%), γ-terpinene (2.6%), p-cymene (1.6%), palmitic acid (1.6%) and xylene (0.1%). Ajwain seed analysis has revealed it to contain fibre (11.9%), carbohydrates (38.6%), tannins, glycosides, moisture (8.9%), protein (15.4%), fat (18.1%), saponins, flavone andmineral matter (7.1%) containing calcium, phosphorous, iron and nicotinic acid. The Ajwain fruits yields 2% to 4% brownish essential oil, with thymol as the major constituent (35% to 60%). The non-thymol fraction (thymene) contains para-cymene, γ-terpenine, α- and β-pinenes, dipentene, α-terpinene, and carvacrol. Minute amounts of caphene, myrcene and α-3-carene also have been found in the plant. Alcoholic extracts contain a highly hygroscopic saponin. From the fruits, a yellow, crystalline flavone and a steroid-like substance have been isolated and also contain 6-O-β-glucopyranosyloxythymol, a glucoside and a yield of 25% oleoresin containing 12% volatile oil (thymol, γ-terpinene, para-cymene and α- and β-pinene [14-17]. The principal oil constituents of *T. ammi* are carvone (46%), limonene (38%) and dillapiole (9%).

In Indian system of medicine, Ajwain is administered as a stomach disorders, a paste of crushed fruits is applied externally for relieving colic pains and a hot and dry fomentation of the fruits applied on chest for asthma. *T. ammi* has been shown to possess Antimicrobial, Hypolipidaemic, Digestive stimulant, Antihypertensive, Hepatoprotective, Antispasmodic, Bronchodilating, Antilithiasis, diuretic, Abortifacient, galactogogic, Antiplatelet-Aggregatory, Antiinflammatory, Antitussive effects, Antifilarial,Gestroprotective, Nematicidal, Anthelmintic, Detoxification of aflatoxins and Ameliorative effect. Therapeutic uses of *T. ammi* fruits include stomachic, carminative, expectorant, antiseptic and amoebiasis, it is also used as Antipyretic, febrifugal and in the treatment of typhoid fever [18-24].

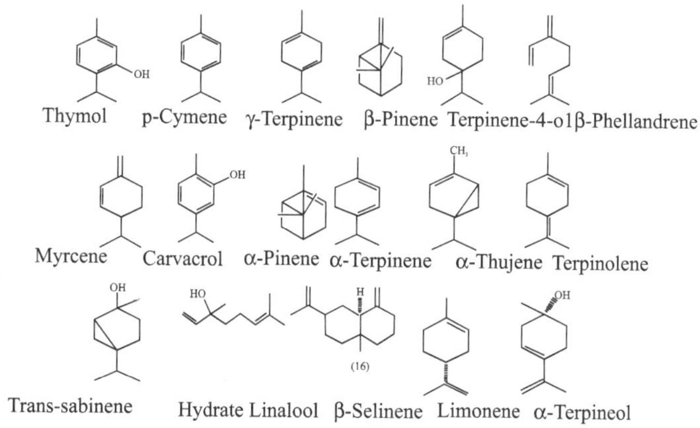

Structure of Chemical constituents occurring in *Trachyspermum ammi*

Traditional uses

Ajwain is very similar to its western relatives in the plant family Apiaceae Cumin, Dill and Parsley, both in the way as it is used in food and medicine. The high concentration of essential oils in Ajwain seeds, primarily thymol, gives them an aroma and flavor resembling thyme, with a stronger bite. Ajwain seeds are used to flavor vegetables and fish in Indian cuisine and are fried in oil or ghee (clarified butter) to mellow the acrid taste. Pale yellow carom oil is widely used as germicide and fungicide. Due to its effects in making the digestive system strong and so metabolism work well, it helps reducing your weight naturally but temporarily. Though the effect on reducing weight may take longer, but it would not be having any side effects on the body, if carom seeds are taken in daily diet. Ajwain oil can work in relieving arthritis pain and symptoms. Carom is the main ingredient used in manufacturing most of the natural herbal products and oils. These oils can work on the inflammations and help to get rid of arthritis related pain in legs and joints. Its effect on inflammation adds value in treating arthritis symptoms. Thymol in carom seeds helps as an antibacterial to fight against bacteria in the digestive system. It can help to relieve excess gas from your body and in turn cure problems with your digestive tract. Due to its fighting power against problems caused by bacteria, Carom seed also helps to cure infections in the intestines. If one has problems with acidity, diarrhoea and flatulence, regular intake of carom seeds will help in regulating the digestive system. Carom seeds to fight against toothache by gargling with carom water to get rid of toothache. Addition of salt in carom water can strengthen weak gums and prevent further toothache. Regular practice of gargling with carom water can keep the bacteria that cause toothache away from mouth [25-26]. Carom seeds can work in chasing away cough, cold and Influenza symptoms. By chewing carom seeds with or without betel leaves can help to control dry throat while coughing. To get relieved from nasal congestion, carom seeds can be smelled by crushing them on palm with thumb of another hand. When the aroma goes inside the nostrils, it fights against the congesting materials in the nasal path and push them away. Carom seeds can be used in controlling occupational or work related asthma. Drinking carom water or mixture of ajwain and jaggery are commonly known home remedies to control asthma related breathing problems and chest congestions. Carom seeds are famously used in Ayurvedic treatments and medications. Ajwain seeds are also known as a digestive aid, and combines well with fennel to relieve gas and bloating. A side dish of ajwain seeds often accompanies food in the Middle East. Ajwain seeds contain about 50% thymol, a well known and antibacterial essential oil, and along with thyme can be used to enhance the immune system to ward off colds and flu and other viral infections. It is also traditionally known as a digestive aid, a relief for abdominal discomfort due to indigestion and an antiseptic. In southern parts of India, dry ajwain seeds are powdered and soaked in milk, which is then filtered and fed to babies. Many assume it relieves colic in babies, and for children it also improves digestion and appetite. Ajwain can be used as digestive mixture in large animals. In India, it is often added to heavy fried dishes to aid digestion. A study conducted using the essential oil suggests that it has some use in the treatment of intestinal dysbiosis. Its benefit comes from being able to inhibit the growth of undesired pathogens while not adversely affecting the beneficial flora. Seeds possesses aromatic, bitter, digestive, diuretic, diaphoretic, expectorant, tonic, antiseptic, antispasmodic properties They are used in treatment of influenza, asthma, coughs, colds, colic, diarrhea, cholera, indigestion, edema, rheumatism. They are also soaked in the lemon juice during night and eaten in the morning to remove eosinophilia from the blood, and extracted essential oils are used as diuretic, carminative and anti-septic. For relieving flatulence, dyspepsia and spasmodic disorders; a teaspoonful of Ajwain seeds with a little amount of rock-salt, mixed with water taken internally. For colic; Ajwain seeds, dry ginger and black salt ground together, the three grams of this powder is taken along with warm water. For flatulence, Ajwain seeds and dried ginger in an equal quantity are soaked into two-and-half times the quantity of lime juice. After draining the water, they are dried and powdered with a little amount of black salt and about 2 grams such powder mixed with warm water and taken internally, 2-3 times a day. For Cholera, flatulent colic, diarrhea, atomic dyspepsia and indigestion; the volatile oil of Ajwain seeds is given internally in a dose of 1-3 drops. For removing phlegm; Ajwain seed powder and buttermilk given internally. For pharyngitis in influenza; Ajwain seeds, clove and a pinch of common salt are chewed for such complaint. For common cold; a tablespoonful of Ajwain seeds crushed and tied in a cloth as a bundle which is then inhaled by the patient and such bundle can be used in nasal congestion, it is covered in the same blanket with the patient during sleeping hours [25-27]. For the acute pharyngitis, sore and congested throat and hoarseness of the voice due to cold or making noise, Infusions of the seeds with common salt are beneficial. Ajwain seeds with the kernel of tamarind seeds act as an effective aphrodisiac; they are prepared by frying an equal quantity of both in pure ghee, dried and then powdered and preserved in airtight container. This is taken at bedtime as a promoter for virility. For an earache, a half a teaspoon of the Ajwain seeds heated in 30ml of milk till the aroma of the seeds permeate the milk, which is then filtered and used as an ear drop. For boils in the ear, 3 grams each of ajwain seeds, with garlic are boiled together in 40 grams of sesame oil until it turns red. The oil is then strained while cooling to body temperature and used as ear drops. A habit of chewing Ajwain seeds prevents bad breath. For bronchial asthma, Ajwain seeds are tied in the cotton cloth, heated in a frying pan and applied on the chest and neck when still warm.

Culinary Uses

Ajwain is also known as carom seeds or ajowan caraway. It is an Indian spice and its ayurvedic medicines formulated with these are used in digestive ailment, mental diseases and respiratory disorders. It is also a common home remedy used for a variety of health conditions such as abdominal pain, cramps, intestinal gas, indigestion, vomiting and abdominal distension, and diarrhea, loose stool, breathing trouble and heaviness in the abdomen after a meal. Ajwain with its characteristic aromatic smell and pungent taste is widely used as a spice in curries. Its seeds are used in small quantities for flavoring numerous foods, as preservatives, in medicine and for the manufacture of essential oil in perfumery. The aromatic seeds are used in adding flavor to a number of desi drinks, curries and even breads like parathas. It is also revered in Ayurveda for its numerous health benefits. But not a lot of people know about ajwain leaves. Although these leaves come from different plant as the true ajwain plant, the succulent leaves are still known as ajwain leaves in the Indian subcontinent. The plant that the leaves are a part of is also known as the 'Indian Borage,' which is also called the ajwain plant sometimes. The leaves of this plant are bright green in color and are broad and pulpy. They have a layer of very fine and soft hair atop them. The reason these leaves are known as ajwain leaves despite being a part of a completely different plant (*Plectranthus Amboinicus*), is that they have a smell that is similar to that of carom seeds. In Kannada, the plant is known as 'saveer sambar soppu' which literally translates to 'thousand utility leaf.' Ajwain leaves can be boiled with water and made into a warm concoction to remedy persistent cold and cough. Ajwainor carom seeds have great importance in Indian cooking that provides flavor and fragrance to food recipes. The leaves have a number of uses and can be added to dishes to add a distinctive flavor and taste to them. Ajwain is very common in Indian households. The aromatic seeds are used in adding flavor to a number of desi drinks, curries and even breads like parathas . It also provides a unique taste to chapatis and recipes. Ajwain leaves can be added to a spiced besan (gram flour) batter and then deep-fried to make delicious and flavorful pakodas, which are known as omavalli bajji. These pakodas can be enjoyed hot with ketchup or any other yogurt dip. Ajwain leaves can be sautéed ground and then added to some creamy yogurt to make a delicious and flavorful dip. The chutney can be enjoyed with pakodas, chips, crisps or even with parathas. Ajwain leaves can be added to any fruit or vegetable juice of choice to add flavor and nutrition to the drinks and also more palatable and flavorful. Ajwain leaves are said to have a number of health benefits, including remedying stomach problems and for improving appetite and digestion. These amazing leaves enhance taste and flavor of everyday dishes and help cure for everyday home remedies.

Conclusion

Ajwain is traditional potential herbs possessing stimulant, antispasmodic and carminative properties. It is an important remedial agent for flatulence, atonic dyspepsia and diarrhoea. The seed of ajwain is bitter, pungent and it acts as anthelmintic, carminative, laxative, and stomachic. It also cures abdominal tumors, abdominal pains and piles. Seeds comprise of an essential oil containing about thymol which is a strong germicide, anti-spasmodic and fungicide. Thymol is also used in toothpaste and perfumery. The fruit possesses stimulant, antispasmodic and carminative properties and is used traditionally as an important remedial agent for flatulence, atonic dyspepsia, diarrhea, abdominal tumors, abdominal pains, piles, bronchial problems, lack of appetite, galactogogue, asthma and amenorrhea. Medicinally, it has been proven to possess various pharmacological activities like antifungal, antioxidant, antimicrobial, antinociceptive, cytotoxic, hypolipidemic, antihypertensive, antispasmodic, broncho-dilating actions, antilithiasis, diuretic, abortifacient, antitussive, nematicidal, anthelmintic and antifilarial. Further, studies reveal the presence of various phytochemical constituents mainly carbohydrates, glycosides, saponins, phenolic compounds, volatile oil (thymol, γ-terpinene, para-cymene and α- and β-pinene), protein, fat, fiber and mineral matter containing calcium, phosphorous, iron and nicotinic acid. This review is an attempt to provide well assembled scientific data on the behalf of *Trachyspermum ammi.* These studies reveal that *T. ammi* is a source of medicinally active compounds and have various pharmacological effects; hence, it is encouraging to find its new therapeutic uses.

REFERENCES

1. Dhiman P, Soni K, Singh S (2014) Medicinal Value of Carom Seeds – An Overview PharmaTutor, 2(3), 119-123.
2. Choudhury S. (1998) Composition of the Seed Oil of Trachyspermumammi (L.) Sprague from Northeast India. J Essent Oil Res 10: 588-590.
3. Ishikawah T, Sega Y, Kitajima J (2011) Water-soluble Constituents of Ajowan. Chem Pharm Bull 2001; 49: 840-844.
4. Garg S (1998) A New glucoside from Trachyspermumammi. Fitoterapia 6: 511-512.
5. Nagalakshmi S (2000) Studies on Chemical and Technological aspects of Ajowan (Trachyspermumammi syn. Carumcopticum) J Food SciTechnol 37: 277-281.
6. Gilani AH, Jabeen Q, Ghayur MN, Janbaz KH, Akhtar MS (2005) Studies on theantihypertensive, Antispasmodic, Bronchodilator and Hepatoprotective Activities of the Carumcopticum Seed extract. J Ethnopharmaco l98(12): 127-135.
7. Srivastava KC (1988) Extract of a spice-omum (Trachyspermumammi)-showsantiaggregatory effects and alters Arachidonic Acid Metabolism in Human Platelets. ProstaglandLeukotrie Essen Fatty Acids 33(1): 16-20.
8. Thangam C, Dhananjayan R (2003) Antiinflammatory Potential of the Seeds of CarumCopticum Linn. Ind J Pharmacol 35: 388-391.
9. Jeet K, Devi N, Thakur N, Tomar S, Shalta L, Thakur R (2012) Trachyspermumammi (Ajwain): A Comprehensive Review Kamal Int Res J Pharm 3 (5): 133-138.
10. Jabbar A, Iqbal Z, Khan MN (2006) In vitro Anthelmintic Activity of *Trachyspermum ammi* Seeds. Pharmacog Magaz 2: 126-129.
11. Mathew N, Bhattacharya SM, Perumal V, Muthuswamy K (2008) Antifilarial Lead Molecules Isolated from *Trachyspermum ammi*, Molecules 13: 2156-2168.
12. Ramaswamy S, Sengottuvelu S, Haja SS, Jaikumar S, Saravanan R, Prasadkumar C, Sivakumar T (2010) Gastroprotective Activity of Ethanolic Extract of *Trachyspermum ammi* Fruit. Int J Pharma Bio Sci 01(01): 1-15.
13. Katasani D, Srinu B, Bala R (2011) Phytochemical Screening, Quantitative Estimation of Total Phenolic, Flavanoids and Antimicrobial Evaluation of *Trachyspermum ammi*. J Atoms Molecules 1(1): 1-8.
14. Dubey S, Kashyap P (2015) *Trachyspermum ammi*: A Review on its Multidimensional Uses in Indian Folklore Medicines. Res J Med Plants, 9: 368-374. doi: 10.3923/rjmp.2015.368.374
15. Saini N, Singh GK, Nagori BP (2014) Physicochemical Characterization and Spasmolytic Activity of Essential Oil of Ajwain (*Trachyspermum ammi* L.) from Rajasthan. Int J Pharmacol Screen Meth 4(1): 49-55.
16. Murthy PS, Borse BB, Khanum H, Srinivas P(2009) Inhibitory effects of Ajowan (*Trachyspermum ammi*) ethanolic extract on A. ochraceus Growth and Ochratoxin Production. Turk J Biol 33: 211-217.
17. Singh, G, Maurya S, Catalan C, M.P. de Lampasona (2004) Chemical Constituents, Antifungal and Antioxidative effects of Ajwain Essential Oil and its Acetone extract. JAgri Food Chem 52: 3292-3296.
18. Tambe M, Mahadik S (2020) The Anthelmintic Activity of Leaves of *Trachyspermum ammi*.Int J ScientEng Res 11 (9): 1752-1756.
19. Bairwa R, Singhal M, Sodha RS, Rajawat BS,Tiwari AK (2011) Medical uses of *Trachyspermum Ammi*.: A Review. Pharmacologyonline 2: 477-485.
20. Garg S (1998) A New Glucoside from *Trachyspermum ammi*. Fitoterapia 6: 511-512.
21. Nagalakshmi S (2000) Studies on Chemical and Technological aspects of Ajowan (*Trachyspermum ammi* syn. Carumcopticum) J Food SciTechnol 37: 277-281.

22. Choudhury S (1998) Composition of the Seed Oil of *Trachyspermum ammi* (L.) Sprague from Northeast India. J Essent Oil Res 10: 588-590.
23. Dwivedi SN, Mishra RP, Alava S (2012) Phytochemistry, Pharmacological Studies and Traditional benefits of *Trachyspermum ammi* (Linn.) Sprague. Int J Pharm Life Sci3(5): 1705-1709.
24. Ashraf M, Bhatty MK (1975) Studies on Essential Oils of the Pakistan species of *Trachyspermum ammi* ajwain Seed Oil. Pak J SciInd Res 18(1): 232-235.
25. Chauhan HB, Kumar G, Ali M (2012) A Review on Phytochemical Constituents and Activities of *Trachyspermum ammi* (L.) Sprague fruits. Am J Pharm Tech Res 2012; 2(4): 329-340.
26. Singh G, Maurya S, Catalan C, De Lampasona MP (2004) Chemical Constituents, Antifungal and Antioxidative effects of Ajwain Essential Oil and its Acetone extract. J Agric Food Chem 2004; 52(11): 3292-3296.http://dx.doi.org/10.1021/jf035211c
27. Saraswat N, Sachan N, Chandra P (2020) A Review on Ethnobotanical, Phytochemical, Pharmacological and Traditional Aspects of Indigenous Indian Herb *Trachyspermum ammi* (L). 6 (3):172-187.doi: 10.2174/2215083805666191107115544

CHAPTER

2

Chemical Constituents and Pharmacological Properties of Anise Seeds (*Pimpinella anisum* L.)

Pimpinella anisum (anise), belonging to Umbelliferae family, is an aromatic plant which has been used In Iranian traditional medicine (especially its fruits) as carminative, aromatic, disinfectant, and galactagogue. *Pimpinella anisum* is a plant rich in volatile oils, which are employed in the folk medicine. So far, different studies were performed on aniseeds and various properties such as antimicrobial, antifungal, antiviral, antioxidant, muscle relaxant, analgesic and anticonvulsant activity as well as different effects on gastrointestinal system have been reported of aniseeds. It can also reduce morphine dependence and has beneficial effects on dysmenorrhea and menopausal hot flashes in women. In diabetic patients, aniseeds showed hypoglycemic and hypolipidemic effect and reduce lipid peroxidation. The most important compounds of aniseeds essential oil were trans-anetole, estragole, γ-hymachalen, para-anisaldehyde and methyl cavicol.

Keywords: Galactagogue, Anethole, Hypoglycemic effect, Antifungal, Analgesic.

Introduction

Pimpinella anisum L., an annual herb belonging to the Umbelliferae family, is one of the oldest medicinal plants. It is an annual grassy herb with 30-50 cm high, white flowers, and small green to yellow seeds, which grows in the Eastern Mediterranean Region, West Asia, the Middle East, Mexico, Egypt, and Spain. *P. anisum* is primarily grown for its fruits (aniseeds). Anise is grown for fruit (*Anisi fructus*), containing essential oil (Anisiaethroleum) with trans-anethole which is a dominant compound and has a characteristic sweet taste and smell. *Pimpinella anisum* has been used as carminative, aromatic, disinfectant, and galactagogue [1-3]. Anise seed contains volatile oil, fixed oil, proteins, mucilage and starch. Essential oil of Anise seeds contains eugenol trans-anethole, anisaldehyde estragole, coumarins, scopoletin, umbelliferon, estrolterpene hydrocarbons polyenes and polyacetylenes, methyl chavicol anisaldehyde. Aniseeds contain 1.5-5% essential oil and used as flavouring, digestive, carminative, and relief of gastrointestinal spasms. Consumption of aniseed in lactating women increases milk and also reliefs their infants from gastrointestinal problems. Anise seeds are used as analgesic in migraine and also as carminative, aromatic, disinfectant, and diuretic in traditional medicine [4]. Aniseed has warm and dry nature and can increase milk production, menstruation, urine, and sweat secretion and also making good complexion. It is also effective in polishing of teeth. In some traditional texts, anise is mentioned for melancholy, nightmare, and also in treatment of epilepsy and seizure. Aniseed or anise essential oil is derived from anise or aniseed. More often than not, this oil is confused with star anise essential oil but that oil comes from star anise plant, scientifically known as *Illicum verum*. The plant is prevalent in the Mediterranean regions and it undoubtedly has a long historical record. In fact, it was introduced to northern Europe by the Romans after they discovered that the aniseed herb could be used as a digestive, specifically added to cakes which contained other digestive seeds like cumin and fennel, eaten after meals. Early settlers brought it to North America. Its essential oil possesses a very distinctive aroma that resembles that of black licorice and it is widely known for its digestive benefits. However, aniseed oil also contains other potent health benefits [4-7].

Chemical Constituents

The chemical constituents of aniseed extract obtained by Supercritical extraction using CO_2 were determined by GC-MS. The major compounds were anethole (~90%), γ-himachalene (2-4%), p-anisaldehyde (<1%), methyl chavicol (0.9-1.5%), cis-pseudoisoeugenyl 2-methylbutyrate (~3%), and trans-pseudoisoeugenyl 2-methylbutyrate (~1.3%). A new terpene hydrocarbon called neophytadiene was isolated from aniseed. 4-(β-D - glucopyranosyloxy) benzoic acid which is one of the phenolic glycosides of the Umbelliferae family was also isolated from aniseed. Four aromatic compound glucosides, an alkyl glucoside, and a glucide were isolated as new compounds from the polar portion of methanolic extract of anise fruits. The structures of the new compounds were clarified as (E)-3-hydroxy- anethole β-D-glucopyranoside, (E)-10-(2-hydroxy-5-methoxyphenyl) propane β-D-glucopyranoside, 3-hydroxyestragole β-D-glucopyranoside, methyl syringate 4-O-β-D -glucopyranoside, hexane-1,5-diol 1-O-β-D-glucopyranoside, and 1-deoxy-l-erythritol 3-O-β D-glucopyranoside. Isolation and structure elucidation of flavonoid constituents from anise, caraway, coriander, and fennel by means of chromatography on cellulose columns lead to isolation of quercetin 3-glucuronide, rutin, luteolin 7- glucoside, isoorientin, and isovitexin as crystalline compounds and apigenin 7-glucoside and a luteolin glycoside as noncrystalline compounds from anise. Pectin substances isolated from the *Pimpinella anisum* herbs, was found that pectin substances are practically not toxic and exhibit pronounced laxative effect. Water Soluble Polydaccharide Compounds isolated from the *Pimpinella anisum* herbs contain two monosaccharides-glucose and ramnose [8-11].

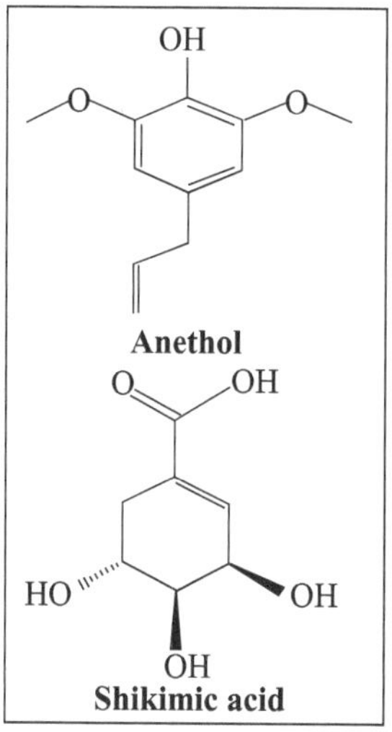

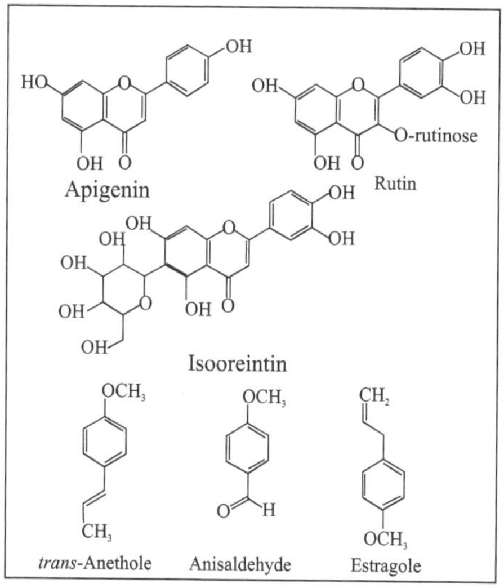

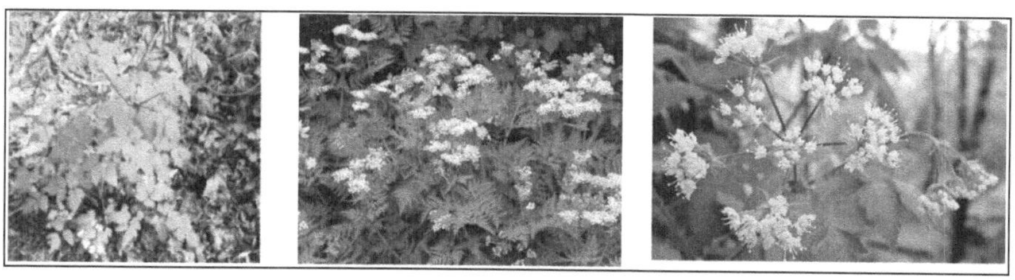

Anise Plant and Inflorescence

Pharmacological Aspects

Anise is used in folk medicine in many countries for treatment of digestive, respiratory and neurological diseases, as well as natural estrogen. It has been found recently to have anti-cancer, antioxidant and antimicrobial properties, and in many countries anise is included in the pharmacopeias as the official drug. Anise is generally recommended as a carminative, digestive agent and improves the regulation of digestion. Experiments showed that anise, in combination with other plants is a safe and efficient alternative therapy for chronic constipation. Also, it was found that anise increases the secretion of salivary glands leading to an increase of pH in the mouth. Furthermore, it can be used for mechanically rinsing the oral cavity, thereby removing dental plaque. Apart from possessing antibacterial activity, anise is effective in the suppression of bacteria which cause dental caries. Anise fruit extract significantly decreases the gastric acid secretion and acidity and thereby inhibits the formation of ulcers in the stomach. Additionally, it possesses anti-diabetic activity, i.e. anise significantly increases glucose absorption in the small intestine, while having no effect on the amount of the water absorbed from the colon. In addition, anise significantly reduces the diuresis [12-14]. The introduction of anise in the diet ensures that the glucose is available to cells and that water is conserved in the body thus preventing dehydration. In many countries, anise is recommended for the treatment of the respiratory tract. Experiments have shown the bronchodilatory and anti-inflammatory effect of anise, thus confirming its effectiveness in the treatment of bronchial asthma. Also, anise is used throughout the world in the treatment of neurological diseases. Studies have found that the plant works as an antiepileptic and as an analgesic. Anise is an herb that has been used for centuries as an estrogenic agent. In women with symptoms of primary dysmenorrhoea the application of anise leads to a reduction of the bleeding period and menstrual pain. In postmenopausal women it effectively reduces hot flashes. In addition, anise acts preventively on osteoporosis caused by estrogen deficiency as it retains calcium in the bones. By using modern scientific methods it has been found that the reactive oxygen species cause oxidative damage to biomolecules, which as a result form many acute and chronic diseases such as atherosclerosis, cancer, aging, neurodegenerative diseases, diabetes, myocardial infarction, apoplexy, chronic inflammation, etc. Anise shows high antioxidant activity. Furthermore, it can be classified as a food for prevention and treatment of cancer, because it was found to have cytostatic activity on human prostate cancer cells and is safe for normal cells [15-16]. Numerous studies found a wide range of anise effects on microorganisms. It works on bacteria as gram positive and gram-negative, which indicates a high antibacterial potential of this plant, especially if we take into account production costs, availability and efficiency. It can be concluded that the extract is effective and inexpensive alternative to synthetic antibiotics. Additionally, in contrast to synthetic antibiotics, bacteria do not develop resistance to phytochemicals. A large number of fungi on which the anise essential oil has antifungal effects are confirmed. The same effect was observed on viruses such as *Herpes simplex* virus, cytomegalovirus, measles viruses and amoebas (*Entamoeba histolytica*) that cause dysentery. All this classifies anise as a functional food against infectious diseases [17-19].

Traditional benefits of Anise Seed Products

Anise seed as well its oil has discovered application in several traditional medications because of their exclusive health endorsing as well as disease stopping functions. A concoction of seeds in hot water is used as a carminative, antiseptic, diuretic, digestive and a folk remedy to insomnia and constipation. Furthermore, several therapeutic effects including those on digestive disorders, gynecologic, and also anticonvulsant, anti-asthma and dyspnea have been described for the seeds of *Pimpinella anisum*. Stir a teaspoon of crushed anise seeds in the cup of boiling water. Steep for Ten minutes. Drink the tea after having a huge meal. Furthermore the tea relax you, anise helps digestion of food, puts a stop to indigestion and contains an anti-flatulence agent. Use the essential oil of anise just as one expectorant. The oil behaves as a decongestant simply by favorably affecting secretory cells within the respiratory system. Anise can also be frequently present in cough syrups as well as cough drops because of its anti-microbial qualities [20-21]. Add anise seeds within sweet foods just like pastries, cakes as well as cookies. The moderate liquorice taste boosts the sweetness. In cooking, mix anise along with cinnamon. Their tastes enhance one another. The fairly sweet, powerful odor attracts fish. Combine anise along with coriander, fennel seed as well as sugared vodka. It seems sensible a fairly sweet liqueur known as anisette. Anise preparations are a fantastic treatment for asthma, bronchitis cough in addition to digestive complaints just like flatulence, bloating, colicky stomach pain, nausea as well as indigestion. The essential oil includes 75-90% anethole that has a noticed estrogenic effect. The decoction extracted from the seeds frequently is recommended within the breastfeeding mothers to enhance breast-milk manufacturing. Anise seed water is extremely useful in reducing running nose symptom in babies. The seeds usually are chewed right after a meal in India to invigorate the breath [22-23].

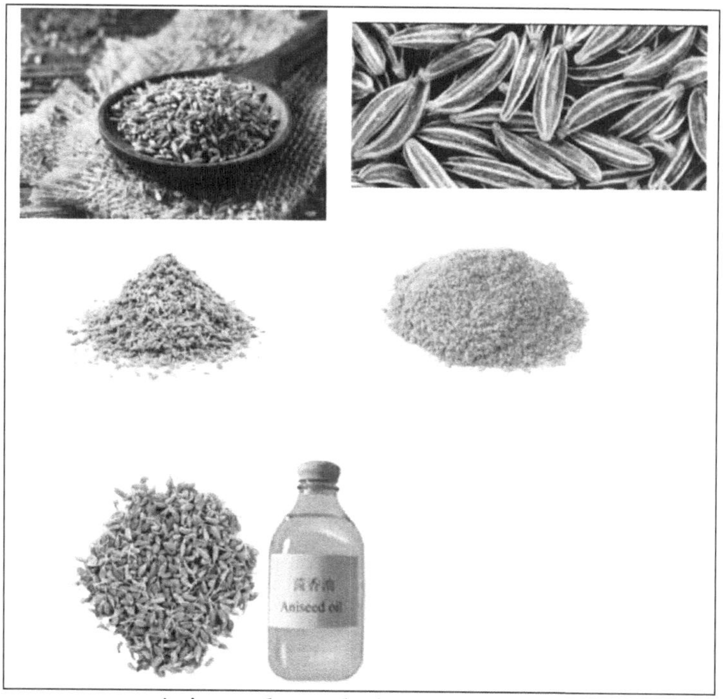

Anise seeds, crushed seeds, powder, oil

Culinary Uses

Aniseed has similar uses to that of fennel seeds but is a popular option for making sweet dishes such as smoothies, desserts, cookies, cakes and drinks. Anise is the preferred spice used to add liquorice flavour to candy and liqueur. Anise is used widely as a flavouring for dairy products, gelatins, puddings, meats, and candies. Both Fennel seeds and Aniseed spice is used as breathe fresheners. Anise seeds, oil and also fresh young foliage is utilized in cooking. The taste is increased by dry-frying the seeds. Anise is utilized in delicious as well as fairly sweet dishes in which it imparts sweet-aromatic taste to number of foods. The entire seeds as well as often-times newly grounded powder included with the recipes in the last moment to restrict the evaporation of essential volatile oils inside them. This sensitive spice is now being utilized as flavoring base for soups, sauces, breads, cakes, biscuits as well as confectionary. Popular aniseed flavor drinks consist of prenod, frenchpastis, spanishojen etc. Anise seeds along with its oil have been around in use in the preparation of sweet dishes in several Parts of Asia. It is utilized like a flavoring base within the preparation of herbal tea; along with liquor known as anisette. Star anise (bajiao) is probably the most significant spices in Chinese cuisine, and it's also the dominating flavor in Chinese five-spice powder together with cloves, cinnamon, huajiao (Sichuan pepper) and ground fennel seeds. In the food industry, anise is used as flavoring and aromatic agent for fish products, ice cream, sweets, and gums.

Conclusion

Pimpinella anisum is one of the medicinal plants which have been used for different purposes in traditional medicine of Iran. So far, different studies were performed on the extracts and essential oil of *Pimpinella anisum* to identify the chemical compounds and pharmacological properties of this plant, and various properties such as antimicrobial, antifungal, antiviral, antioxidant, and insecticidal effects have been reported of aniseeds. The findings also revealed that aniseeds can cause gastric protection, muscle relaxant, and affect digestive system. In diabetic patients, it has hypoglycemic and hypolipidemic effects and reduces lipid peroxidation. Aniseed also has beneficial effects on dysmenorrhea and menopausal hot flashes in women. The most important compounds of aniseeds essential oil were trans-anethole, estragole, γ-hymachalen, *p*-anisaldehyde, and methyl chavicol.

REFERENCES

1. Ahmad AF, Youssef MSH (2015) Chemical Composition and Bioactive Properties of *Illicium verum* (star-anise) extracts Prepared by different methods J Che Biol Phy Sci B 5(2;): 1160-1170.
2. Review of Pharmacological Properties and Chemical Constituents of *Pimpinella anisum* Asie Shojaii* and MehriAbdollahiFard MA (2012) ISRN Pharm. 2012: 510795. doi: 10.5402/2012/510795.

3. Özcan MM, Chalchat JC. Chemical Composition and Antifungal effect of Anise (*Pimpinella anisum* L.) Fruit Oil at Ripening Stage. *Annals Microbiol.* 2006; 56(4): 353-358.
4. Gulcin I, Oktay M, Kirecci E, Kufrevioglu OI. Screening of Antioxidant and Antimicrobial Activities of Anise (*Pimpinella anisum* L.) Seed extracts. Food Chem. 2003; 83(3): 371-382.
5. Orav A, Raal A, Arak E. Essential Oil Composition of *Pimpinella anisum* L. Fruits from various European Countries. Nat Prod Res. 2008; 22(3): 227-232.
6. Embong MB, Hadziyev D, Molnar S. Essential Oils from Spices Grown in Alberta. Anise oil (*Pimpinella anisum*) Canadian J Plant Sci. 1997; 57: 681-688.
7. Rodrigues VM, Rosa PTV, Marques MOM, Petenate AJ, Meireles MAA. Supercritical Extraction of Essential Oil from Aniseed (*Pimpinella anisum* L) using CO_2: Solubility, Kinetics, and Composition Data. J Agri Food Chem. 2003; 51(6): 1518-1523.
8. Burkhardt G, Reichling J, Martin R, Becker H. Terpene Hydrocarbons in *Pimpinella anisum* L. Pharmaceutisch Weekblad. 1986; 8(3): 190-193.
9. Dirks U, Herrmann K. 4-(β-d-glucopyranosyloxy) Benzoic Acid, a Characteristic Phenolic Constituent of the Apiaceae. Phytochem. 1984; 23(8): 1811-1812.
10. Fujimatu E, Ishikawa T, Kitajima J. Aromatic Compound Glucosides, Alkyl Glucoside and Glucide from the Fruit of Anise. Phytochem. 2003; 63(5): 609-616.
11. Kunzemann J, Herrmann K. Isolation and Identification of Flavon (ol)-O-glycosides in caraway (Carumcarvi L.), fennel (*Foeniculum vulgare* Mill.), anise (*Pimpinella anisum* L.), and Coriander (Coriandrumsativum L.), and of Flavon-C- glycosides in Anise—I. Phenolics of spices. Zeitschriftfür Lebensmittel-Untersuchung und-Forschung. 1977; 164(3): 194-200.
12. Singh G, Kapoor IPS, Singh P, Heluani CSD, Catalan CAN. Chemical Composition and Antioxidant Potential of Essential Oil and Oleoresins from Anise Seeds *(Pimpinella anisum L.) Int J Essen Oil Therapeut.* 2008; 2(3): 122-130.
13. Rajeshwari CU, Abirami M, Andallu B. In vitro and in vivo Antioxidant Potential of Aniseeds (*Pimpinella anisum*) *Asian JExpBiol Sci.* 2011; 2(1): 80-89.
14. Kosalec I, Pepeljnjak S, Kustrak D. Antifungal Activity of Fluid extract and Essential Oil from Anise Fruits (*Pimpinella anisum* L., Apiaceae). PubMed. 2005; 55(4): 508-515.
15. Ansari S, Musarrat M, Patel MF, Ara J, Khan TS, Shaikh S, Salar S. Review of Anisoon (*Pimpinella anisum* Linn.) with Unani Perspectives and modern Pharmacological uses. Indian Journal of Unani Med. 2021; XIV(2): 135-141 https:// doi.org/10.53390/ijum.v14.i2.11
16. Wozniak KS, Walasek M, Ludwiczuk A, Glowniak K. Isolation of Terpenoids from *Pimpinellaanisum* Essential Oil by High-performance Counter-current Chromatography. J Sep Sci. 2013; 36(16): 2611-2614 https://doi.org/10.1002/jssc.201300407 20.
17. Kolisnyk S, Khanin V, Umarov U, Ugli A, Koretnik O. Study of the Monosaccharide Composition of Water-soluble Polysaccharide Complexes and Pectic Substances of *Pimpinella anisum* Herbs. Sci Rise Pharmaceut Sci. 2020; 3 (25), 33-38. doi: https://doi.org/10.15587/2519-4852.2020.2067
18. Acimovic M, Dojcinovic N. A Review of Pharmacological Properties of Anise (*Pimpinella anisum* L.). Lekovite Sirovine. 2014; 34(34): 3-17. doi: 10.5937/leksir1434003A
19. Özcan MM, Chalchat JC. Chemical Composition and Antifungal Effect of Anise (*Pimpinella anisum* L.) Fruit Oil at Ripening Stage. Annals of Microbiol. 2006; 56(4): 353-358.
20. Gulcin I, Oktay M, Kirecci E, Kufrevioglu OI. Screening of Antioxidant and Antimicrobial Activities of Anise (*Pimpinella anisum* L.) Seed extracts. Food Chem. 2003; 83(3): 371-382.

CHAPTER 3

Health benefits of Bay Leaves *(Laurus nobilis* L.)

ABSTRACT

Laurus nobilis essential oil benefits are well-regarded in aromatherapy due to its unique phytoconstituents. *Laurus nobilis* essential oil benefits can be attributed to its properties like anti septic, antibiotic, antineuralgic, antispasmodic, analgesic, aperitif, astringent, cholagogue, emenagogue, febrifuge, insecticide, sedative, stomachic, sudorific and tonic. Essential oil from the bay leaves contains mostly cineol; furthermore, eugenol, chavicol, acetyl eugenol, methyl eugenol, α- and β-pinene, phellandrene, linalool, geraniol, and terpineol are also found. Caffeic acid and rutin are both important organic compounds, found in bay leaves, that helps in CVDs. Rutin strengthens capillary walls in the heart and the body's extremities, while caffeic acid can help eliminate LDL or bad cholesterol from the cardiovascular system. Linalool is often associated with thyme and basil, but it is also present in bay leaves. The plant shows a rich content of metabolites including proteins, free sugars, organic acids, PUFA and tocopherols and exhibit a biological potential with a wide range of bioactivity including antimicrobial and antioxidant properties. This review is aimed to contribute to the knowledge of the plant by providing a critical overview of the botanic characteristics, the traditional uses, the plant chemistry and the biological activities.

Keywords: Anti neuralgic, Antispasmodic, Astringent, Cholagogue, Cineol CVDs. Caffeic acid.

Introduction

Laurus nobilis L. commonly known as bay belonging to the family Lauraceae is evergreen hardy multi branched tree with smooth bark used in foods, drugs and cosmetics. Bay is cultivated throughout the world mainly in tropical and sub-tropical Asia, Australia, Pacific region and South Asia. *Laurus* is also known as sweet bay, bay laurel, Grecian laurel, true bay and bay tree. In India it is found in Uttarakhand and Himachal Pradesh along the Western Himalaya and also in Sikkim, Assam, Mizoram and Meghalaya and is cultivated in many warm regions of the world, particularly in Southern Europe and around the shores of the Mediterranean Sea. Turkey, Algeria, France, Greece, Morocco, Portugal, Spain, Belgium, Mexico, Central America and the Southern United States are the commercial production centers of bay. Turkey is one of the main producers and suppliers of bay leaves [1-3]. This tree attains height upto 10m. It has alternate, narrowly oblong-lanceolate leaves. The flowers are small and four lobed; the male has 8-12 stamens and female 2-4 staminodes. The fruit is 10-15 mm, ovoid and black when ripe. These are aromatic and fragrant plants yielding fixed and volatile oil as well as camphor. *Laurus nobilis* is a plant of industrial importance, used in foods, drugs, and cosmetics. The dried leaves and essential oils are used extensively in the food industry for seasoning of meat products, soups and fishes. Its antimicrobial and insecticidal activities are other factor for which bay is used in the food industry as a food preservative. The fruits contain both fixed and volatile oils, which are mainly used in soap making. Traditionally it is used in rheumatism, dermatitis, gastrointestinal problems such as epigastric bloating, impaired digestion, eructation, and flatulence. Chemically it has found to contain sesquiterpene lactones such as epigazaniolide, gazaniolide, spirafolide, costunolide, reynosin, santamarine, flavonoid glycosides, and essential oil. It has been reported to possess wound healing, neuroprotective, antioxidant, antiulcerogenic, anticonvulsant, antimutagenic, antiviral, anticholinergic, antibacterial, antifungal activities [4-6]. Recently it is used in treating diabetes and preventing migraine. *Laurus nobilis* is traded as sweet bay leaf and true Romanor Turkish laurel. Bay essential oil can be extracted from various parts of plant and chiefly consisted of 1, 8 Cineole, sabinene, α-pinene and p-Cymene. This compound can help lower the level of stress hormones in the body, especially when used in aromatherapy. Excess stress hormones can be dangerous for long-term health, so bay leaves can help you calm down and remain relaxed even in your high-anxiety moments. The components in the essential oil can also be used in many traditional medicines in the treatment of arthritis, muscle pain, bronchitis, and flu-symptoms. This review highlighted chemical composition and biological activities of *Laurus nobilis* [5-7].

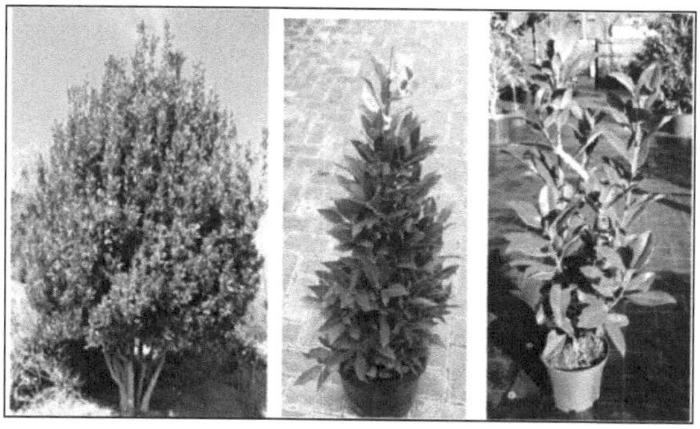

L. nobilis **trees**

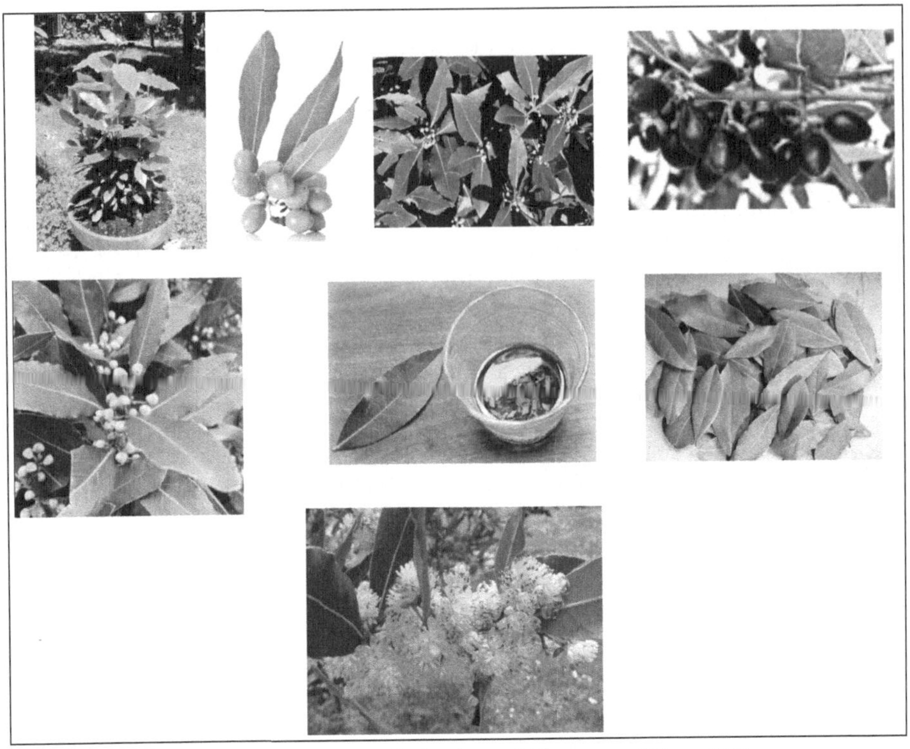

Leaves (green & dried), buds and Flowers of *L. nobilis*

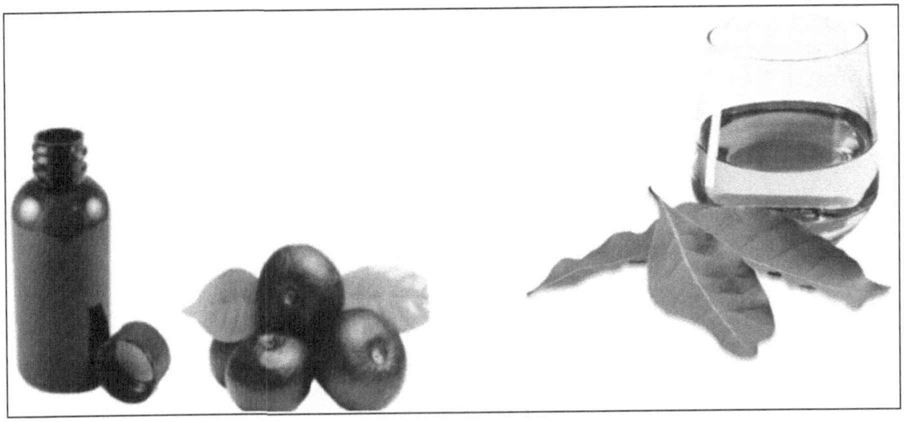

Bay leaf (*L. nobilis*) Nutritional value/100g

Principle	Nutrient Value	Percentage of RDA
Energy	313 Kcal	15.5%
Carbohydrates	74.97 g	57%
Protein	7.61 g	13%
Total Fat	8.36 g	29%
Cholesterol	0 mg	0%
Dietary Fiber	26.3 g	69%
Vitamins		
Folates	180 mcg	45%
Niacin	2.005 mg	12.5%
Pyridoxine	1.740 mg	133%
Riboflavin	0.421 mg	32%
Vitamin A	6185 IU	206%
Vitamin C	46.5 mg	77.5%
Electrolytes		
Sodium	23 mg	1.5%
Potassium	529 mg	11%
Minerals		
Calcium	834 mg	83%
Copper	0.416 mg	46%
Iron	43 mg	537%
Magnesium	120 mg	30%
Manganese	8.167 mg	355%
Phosphorus	113 mg	16%
Selenium	2.8 mcg	5%
Zinc	3.70 mg	33%

Source: USDA: National Nutrient data Base

Chemical Constituents

Essential oils are generally derived from one or more plant parts, such as flowers, leaves, stems, bark, wood, roots, seeds or fruits and the yield of the essential oil varies among different parts of the same plant. The main components of *L. nolilis* reported were α-eudesmol, β-elemene and β-caryophyllene in flowers, (E)-β-ocimene and biclyclogermacrene in fruits, (E)-β-ocimene and germacrene D in buds. The ethanolic extract of bay seed analyzed by gas chromatography and mass spectrometry (GC-MS) showed 1,8-cineole, an oxygenated monoterpene. Other predominant compounds of were α-thujene, α-pinene, βpinene, D-limonene and o-cymene. The components present in bay leaf essential oil were 1,8 cineole, Tricyclene, limonene, γ-Terpinene, Sabinene, α-Pinene, Eugenol, Linalool, p-Cymene, α-Phellandrene, Camphene, β-Pinene, Camphor, Terpinene-4-ol, α-Terpineol, α-Thujene, Myrcene, α-Terpinene, Terpineolene, Sabinol, Borneol, γ-Cadinene, β-Elemene, Germacrane A, Germacrane D-4-ol, -Humulene [7-10].

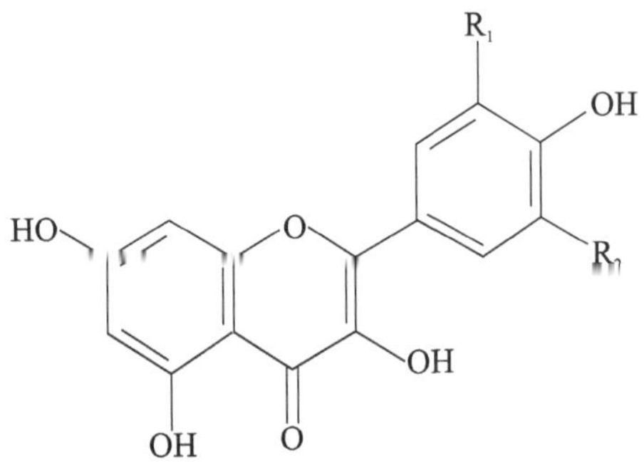

Flavonol	R1	R2
Kaempferol	H	H
Quercetin	OH	H
Isorhamnetin	OMe	H

Main chemical flavonoids occurring in leaves of *L. nobilis*

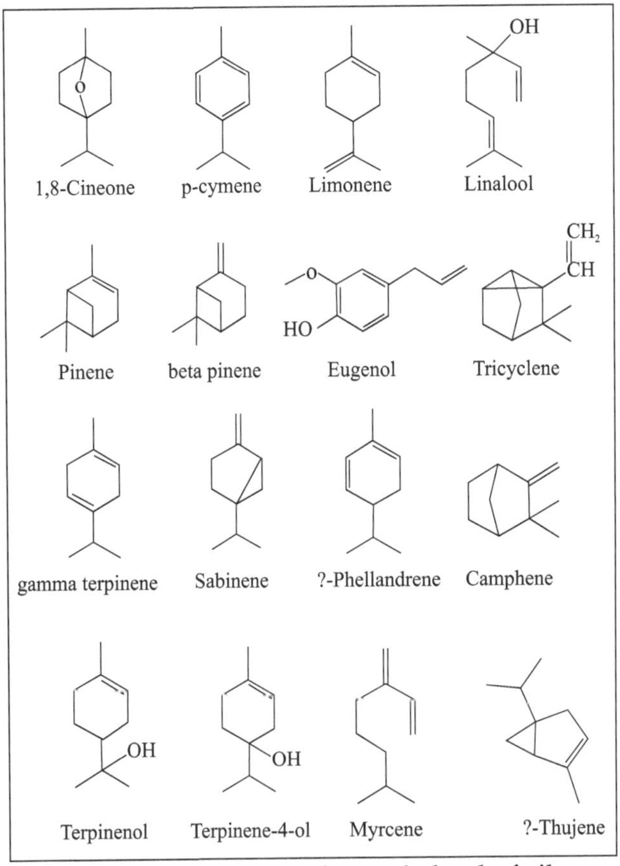

Structure chemical constituents in bay leaf oil

Bay Leaf Oil Benefits and Uses

Bay leaf oil is a type of essential oil made from the leaves of the bay laurel, also called sweet bay (*Laurus nobilis*). Another species, the West Indian bay leaf (*Pimenta racemosa*), also allows for the extraction of the essential oils in the leaves and the production of an oil with the same name. Bay leaf oil is the oil extracted from the leaves of the bay laurel, *Laurus nobilis*.

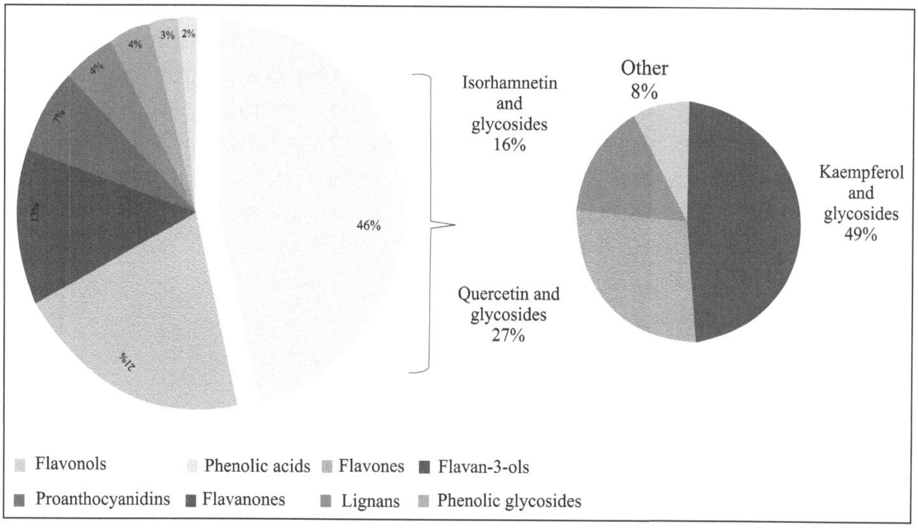

It is an essential oil, meaning it is meant for external use only and should not be ingested. It is obtained from the mature, fresh leaves of the bay laurel tree through a process called steam distillation. The process allows for the extraction of the main essential oil constituents from the leaves [11-12]. The essential oil constituents are responsible for the particular aroma of bay leaves and a source of varied health benefits. The uses of bay leaf oil cover a range of health aspects and primarily include benefits for nerve and muscle pain and joint swelling and pain. Some of the less known benefits and uses of bay leaf oil are a natural decongestant action, antibacterial and antifungal effects, astringent properties as well as a mild sedative quality that contributes to lowering stress and anxiety levels. Bay leaf oil is added to bath water, soap and other skin and hair-products. In hair care, it is used for strengthening hair, maintaining scalp health, controlling dandruff, combating dullness and restoring shine. Some of the aromatic compounds that give bay leaf oil its characteristic scent exhibit analgesic properties and can help relieve arthritis-related joint inflammation and pain. Limonene, linalool, myrcene, estragol, eugenol, alpha-pinene, beta-pinene, phellandrene are the most prominent aromatic compounds in the oil with proven pain-relieving properties. Myrcene is of particular interest because it has been shown to pass the skin barrier and reach the bloodstream, which could be one explanation for the reduction in swelling and pain relief observed with the use of the oil for joint pain management. Still, bay leaf oil for joint pain should be used cautiously (in small amounts, diluted in a carrier oil) [11-14]. One of the best bay leaf oil uses is for treating neuralgia, or nerve pain. Neuralgia is essentially pain along the course of one or more nerves. Even at modest intensity, it can be debilitating and interfere with daily life. Applying very small amounts of bay leaf essential oil diluted in a carrier oil such as olive oil onto the affected area and massaging it onto the skin can help provide temporary relief. Once again, the biologically active compounds responsible for the analgesic action of the oil are limonene, linalool, myrcene, estragol, eugenol, alpha-pinene, beta-pinene, phellandrene. In addition to pain-relieving properties, many of the aromatic compounds extracted in bay leaf oil (eugenol, estragol etc.) also exert an antispasmodic action, recommending the oil for use in the treatment of muscle cramps and spasms [14-16].

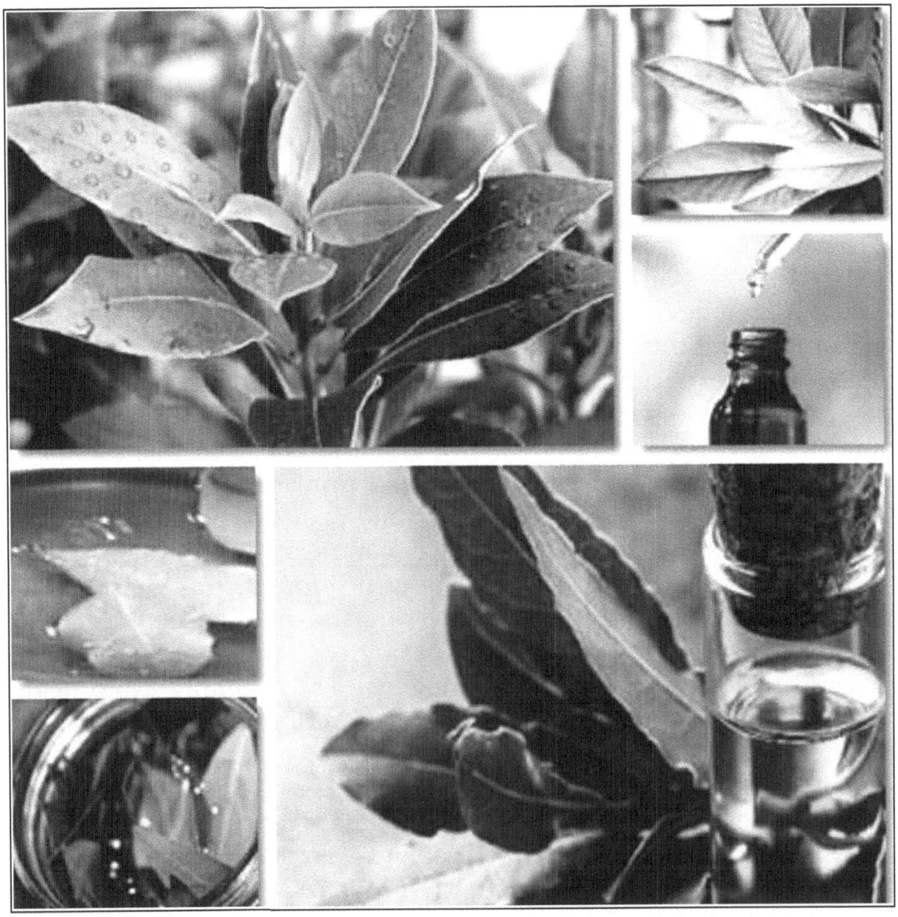

The oil is to be used for massaging the affected area. Complementary to the antispasmodic effects of the active constituents, the massage serves to stimulate circulation, increasing the absorption of the active constituents into the skin for a stronger antispasmodic effect. The analgesic effects of the oil further help in the treatment of muscle aches and pain. This particular property is also at the root of the recommending bay leaves, bay leaf tea and even oil for relieving cough in common cold and flu infections. Studies show eugenol in bay leaf oil has antibacterial activity and is effective against a range of Gram-positive and Gram-negative bacteria as well as holds antifungal properties. For example, in vitro studies show eugenol inhibits bacteria such as *Escherichia coli* , *Staphylococcus aureus* , *Pseudomonas aeruginosa*, *Klebsiella pneumoniae*, *Helicobacter pylori*, *Salmonella typhi* and *Candida albicans*, pathogens that cause infections of the skin, respiratory system, digestive tract and more. Other aromatic compounds also hold antibacterial and antifungal properties. Bay essential oil actively inhibits the growth of bacteria and fungi, preventing infections of the skin [16-18]. When used in massage therapy, it moisturizes the skin and prevents drying that could predispose to infections. As an astringent, it can help with faster wound healing. However, given that it can act as an irritant, it is always recommended to use it in combination with a carrier oil such as olive oil. Bay leaf essential oil is a great choice for an aromatherapy oil to use in a diffuser. Infusing the air with warm, spicy, earthy, herbal bay leaf notes can promote relaxation and induce calm. Moreover, the aromatic compounds myrcene has mild sedative properties and further contributes to restoring a feeling of calm, reducing stress and lowering anxiety levels. Bay leaf oil lends itself to topical use and one of its best applications is maintaining scalp health. Applying a few drops of bay leaf oil diluted in a carrier oil such as olive on the scalp and massaging it for several minutes can help improve circulation to the root of the hair as well as combat dryness and even dandruff. Two of the most common causes of dandruff are dry scalp and fungal infections and bay leaf oil both moisturizes the scalp and has antifungal properties which recommends it for use for scalp health. Bay leaf essential oil is called a hair tonic because of its moisturizing action. Aromatic essential oils and fatty acids nourish hair and help restore shine. Regular application in combination with a carrier oil can help combat dryness, strengthen hair and improve scalp health for better-looking, healthier hair. Both bay leaves and the oil obtained from them can be used to repel bugs and roaches and other insects. Eucalyptol, the main aromatic compound in the oil, is a proven insect repellent, but other compounds are also toxic at certain concentrations and, as a result, may also hold similar insect-repellent properties [17-20].

Glycosides *Laurus nobilis* leaves yielded four nonpolar flavonoids kaempferol-3-O-α-L-(3″, 4″-di-E-p-coumaroyl)-rhamnoside, kaempferol-3-O-α-L-(2″,4″-di-E-pcoumaroyl)-rhamnoside, kaempferol-3-O-α-L-(2″-4″-

coumaroyl)- rhamnoside and a new product kaempferol-3-O-α-L-(2″,4″-di-Z-p-coumaroyl)-rhamnoside. Five new mega stigmane glucosides name dlaurosides A–E and a new phenolic glucoside were isolated from the methanolic extract of *L. nobilis* L. leaves. Kaempferol- 3-hamnopyranoside, and kaempferol-3, 7- di-rhamnopyranoside were isolated from *Laurus nobilis* aqueous ethanolic extract. Anthocyanin, the major anthocyanins were characterized as cyanidin 3-O-glucoside and cyanidin 3-O-rutinoside. Furthermore, two minor anthocyanins were detected and identified as 3-O-glucoside and 3-Orutinoside.

Traditional and Culinary uses

Traditionally, bay leaves are picked and dried slowly under the shade away from direct sunlight to retain their volatile essential oils. In the spice stores, one might come across different kinds of bay leaf preparations. Dried bay laurel berries are also being used as a flavoring item in dishes Discovered in the twentieth century, with a masculine and spicy aroma, *Laurus nobilis* essential oil is pleasant to use during fall and winter. *Laurus nobilis* essential oil benefits are enormous. From its application as hair growth tonic to keeping dandruff at *Laurus nobilis*, it possesses a lot of therapeutic properties. Being a stimulant of the digestive system, respiratory passages, circulatory system and the lymphatic functions, *Laurus nobilis* leaf has been a trusted traditional remedy for keeping numerous health conditions at *Laurus nobilis*. Pleasantly aromatic bay leaf or bay-laurel is one of the well-recognized culinary leaf-spices in use since the earliest times. In the legends, bay laurel is depicted as the tree of the *Sun god,* under the celestial sign of *Leo*. Bay leaves give off a pleasing and sweet aroma when added to the recipes. Wilted and dried leaves indeed are strongly aromatic and can be stored for months. Its dried fruit (berries) can also be employed as a flavoring agent in the cuisine. Medicinally, the benefits of the bay leaf and its berries are plentiful. Infusions of herb parts are reputed to soothe stomach ulcers and help relieve flatulence and colic pain. Glossy, dark-green bay leaves can be used fresh. However, they are at their best after being allowed to wilt under the shade for few days till their bitterness has gone, but the leaves still retain their pleasing aroma. Besides being quite strongly flavored, the laurel leaves are leathery in texture and tough to chew and swallow [18-22]. Laurel trees leaves have been a part of the culinary and medicinal world for thousands of years, dating to at least the ancient Roman times. There are many types of plants containing leaves referred to as "bay leaves", but the true bay leaf is scientifically known as *Laurus nobilis.* Many other leaves have a similar appearance and aroma like true bay leaves, but not the same nutrient content. Commercial essential oils generally obtained by hydrodistillation or steam distillation are commonly employed by the pharmaceutical and food industries. In Indian cuisine, bay laurel leaves are sometimes used in place of Indian bay leaf although they have a different flavour. They are most often used in rice dishes like biryani and as an ingredient in garam masala. Bay (laurel) leaves are frequently packaged as *tezpattÊ* (the Hindi term for Indian bay leaf) creating confusion between the two herbs. In the Philippines, dried bay laurel leaves are used in several Filipino dishes such as menudo, beef pares, and adobo. Bay leaves were used for flavouring by the ancient Greeks. They are a fixture in the cooking of many European cuisines (particularly those of the Mediterranean), as well as in the Americas. They are used in soups, stews, brines, meat, seafood, vegetable dishes, and sauces. The leaves also flavour many classic French and Italian dishes. The leaves are most often used whole (sometimes in a *bouquet garni*) and removed before serving (they can be abrasive in the digestive tract). Bay leaves can also be crushed or ground before cooking. Crushed bay leaves impart more fragrance than whole leaves, but are more difficult to remove and thus they are often used in a muslin bag or tea infuser. Ground bay laurel may be substituted for whole leaves, and does not need to be removed but it is much stronger. The uses of bay leaves include grinding the leaves into a spice to flavor soups and stews, but they are most commonly added in their whole form as a flavoring for certain Italian dishes. They are removed from the dish prior to consuming or used as a garnish. Whole leaves are not commonly consumed. There is no extensive range of culinary applications for bay leaves, although extracts of these leaves have numerous medical uses. [19-23]

Conclusion

Laurus nobilis L., known as bay, sweet bay, bay laurel, Roman laurel or daphne is an evergreen Mediterranean shrub whose leaves have traditionally been used in cuisines and folk medicine due to their beneficial health effects, which can nowadays be scientifically explained by various biological activities of the leaf extracts. Many of these activities can be attributed to phenolic compounds present in *L. nobilis* leaves which include flavonoids, phenolic acids, tannins (proanthocyanidins) and lignans. The presence of large amount of the biologically active compounds methyl eugenol for food use and 1,8-cineole for medicinal use can contribute to their pharmacological properties, muscle relaxant effect, and anti-inflammatory activity, respectively. It has astringent, diuretic, and appetite stimulant properties. The lauric acid in the bay laurel leaves has insect repellent properties. Laurel leaves, due to a wide range of structurally diverse bioactive molecules and their antioxidant, antimicrobial, anti-inflammatory, and other health beneficial properties, are an excellent base for the production of high-quality extracts with potential applications in the food, pharmaceutical, and cosmetic industries. Insights into the biopotential of laurel require new approaches in the production of plant extracts, and consequently, the use of advanced green techniques that allow the development of formulations and high value-added products with improved biological properties and actions.

REFERENCES

1. Marzouki H, Piras A, Salah KB, Medini H, Pivetta T; Bouzid, S, Marongiu B, Falconieri D. Essential Oil Composition and Variability of *Laurus nobilis* L. Growing in Tunisia, Comparison and Chemometric Investigation of different Plant Organs. Nat Prod Res. 2009; 23 (4): 343-54.
2. Fiorini C, Fourasté I, David B, Bessière JM. Composition of the Flower, Leaf and Stem Essential Oils from *Laurus nobilis*. FlavFragra J. 1997; 12(2): 91-93.
3. Caputo L, Nazzaro F, Souza LF, Aliberti L, Martino LD , Fratianni F, Coppola R, Feo VD. *Laurus nobilis*: Composition of Essential Oil and its Biological Activities Molecules. 2017; 3; 22(6): 930-933. doi: 10.3390/molecules22060930.
4. Kilic A, Hafizoglu H, Kollmannsberger H, Nitz S. Volatile Constituents and Key Odorants in Leaves, Buds, Flowers, and Fruit of *Laurus nobilis* L. J.Agri Food Chem. 2004; 52: 1601-1606. doi: 10.1021/jf0306237.
5. Dahab RA., Kasabri V, Afifi F. Evaluation of the Volatile Oil Composition and Antiproliferative Activity of *Laurus nobilis* L. (Lauraceae) on Breast Cancer Cell Line Models. Rec Nat Prod. 2014; 8: 136-147.
6. Caputo L, Nazzaro F, Souza LF, Aliberti L, Martino LD, Fratianni FF, Coppola R, Feo VD. *Laurus nobilis*: Composition of Essential Oil and its Biological Activities. 2017; 3; 22(6): 930. doi: 10.3390/molecules22060930.
7. Derwich E, Benziane Z, Boukir A. Chemical Composition and Antibacterial Activity of Leaves Essential Oil of *Laurus nobilis* from Morocco. Australian J Basic Appl Sci. 2009, 3 (4): 3818-3824.
8. Dadalioglu I, Evrendilek GA. Chemical Compositions and Antibacterial Effects of Essential Oils of Turkish Oregano (*Origanum minutiflorum*), Bay Laurel (*Laurus nobilis*), Spanish Lavender (*Lavandula stoechas* L.), and Fennel (*Foeniculum vulgare*) on Common Foodborne Pathogens. J Agri Food Chem. 2004, 52 (26): 8255-8260.
9. Chaudhry, NMA, Tariq P. Bactericidal Activity of Black Pepper, Bay Leaf, Aniseed, and Coriander against Oral Isolates. Pak J Pharmaceut Sci. 2006; 19 (3): 214-218.
10. Acqua SD, Cervellati R, Speroni E, Costa S, Guerra MC, Stella L, Innocenti G. Phytochemical Composition and Antioxidant Activity of *Laurus nobilis* L. Leaf Infusion. J Med Food. 2009; 12 (4): 869-876.
11. Márquez, DBM, Ávila GCM, Paz JEW, Cerda, RB, Herrera, RR, Aguilar CN. Ultrasound-assisted Extraction of Phenolic Compounds from *Laurus nobilis* L. and their Antioxidant Activity. Ultrasonics Sonochem 2013; 20 (5): 1149-1154.
12. Khan A, Zaman G, Anderson RA. Bay Leaves Improve Glucose and Lipid Profile of People with Type 2 Diabetes. Journal of Clinical Biochemistry and Nutrition 2009; 44 (1): 52-56.
13. Sayyah M, Saroukhani G, Peirovi A, Kamalinejad M. Analgesic and Anti-inflammatory Activity of the Leaf Essential Oil of *Laurus nobilis* Linn. 2003; 17(7): 733-736. https://doi.org/10.1002/ptr.1197
14. Dobroslaviæ E, Repajiæ M, Uzelac VD , Garofulic IE. Isolation of *Laurus nobilis* Leaf Polyphenols: A Review on Current Techniques and Future Perspectives. Foods. 2022; 16; 11(2): 235. doi: 10.3390/foods11020235.
15. Anzano A, de Falco B, Grauso L. *et al.* Laurel, *Laurus nobilis* L.: A Review of its Botany, Traditional uses, Phytochemistry and Pharmacology. Phytochem Rev 2022; 21, 565-615. https://doi.org/10.1007/s11101-021-09791-z
16. Basak, S, Candan F. Effect of *Laurus nobilis* L. Essential Oil and its Main Components on á-glucosidase and Reactive Oxygen Species Scavenging Activity. Iran J Pharm Res. 2013, 12, 367-379.

17. Usmani QI, Ahmad A, Jamaldeen FN. *Laurus nobilis* L., (Habb-ul-Ghar), A Review on Phytochemistry, Pharmacology and Ethnomedicinal Uses. J Drug Deli Therapeut. 2021; 11(5): 136-114.
18. Chahal KK, Kaur M, Bhardwaj U, Singla N, Kaur A. A Review on Chemistry and Biological Activities of *Laurus nobilis* L. essential Oil. Journal of Pharmacog Phytochem. 2017; 6(4): 1153-1161.
19. BozanB, KarakaplanU. Antioxidants from laurel (*Laurus nobilis* L.) berries: Influences of Extraction Procedure on yield and Antioxidant Activity of extracts. ActaAlim. 2007; 36: 321-328.
20. Kilic A, Hafizoglu, H, Kollmannsberger H, Nitz S. Volatile Constituents and Key Odorants in Leaves, Buds, Flowers, and Fruits of *Laurus nobilis* L. J Agri Food Chem. 2004; 52: 1601-1606.
21. Gülçin I. Antioxidant Activity of Caffeic Acid (3, 4-dihydroxycinnamic acid). Toxicol. 2006; 217 (2-3): 213-220.
22. Mansour O, Darwish M, Ismail G, Douba ZA , Ismaeel A, Eldair KS. Review Study on the Physiological Properties and Chemical Composition of the *Laurus nobilis*. The Pharmaceut Chem J. 2018:5(1): 225-231.
23. Olga K, Irina P, Yuliia F, Kateryna S, Component Composition of Essential Oil Shoots and Leaves of *Laurus Nobilis* L. Ukrainian Origian Science Rise. Pharmaceut Sci. 2021; 4(32): 50-58. https://doi.org/10.15587/2519-4852.2021.239335

CHAPTER 4

An Appraisal of Ethnopharmacological relevance and Phytoconstituents of Black Cardamom (*Amomum subulatum* Roxb.)

ABSTRACT

Amomum subulatum is also known as 'Badi Elaichi' is an aromatic and medicinal spice, used as a flavoring agent in various dishes. It is also known as Queen of spices. It is a native of the Eastern Himalayan region. Traditionally, black cardamom has been utilized as a preventive and remedial measure for throat problems, blockage of lungs, irritation of eyelids, stomach-related problems and in the treatment of aspiratory tuberculosis. It is considered as a conclusive drug in the traditional medicinal system like Unani and Ayurveda since ancient times. The present traditional knowledge highlights the effectiveness of *A. subulatum* possessing biological activities like anti-inflammatory, anti-ulcer, anti-oxidant, anti-microbial and cardio-adaptogen. The chemical constituents of various extracts of *A. subulatum* revealed the presence of carbohydrates, flavonoids, amino acids, steroids, triterpenoids, glycosides, tannins, anthocyanin's, aurone, flavanone alkaloids, fixed oil and fats. The chemical constituents of the Badi Elaichi are 1,8-cineole around (65-80%) and the other phytochemicals are Terpenyl acetate (traces to five percent), The distribution of the essential oil of black cardamom is 1,8-cineole (65 to 80%) and limonene (10.3%) as a significant constituent. The monoterpene hydrocarbon present is 5 to 17% of which limonene, sabinene, terpinenes and pinenes are major components. The terpinols contain around 5 to 7% of the oil.

Keywords: Terpenyl acetate, 1,8-cineole, Cardioadaptogen, Antiinflamtory, Limonene.

Introduction

Amomum subulatum Roxb. (Large Cardamom) is a perennial herbaceous crop, cultivated in swampy places across hills around water streams. It has been used as flavouring agent to various dishes indigenous to the Eastern

Himalayan region particularly Nepal, Bhutan, and India. Sikkim State of India is the largest producer of cardamom that is around 50% of the world's production. Its fruits are widely used as a spice. It is a part of official ayurvedic formulations used in folklore medicine. *A. subulatum* has been used in ayurvedic formulations to treat various lung conditions such as cough, lung congestion, and pulmonary tuberculosis. Black Cardamom is also known as "Black gold" or "Queen of spices" is a high market value plant that is utilized as an enhancing agent in different food items. [1-4] Because of its pleasant fragrance, it has been utilized as a significant ingredient in blended flavors for seasoning vegetables, numerous food arrangements and pickles, in the world mainly in China, India, Nepal, Bhutan. The seed is used for commercial practice. It is also used in the treatment of teeth and gums infection, as medicine for stomach problems and in malaria, and also used as an antidote against snake and scorpion venom. Great cardamom is used in the Ayurveda and Unani medicinal systems to cure diseases including heartburn, vomiting, rectal infections, looseness of the bowels, liver blockage, gastrointestinal issues, and genitourinary grumblings. Black Cardamom helps in improving the metabolic conditions when added to the eating routine. Black cardamom helps to enhance the functioning of the liver. [5-9]

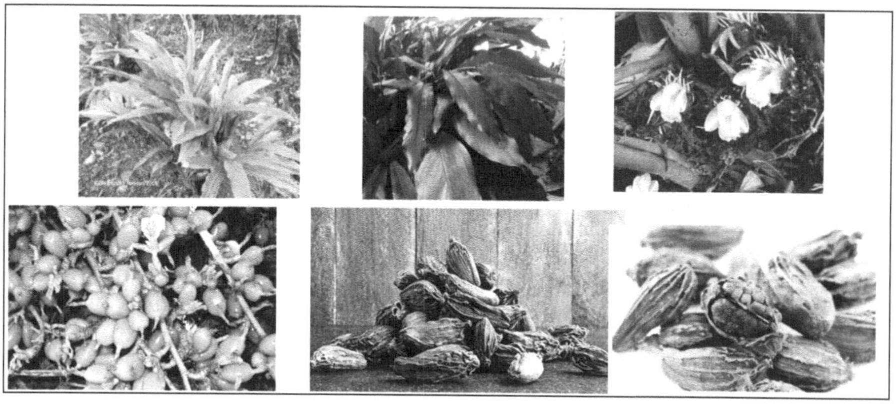

Black Cardamom plant leaves, flowers, unripe & ripened fruits

Phytochemical constituents of BadiElaichi

Qualitative chemical examinations of various extracts of *A. subulatum* revealed the presence of carbohydrates, flavonoids, amino acids, steroids, triterpenoids, glycosides, tannins, anthocyanins, aurone, flavanone and alkaloids, fixed oil and fats. *A. subulatum* composition varies with variety, region and age of the product. The fruit on average comprises 70% seeds and 30% skin (Pruthi, 1993). Seeds contains 8.6% moisture, 5% total ash value, 1.5% ash insoluble in acid, 3.5% water soluble ash value, 4.88% alcohol extract, 4% non-volatile ether extract and 91.4% of total solid. Volatile oil content varies between 1.95 to 3.32% in different varieties of the cardamom.

In is reported that cardamom seeds contain Copper (7.4 mg. kg^{-1}), Nickel (<0.006 mg.kg^{-1}), Zinc (57.6 mg.kg^{-1}), Lead (<0.015 mg.kg^{-1}), Cobalt (5.4 mg.kg^{-1}), Cadmium (0.2 mg.kg^{-1}), Iron (111.2 mg.kg^{-1}) and Chromium (<0.003 mg.kg^{-1}). The composition of the essential oil of large cardamom are 1,8-cineole (65 to 80%) and limonene (10.3%) as a major constituent. The monoterpene hydrocarbon content is in the range of 5 to 17% of which lamonene, sabeinene, the terpinenes and the pinenes are significant components. The terpinols comprise ~5 to 7% of the oil. The high cineole and low terpenyl acetate probably account for the very harsh aroma of this spice in comparison with that of true cardamom. The seed of the cardamom contain mainly essential oil, flavonoids, carbohydrates and fats. [10-14] Total phenolic content in seed was found to be 0.00366% w/w (weight by weight) which has been reported as gallic acid while total flavonoid content in seed was observed to be 0.0361% w/w. The extract of seeds also contains few glycosides such as subulin, petunidin-3,5-diglucoside, leucocyanadin-3-O-β-D-glucopyranoside along with cardamom and alpinetin. Steam distillation of seed contains essential oil having cineole as principal constituent. Other constituents are α- and β-pinene, sabinene, p-cymene, terpinen-4-ol, α- and β-terpineol, nerolidol, terpinene, terpinyl acetate and bisabolene. Protocatechualdehyde, 1,7-bis(3,4-dihydroxyphenyl) hepta-4E, 6E-dien-3-one, Protocatechuic acid, and 2, 3, 7-trihydroxy-5-(3,4- dihydroxy-E-styryl) -6, 7, 8, 9- tetrahydro - 5H –benzocycloheptene, are isolated from greater cardamom. Protocatechualdehyde and protocatechuic acid possess have potent antioxidant activity. The high cineole and low terpenyl acetate derivatives are responsible for the aroma of this spice. The seed of cardamom contains primarily essential oil, flavonoids, carbohydrates and fats. [15-22]

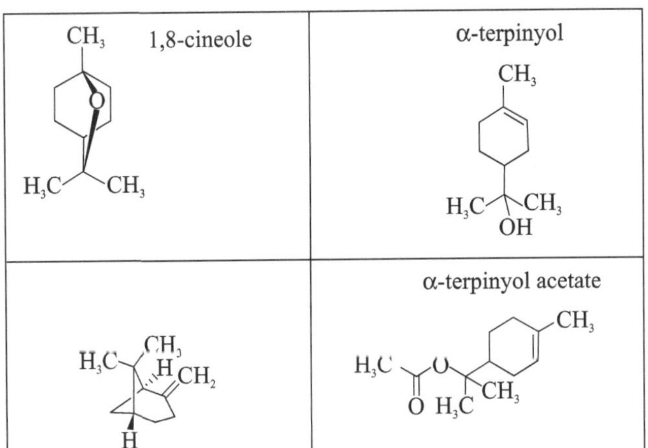

Chemical structures of major constituents occurring in black cardamom

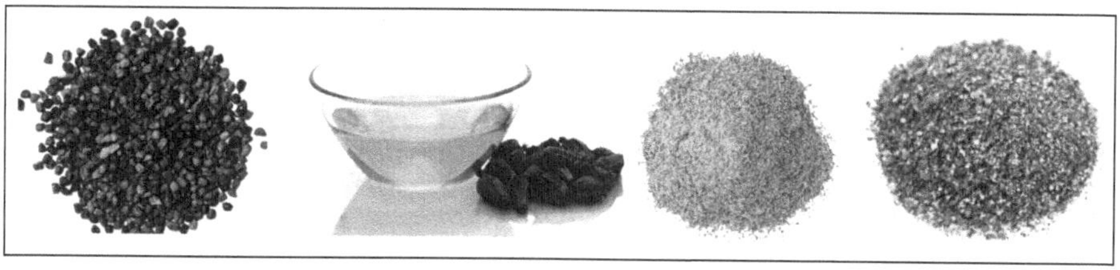

Seeds, Coarse ground and powder of Black cardamom

Ethnopharmacological Relevance

Traditionally, black cardamom has been utilized as a preventive and remedial measure for throat problems, blockage of lungs, irritation of eyelids, stomach-related problems and in the treatment of respiratory tuberculosis. From ancient times, black cardamom seeds have been utilized to fix dyspnoea, hack, thirst, vomiting, infection of the mouth, nausea, tingling, acid reflux, biliousness, stomach torments and rectal infections in rural areas and cities too. *A. subulatum* seeds and fruits are used in the preparation of food items as flavors consistently around the world and prevent gastrointestinal problems, respiratory issues. It increases the palatability and flavor to make food more edible. Residues of charred leaves are used with mustard oil and taken twice for sexually transmitted diseases and hack. "Alui" a formulation prepared from the combination of cumin and black cardamom is utilized for the treatment of malaria. The seed decoction is helpful as a gargle in infection of the teeth and gums while the pericarp is helpful in cerebral pain and stomatitis [23-26]. The seeds are additionally helpful as an antidote against snake and scorpion venom. It is a significant constituent in Arabic coffee. They own coffeepots that can keep a few cardamom seeds in their spouts and use cardamom in blend form with different flavors in their dishes. Scandinavian nations utilize cardamom in biscuits and sweetbreads. Black cardamom in Ayurveda: Badi Elaichi is an herb that reduces Vata (air component) and Kapha (earth and water component) and increases pitta (digestion and metabolism) component of human body. In the Ayurvedic medicinal system, it is utilized as a carminative, diuretic, stomachic and stomach related, and for colds and heart stimulation. Cardamom has been utilized in traditional medication against kidney and urinary problems, and as a gastrointestinal defensive. Cardamom oil has revealed calming and antibacterial uses. In India, black cardamom (*A. subulatum*) is comprehensively used to treat contaminations of the teeth and gums and to treat throat inconvenience, blockage of the lungs and pneumonic tuberculosis, asthma, coronary illness, aggravation of the eyelids and stomach related problems. At the point when mixed with neem and camphor, cardamom is utilized as a nasal readiness to treat colds. Implantation of cardamom can be utilized as a rinse to mitigate sore throats, which has prompted its utilization in hack desserts. Cardamom is also utilized as a remedy for the treatment of both snake and scorpion toxins and food contamination. In traditional Chinese medication, it is utilized to treat stomachache, stoppage, loose bowels, and other processing issues. Cardamom seeds when mixed with milk, are used for bladder related issues. The seeds are famously accepted to be a Spanish fly. Large cardamom has been used as preventive as well as a curative for throat trouble, congestion of lungs, inflammation of eyelids, digestive disorders and in the treatment of pulmonary tuberculosis. It is also useful in treatment of flatulence, loss of appetite, gastric troubles, congestion and liver complaints [27-29]. The seeds are reported an official drug in Ayurvedic. Seeds and fruits of *A. subulatum* are added to cooked food items as spices by the general population on a daily basis and can play a preventive role in the occurrence of respiratory problems, and through increasing palatability and flavor of foods make them more serve to maintain good health. A preparation called "Alui" is prepared for the treatment of malaria by administering the mixture of cumin (*cuminium cyminum*) and large cardamom. The teeth and gums while the pericarp is useful in headache, stomatitis and snake bite. Seeds and fruits were found to be useful in prevention of hyperlipidaemia. Ashes of burned leaves are mixed with mustard oil and taken twice daily for cough and sexually transmitted diseases. Essential oil, oleoresin, encapsulated flavour, cardamom cola, flavoured biscuits and flavoured liquors are some of the products developed for diversifying the uses of large cardamom. Cardamom cola is prepared by blending caramel acid, large cardamom flavour and carbonating the mixture. [30-32]

The seeds are aromatic and pungent, with a sharp, pleasant taste; they are similar in properties to the true cardamom for which they are often substituted both as a spice and as a masticatory or as an ingredient of chewing preparation. In South India, large cardamom is used in the preparation of snuff and agarbatties. Medicinally, the seeds are credited with stimulant, stomachic, alexipharmic and astrigent properties, and are prescribed for the treatment of indigestion, vomiting, biliousness, abdominal pains and rectal diseases. A decoction of the seeds is used as a gargle in affections of the teeth and gums. With melon seeds, they are used as a diuretic in cases of gravel of the kidneys. They promote elimination of bile and are useful in congestion of liver; they are also used in gonorrhoea. In large doses (30 grains) with quinine, they are useful in neuralgia. The pericarp is useful in headache and heals stomatitis. The aromatic oil extracted from the seeds is applied to the eyes to allay inflammation. In Ayurvedic and Unani medicines large cardamoms are used as a preventive as well as a curative for throat troubles, congestion of lungs, inflammation of eyelids, digestive disorders and in the treatment of pulmonary tuberculosis. [28, 31-34]

Conclusion

Large cardamom is very popular since prehistoric time. It is more valued due to its acceptable taste, flavor and aroma. It has been reported to possess valuable therapeutic properties. Fruits of *Amomum subulatum* are prescribed mainly to treat indigestion, vomiting, biliousness, acne, gout, spasm and cardiac arthymia. Besides, it has been used as an insecticide. *Amomum subulatum* Roxb is commonly known as, Badi Elaichi or Greater Cardamom is a well-known Indian medicinal plant widely used in the treatment of many clinical conditions. The major constituent of large cardamom is volatile oil (2-4%). It is the principal aroma-giving compound and 1, 8-cineole is the major active compound, in an extent 60 to 80% of the total volatile oil. The monoterpene hydrocarbon contentrange is from 5 to 17%, out of which lamonene, sabeinene, and pinenes are significant components. Terpinols comprise ~5 to 7% of the oil. Seeds and dry ripe fruit are used for its therapeutic actions such as stimulant, laxative, aromatic, carminative and gastro-protective, cardio-protective properties. Keeping in view the medicinal properties of *A. subulatum* Roxb an attempt has been made to give overview on the processing technology, chemistry, bioactivity and therapeutic uses of large cardamom and its components.

REFERENCES

1. Choudhary S, Madhusudan S, Walia B, Chaudhary G. Black Cardamom (*Amomum sabulatum*): A Review Int J Curr Res.2021: 13(4): 17027-17032.doi: https://doi.org/10.24941/ijcr.40962.04.2021
2. Makhija P, Handral HK, Mahadevan G, Kathuria H, Sethi G, Grobben B. Black Cardamom (*Amomum subulatum* Roxb.) Fruit Extracts Exhibit Apoptotic Activity against Lung Cancer Cells. J Ethnopharmacol. 2022; 6(287): 114953. doi: 10.1016/j.jep.2021.114953
3. Bisht VK, Negi JS, Bhandari AK, Sundriyal RC. *Amomum subulatum* Roxb: Traditional, Phytochemical and Biological Activities-An Overview. Afri J Agri Res. 2011; 6(24): 5386-5390.doi: 10.5897/AJAR11.745
4. Alam K, Pathak D, Ansari SH. Evaluation of Anti-Inflammatory activity of *Amomium Subulatum* Fruit Extract. Int J Pharmaceu. Sci. Drug. Res.2011; 3(1): 35-37.
5. Aneja KR, Joshi R. Antimicrobial Activity of *Amomum subulatum* and *Elettaria cardamomum* against Dental Carries Causing Microorganisms. EthnobotLeaflets. 2009; 13: 840-849.
6. Bisht VK, Purohit V, Negi JS, Bhandari AK. Introduction and Advancement in Cultivation of Large Cardamom (*Amomum subulatum* Roxb.) in Uttarakhand, India. ResJ Agri Sci.2010; 1(3): 205-208.
7. Jafri MA, Farah KJ, Singh S. Evaluation of the Gastricantiulcerogenic effect of Large Cardamom (Fruits of *Amomum subulatum* Roxb.). J. Ethnopharmocol.2001; 75: 89-94.
8. Kikuzaki H, Kawai Y, Nakatani N. Diphenyl-2-picrylhydrazylradical-scavenging Active Compounds from Greater Cardamom (*Amomum subulatum* Roxb.). J. Nutr. Sci. Vitaminol. 2001; 47(2): 167-171.
9. Kumar U, Kumar B, Bhandari A, Kumar Y. Phytochemical Investigation and Comparison of Antimicrobial Screening of Clove and Cardamom. Int JPharmaceutSci Res., 2010;1(12): 138-147.

10. Lakshmi V, Chauhan JS. Chemical Examination of the Seeds of *Amomum subulatum*. J IndChem Soc.1976; 53: 633-636.
11. Patra NK, Siddiqui MS, Akhila A, Nigam MC, Naqvi AA. Chemical Composition of the Volatile Oil from the Pericarp (Husk) of Large Cardamom (*Amomum subulatum* Roxb.) Pafai J. 1982; 4(4): 29-31.
12. Shukla SH, Mistry HA, Patel VG, Jogi BV. Pharmacognostical, Preliminary Phytochemical Studies and Analgesic Activity of *Amomum subulatum* Roxb. PharmSciMonit. 2010; (1): 90-102.
13. Verma SK, Rajeevan V, Bordia A, Jain V. Greater Cardamom (*Amomum subulatum* Roxb.)–A Cardio-adaptogen against Physical stress. J Herb Med Toxicol.2010; 4(2): 55-58.
14. Parveen U, Maaz M, Mujeeb M, Jahangir U. Biological and Therapeutic uses of *Amomum subulatum*, Roxb. A Review. Eur J Biomed Pharmaceut Sci. 2018; 5(1): 167-176
15. Gautam N, Bhattarai RR, Khanal BKS, Oli P. Technology, Chemistry and Bioactive Properties of Large Cardamom (*Amomum subulatum* Roxb.): An Overview. Int J ApplSciBiotechnol. 2016; 4(2): 139-149.
16. Gautam N. Technology, Chemistry and Bioactive Properties of Large Cardamom (*Amomum subulatum* Roxb.): An Overview. IntJApplSciBiotechlol. 2016; 139-149.
17. Rout PK, Sahoo D, Jena KS, Rao YR. Analysis of the Oil of Large Cardamom (*Amomum subulatum* Roxb.) Growing in Sikkim. J Essent Oil Res. 2003; 15: 265-266.
18. Karisappa G. Post Harvest Studies In Large Cardamom (*Amomum sublatum*Roxb.). SikkimSciSoc Newsletter 1987; 6(3): 2-10.
19. Bhandari AK, Bhist VK, Negi JS, Baunthiyal M. 1,8-Cineole: A Predominant Component in the Essential Oil of Large Cardamom (*Amomum subulatum* Roxb.). J Medi Plants Res. 2013; 7(26): 1957-1960.
20. Rao YS, Kumar A, Chatterjee S, Naidu R, George CK. Large Cardamom (*Amomum subulatum* Roxb.)– A Review. J Spices Aroma Crops.1993; 2(1&2): 1-15.
21. Nigam S, Purohit R. Chemical Examination of the Essential Oil Derived from the Seeds of *Amomum subulatum* Roxb. Perfumery Essent OilRecord. 1960; 51(3): 121-122.
22. Lawrence BM, Terpenes in Two Amomum species. Phytochem. 1970; 9: 665-667.
23. Lakshmi VCJ. Chemical Examination of the Seeds of *Amomum subulatum*. J IndChem Soc. 1976; 53: 633-635.
24. Kikuzaki HKYNN. Diphenyl-2-picrylhydrazylradical Scavenging Active Compounds from Greater Cardamom (*Amomum subulatum* Roxb.). J NutrSciVitaminol. 2001; 47(2): 167-171.
25. Shukla S, Mistry H, Patel V, Jogi B. Pharmacognostical, Preliminary Phytochemicalstudies and Analgesic Activity of *Amomum subulatum* Roxb. Pharm SciMonit. 2010; 1(1): 90-102.
26. Alam K, Pathak DAS. Evaluation of Anti-Inflammatory Activity of *Amomum subulatum* fruit extract. Int. J PharmaceutSci Drug Res. 2011; 3(1): 35-37.
27. Kumar U, Kumar B, Bhandari A, Kumar Y. Phytochemical Investigation and Comparison of Antimicrobial Screening of Clove and Cardamom. Int J PharmaceutSci Res., 2010; 1(12): 138-147.
28. Aneja KR, Joshi R. Antimicrobial Activity of *Amomum subulatum* and *Elettaria cardamomum* against Dental Caries Causing Microorganisms. Ethnobot Leaflets. 2009; 13: 840-49.
29. Agnihotri S, Wakode S. Antimicrobial Activity of Essential Oil and Various Extracts of Fruits of Greater Cardamom. Indian J Pharm Sci. 2010; 72(5): 657-659.

30. Kikuzaki h, Kawai y, Nakata N. 1,1-Diphenyl-2-picrylhydrazyl radical-scavenging Active Compounds from Greater Cardamom (*Amomum subulatum* Roxb.). J NutrSciVitaminol. 2001; 47(2): 167-71.
31. Singhal PK, Gautam GK, Kumar R, Kumar G. A Review on *Amomum subulatum* and *Elettaria Cardamomum* with their Pharmacological Activity Recent Trends PharmaceutSci Res. 2022; 4(1): 1-6.
32. Sen S, Chakraborty R, Dev B, Mazumder J. Plants and Phytochemicals for Peptic Ulcer: An Overview.Pharmagonosy Rev, 2009; 3(6): 270-279.
33. Satyal P, Dosoky NS, Kincer BL, Setzer WN. Chemical Compositions and Biological Activities of *Amomum subulatum* Essential Oils from Nepal. Nat Prod Commun. 2012; 7(9): 1233-1236.

CHAPTER

5

To Endeavor a Systematic review on the Traditional uses, Phytochemical Composition and Pharmacological Properties of Black pepper (*P. nigrum* L.)

ABSTRACT

Black pepper (*Piper nigrum* L.) is an important healthy food owing to its antioxidant, antimicrobial potential and gastro-protective modules. Black pepper, with piperine as an active ingredient, holds rich phytochemistry that also includes volatile oil, oleoresins, and alkaloids. It has also been extensively explored for its biological properties and its bioactive phyto-compounds. In addition to its culinary uses, pepper has important medicinal and preservative properties, and, more recently, piperine has been shown to have fundamental effects on p-glycoprotein and many enzyme systems, leading to biotransformative effects including chemoprevention, detoxification, and enhancement of the absorption and bioavailability of herbal and conventional drugs. The alkaloid piperine improves the therapeutic value of several drugs, vaccines and nutrients by enhancing bioavailability through inhibiting numerous digestive enzymes. Piperine also aids in digestion through stimulating pancreatic and intestinal enzymes, and enriches cognitive skills and fertility. Furthermore, piperine is recognized as delivering several therapeutic activities distinct from other chemical components. This study endeavors to systematically review précised data on the traditional uses and pharmacological properties of black pepper. Besides, this review presents a summary of the data on the chemical composition of black pepper, including minerals, vitamins, carotenoids and flavonoids, and various therapeutic benefits. Up to date existing information, various metabolites have been isolated from *P. nigrum*. Among them, biologically active alkaloid piperine and the main essential oils constituents including β-caryophyllene, limonene, sabinene, α-pinene, β-bisabolene and α-copaene can serve as a new natural source for use in food, aroma, cosmetics and pharmaceutical industries.

Keywords: Oleoresins, Piperine.

Introduction

Black pepper, the (*Piper nigrum* L.), is a widely used spice, known for its pungent odour. *Piper nigrum* it is a perennial shrub native to southern India, and has been extensively cultivated there and in other tropical regions. Due to its strong pungency, it has valuable medicinal potency. It is one of the world most common kitchen spices and well known for its pungent chemical constituent piperine (1-peperoyl piperidine, which has diverse pharmacological activities. It is commonly known as Kali mirch in Urdu and Hindi, Marich in Nepali, Pippali in Sanskrit, Milagu in Tamil, and Black Pepper, Peppercorn, Green pepper, White pepper, Madagascar pepper in English. *P. nigum* is a woody climbing vine growing to 30 ft and the grayish stem may reach 1.2 cm diameter. Numerous rootlets grow from swollen stem nodes. [1-2] Leaves dark green above and pale green beneath, glossy, ovate and acutely tipped, and range in size from 13-25 cm in length. Elongated, slender spikes or catkins (1.6-2 cm in length) bear minute, white flowers. The flower spikes, each producing from 50-60 single-seeded dark red berries, ~5mm in diameter, always appear on stems opposite the leaves. Different parts of the plant are used for medicinal purposes; however, the part commonly used as the spice black pepper is the cooked and dried unripe berry. Due to some religious value of black pepper, its being popular from ancient time to modern generation. This review is aimed to provide a literature review on recent advancement of chemistry, pharmacognosy, pharmacological activities other general use of *Piper nigrum*. It is widely accepted and most used in different traditional systems of medicine, like the Unani and Ayurvedic systems. Recent scientific researchers have established the presence of many active compounds in this spice that are known to possess specific pharmacological properties.

Almost all spices have aromatic features, regular grindings of spices lead to loss of important aroma compounds and accordingly resulted to considerable loss of aroma and flavor components and deterioration of quality. The dried black pepper fruit is rich in bioactive phytochemical compounds. Piperine is one of the most abundant chemical alkaloids in the black pepper. Other similar alkaloids are also isolated from black pepper such as piperanine, piperettine, piperylinA, piperolein B, and pipericine. However, the pungency of these piperine's analogs are less than the Piperine). Black pepper was also found to have a good quantity of polyphenols. The interesting findings are that, black pepper contains more polyphenols compared with white pepper (White pepper is made from fully ripe pepper berries. They are soaked in water for about 10 days, leading to fermentation. Then their skins are removed, which also removes some of the hot piperine compound, as well as volatile oils and compounds that give black pepper its aroma. As a result, white pepper has a different flavor and heat component than black pepper. The process used and handling of white pepper can introduce different flavor notes as well.). [3-5] Moreover, it is believed that, after eating Black pepper, it hydrolyzed in the gut and liberating these bound polyphenols. Even some studies stated that the Black pepper contains aromatic compounds, flavonoids, alkaloids, amides and lignans. The volatile oils of the Black pepper fruits were analyzed using column chromatography, high resolution gas chromatography and gas chromatography mass spectrometry (GC-MS); up to 46 compounds were identified including δ-cadinol, δguaiene, (Z) (E)- farnesol, (E)-β-ocimene and guaiol. In another study, five phenolic amides were isolated from the black pepper, which revealed high antioxidant activity more effective than some naturally occurring antioxidants of the black pepper in bioactive phytochemical components of promising medicinal importance. The therapeutic efficacy of this individual spice for specific pharmacological actions has also been established by experimental and clinical studies.[6-9]

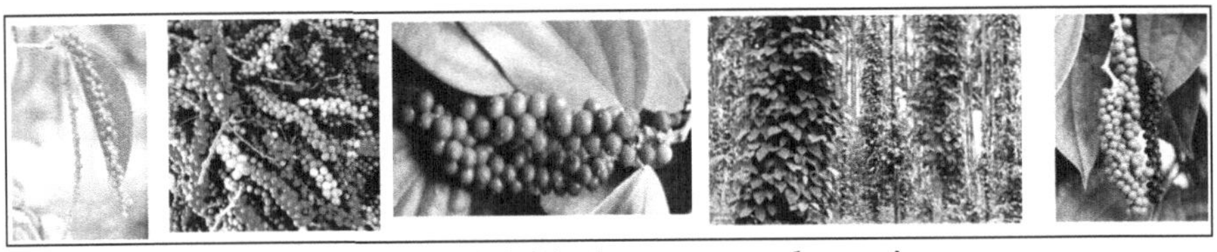

Green and Pink black pepper seeds on vine

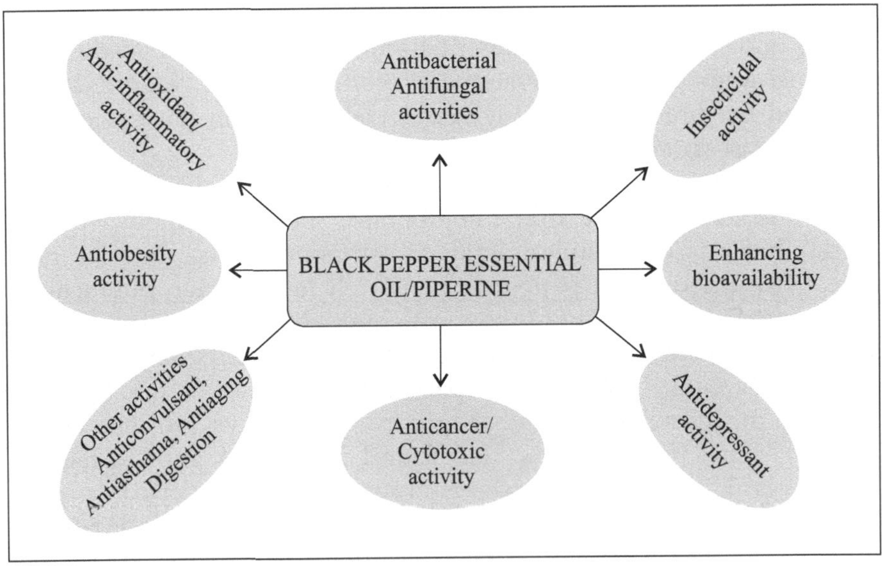

Bioactive chemical compounds of the black pepper

Black pepper is rich in minerals, vitamins and nutrients. The chemical composition of 100 g of black pepper seeds includes carbohydrate 66.5 g, protein 10 g, and fat 10.2 g, as well as a relatively high concentration of minerals such as calcium (400 mg), magnesium (235.8-249.8 mg), potassium (1200 mg), phosphorus (160 mg), and the lower concentration of sodium, iron and zinc. These minerals are essential elements for day-to-day activities of humans. Besides, black pepper also has a significant concentration of vitamins such as Vitamin C, B1, B2 and B3. Nine accessions of Nigeria grown black pepper had a concentration of tannin ranging from 2.11 to 2.80 mg/100 g. In a recent study on black pepper, catechin, Quercetin, myricetin, and carotenoids, namely lutein and β-carotene have also been detected in significant concentration. Several researchers evaluated essential oils (EO), oleoresin and piperine in various parts of black pepper. The EO yield of black pepper berries and leaves have varied from 1.24 to 5.06%, and 0.15-0.35%, respectively. It has been observed that variability of volatile oil and oleoresin content in 14 black pepper accessions ranged from 2.7-5.1% and 7.6-9.4%, respectively. The oleoresin content of black pepper ranged between 4.27 and 12.73% and the characteristic natural alkaloid of black pepper "piperine" ranged from 2.13-5.80% and 0.12-20.86%, in seeds and leaves correspondingly. [10-34]

Chemical Composition	Concentration
Proximate	
Water (g)	8.0
Energy (Kcal)	400.0
Carbohydrate (g)	66.5
Protein (g)	10.0
Fat (g)	10.2
Total Ash (%)	3.43-5.09
Crude fibre (%)	10.79-18.60
Minerals	
Calcium (mg)	400.0
Magnesium (mg)	235.8-249.8
Phosphorus (mg)	160.0
Sodium (mg)	10.0
Potassium (mg)	1200.0
Iron (mg)	17.0[36]
Zinc (mg)	1.45-1.72
Vitamins	
Vitamin C (mg)	27.46-32.53

(Contd...)

Vitamin B1 (mg)	0.74-0.91
Vitamin B2 (mg)	0.48-0.61
Vitamin B3 (mg)	0.63-0.78
Metabolites	
Tannin (mg)	2.11-2.80
Flavonoids	
Catechin (µg)	410.0
Myricetin (µg)	56.0
Quercetin (µg)	13.0
Carotenoids	
Lutein (µg)	260.0
β-carotene (µg)	150.0

Nutritional composition of Black Pepper [Nutrient concentration/100g]

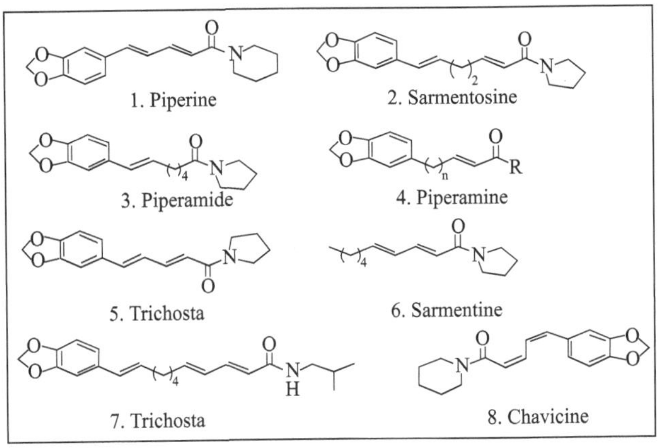

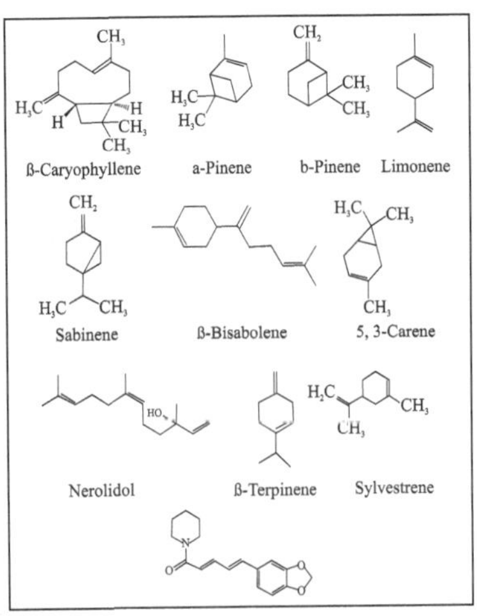

Major chemical constituents of Black pepper seed and essential oil. [15-18]

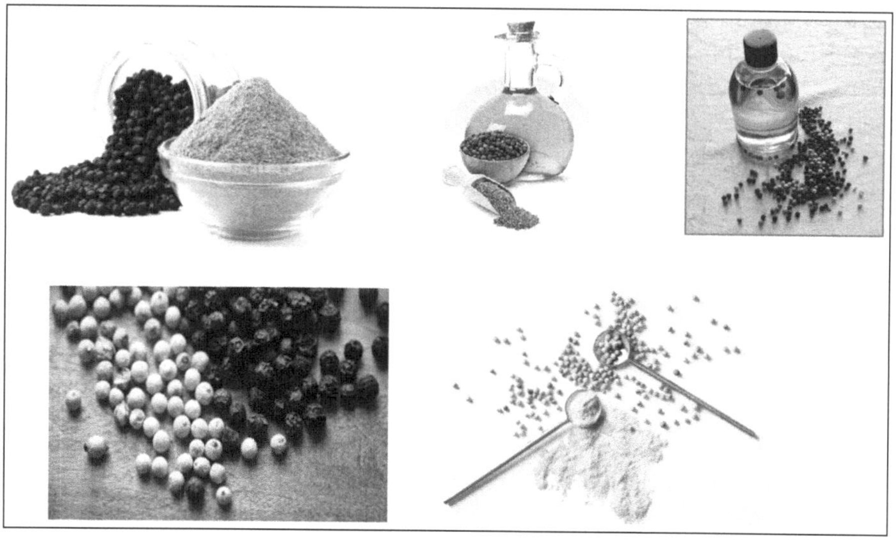

Traditional Medicinal Uses

Traditionally, black pepper has been used in a variety of different remedies and for different purposes. According to Ayurveda, the pungency and heating properties of black pepper work to help metabolize food as it is digested in our system. Its heat works as a stimulant like lighting a fire might. Like many aromatic kitchen herbs, black pepper is considered a carminative in Western herbalism, and in Ayurveda black pepper is known to enkindle *agni,* the digestive fire. These actions are likely due to the taste of black pepper on the tongue triggering the stomach to release hydrochloric acid, which is needed to digest protein, and pepper's ability to stimulate digestive enzymes in the pancreas. This stimulating quality is also used to clear congestion in the respiratory system as well as other processes. In the classical literature, many Unani scholars have mentioned various medicinal uses of black pepper. It has been described for its efficacy in cholera, dyspepsia, flatulence, diarrhea, and other gastrointestinal ailments. It is also a useful ingredient in tooth powders. In "Ilaj-ul-Ghurba" a pill is recommended for syphilis, which is prepared by taking black pepper (*P. nigrum*), *Calotropis gigantea,* and jaggery. Externally, it is applied to boils. It is also used in case of sore throat, alopecia, skin disorders, and piles etc. Finely powdered black pepper and sesame oil well mixed and heated, when applied over the paralytic area, is proved to be very effective. A preparation made with black pepper and leaves of Cassia occidentalis is even good for night blindness. It is also used in the treatment of gonorrhea. The drug is used as an antidote for scorpion sting. The plant *Cissampelo spareira,* in combination with black pepper, has been claimed to be useful in birth control when given immediately after delivery. In Cambodia, it is also used as cure for dysentery. In reference with Dioscorides. It is beneficial for the treatment of cough and chest pain when given in the form of sharbat (Syrup) or lauq (Paste). Along with honey, it is good for diphtheria. The combination of black pepper, onion, and salt, when applied on the bald area, is effective for curing alopecia. When used along with vinegar, it is also good for tooth ache. [10-14]

Health Benefits of Black Pepper

Just a pinch of black pepper when added to any food preparation can enhance its flavor. It is a spice that is known to offer many health benefits. It helps to promote weight loss and even aids in digestion. It is believed that this amazing spice prevents cancer as black pepper detoxifies the body, cleanse the intestine and stomach. Black pepper releases hydrochloric acid in stomach which helps in cleaning the intestines. It prevents constipation and helps to combat occurrence of common cold. Black pepper is used for combating skin exfoliation, skin deformation and helps to keep wrinkles at bay. It is used to combat dandruff, helps in restoring hair growth and makes the hair shiny. Mentioned below are the best health benefits of Black Pepper. Black pepper helps to prevent the occurrence of cancer. Black pepper is credited with piperline and this when combined with turmeric can help in preventing cancer. Black pepper is also loaded with antioxidants, and presence of vitamins like Vitamin A, flavonoids and carotenes helps in combating cancer causing free radicals. Black pepper aids in digestion problem, and when a person consumes raw black pepper, hydrochloric acid is released by the stomach, and this helps in breaking down of proteins. The release of hydrochloric acid in black pepper also helps in cleaning the intestines and helps in combating gastrointestinal diseases. Stomach disorders such as constipation, colon cancer, diarrhoea and other bacterial diseases are prevented when black pepper is consumed daily. Cold and cough can be cured by adding this spice to herbal tea and consumed two or three times a day. Having dishes prepared with black pepper are useful in winter and facilitate removal of phlegm from the body. Black pepper with honey prevents chest congestion. One can add crushed black pepper to warm water along with eucalyptus oil drops and inhale the steam to get rid of chest congestion. Black pepper prevents a skin pigmentation disease called vitiligo. This condition makes the skin turn white. There are many chemical rich medicines available in the market to restore skin color. However, one should know that black pepper is loaded with piperine that helps in restoring the natural color of the skin. This also ensures that the chances of occurrence of skin cancer due to overexposure to chemicals are reduced. Black pepper used for skin rash and skin allergy, you also uses black pepper as scrub to remove dead skin. Skin deformation, like wrinkles, is kept at bay if one adds black pepper to their diet since young age. The occurrence of premature ageing, dark spots are also kept in control if one eats black pepper in raw or cooked form. Eating black pepper makes sure that blood circulation to different parts of the body is improved. This also ensures that skin is rejuvenated. Skin disorders like acne are controlled if one adds black pepper to their diet. The skin exfoliation can be done by crushing some black pepper and applying it over skin. Black pepper is used in the treatment of dandruff in hair. Add curd with black pepper for hair loss problem, one of the effective home remedy. Even black pepper oil used to prevent hair loss and hair regrowth. Black pepper aids in weight loss. The reason is that black pepper is rich in phytonutrients and this helps in breaking down excess fat and improves the metabolism of the body. Black pepper is used in the treatment of depression. When one chews raw black pepper, a mood-inducing chemical is released from the brain, and this fills the mind with a soothing, calm mood. Black pepper is good for prevention of arthritis and joint pains. Black pepper has medicinal properties that help to combat gout. It is useful for people suffering from joint and spinal pain. This wonder spice helps to promote sweating and urination. Thus help to get rid of toxins in the body. Black pepper is good for prevention of arthritis and joint pains. Black pepper has medicinal properties that help to combat gout. It is useful for people suffering from joint and spinal pain. Black pepper is used in many cuisines as a spice globally. It is used extensively during cold and winter seasons and helps to combat respiratory problems. It is used as an aphrodisiac and also in the treatment of erectile dysfunction. Black pepper is found to cause stomach burns when taken in large quantities. When large quantities of black pepper enter the lungs, it may cause death. Black pepper is known to cause burning sensation inside the stomach in certain people, and they should check the quantity of black pepper being consumed before discarding it fully. There are certain cases in which black pepper reacts with medicines. Black pepper may cause some irritation to pregnant women, and may cause some allergies to breast feeding mothers. [31-34]

Discussion and Conclusions

For millennia, spices have been an integral part of human diets and commerce. Recently, the widespread recognition of diet-health linkages bolsters their dietary importance. The bioactive components present in them are of considerable significance owing to their therapeutic potential against various ailments. They provide physiological benefits or prevent chronic ailment in addition to the fundamental nutrition and often included in the category of functional foods. Black pepper (*Piper nigrum*) is one of the most widely used among spices. It is valued for its distinct biting quality attributed to the alkaloid, piperine. Black pepper is used not only in human dietaries but also for a variety of other purposes such as medicinal, as a preservative, and in perfumery. Many physiological effects of black pepper, its extracts, or its major active principle, piperine, have been reported in recent decades. Dietary piperine, by favorably stimulating the digestive enzymes of pancreas, enhances the digestive capacity and significantly reduces the gastrointestinal food transit time. Black pepper essential oil constitutes approximately 0.4-7% of the berry dry weight and is beneficial for the management of rheumatism, cold, tiredness, muscular pains and infection. It was also used as a nerve stimulant to enhance blood circulation. Both white pepper and black pepper contained 2-7% piperine. The volatile oil constituent piperamides and nerolidol exhibited insecticidal activities. β-caryophyllene displayed anesthetic effects, and piperine was used in perfumes. Black pepper has been used for millennia, including plant breeding activities for the development of superior varieties with improved organoleptic and nutritional properties. It has been used in traditional as well as modern medicine. Based on the reviewed literature, *Piper nigrum* (L.) has many favourable chemical properties and beneficial effects. Besides, this review presents a summary of the data on the chemical composition of black pepper, including minerals, vitamins, carotenoids and flavonoids, and various therapeutic benefits. Up to date existing information, >80 metabolites have been isolated from *P. nigrum.* Among them, biologically active alkaloid piperine and the main essential oils constituents including β-caryophyllene, limonene, sabinene, α-pinene, β-bisabolene and α-copaene can serve as a new natural source for use in food, aroma, cosmetics and pharmaceutical industries. Piperine also has a broad spectrum of therapeutic potential and potential for improving the bioavailability of therapeutic drugs and nutrients. BPEO and piperine have many biological effects such as antioxidant, antiobesity, antitumor, antipyretic, anticonvulsant, anti-thyroid, antifungal, antibacterial, insecticidal, hepatoprotective, anti-asthmatic, larvicidal, antihypertensive, anti-inflammatory, antidiabetic, antidiarrheal, bioavailability enhancer, immunomodulator, antiepileptic, antifertility, GI stimulant, lipid metabolism accelerator, anticancer, CNS stimulant, diuretic, aphrodisiac, blood purifier and antiplatelet activities, etc. For centuries, black pepper has been used for traditional medicines to cure cuts and wound injuries. Piperine stimulates a dose-dependent increase in the secretion of gastric acid and interruption of gastrointestinal motility. The oral administration of piperine activates the liver, pancreas and digestive enzymes in the small intestinal mucosa. Furthermore, the addition of piperine in food materials as food flavours may increase the protease, lipase, and pancreatic amylase activities.

REFERENCES

1. Parthasarathy VA, Sasikumar B, Nair RR, George KJ. Black Pepper: Botany and Horticulture. In; Hort Rev. 2007; 33: 173-266.
2. Acharya SG, Momin AH, Gajjar AV. Review of Piperine as A Bio-Enhancer. Am J Pharm Tech Res. 2012; 2: 32-44-48.
3. Agbor GA,Vinson JA, Oben JE, *et al.* Comparative Analysis of the in vitro Antioxidant Activity of White and Black Pepper. Nut Res. 2005; 26(12): 659-663.

4. Ahmad N, Fazal H, Abbasi BH, Farooq S, Ali M, *et al*. Biological Role of *Piper nigrum* L. (Black pepper): A Review. Asian Pacific J Trop Biomed: 2012; S1945-S1953.
5. Damanhouri ZA, Ahmad A. A Review on Therapeutic Potential of *Piper nigrum* L. (Black Pepper): The King of Spices. Medicinal and Aromat Plants. 2014; 3(3): 1-6.
6. Elizabeth TJ, Gassara F, Kouassi AP, *et al*. Spice use in Food: Properties and Benefits. Crit Rev Food SciNutr. 2015; 57(6): 1078-1088.
7. Gorgani L, Mohammadi M, Najafpour GD, *et al*. Piperine-The Bioactive Compound of Black pepper: From Isolation to Medicinal Formulations. Comprehensive Review in Food and Food Safety; 2017; 16: 124-140.
8. Khan M, Siddiqui M. Antimicrobial Activity of Piper Fruits. Nat Prod Rad 2007; 6: 111-113.
9. Liu Q, Meng X, Li Y, *et al*. Antibacterial and Antifungal Activities of Spices. Int J Mol Sci. 2017; 18(6): 1283.
10. Meghwal M, Goswami TK. *Piper nigrum* and piperine: An Update. Phytother Res. 2013; 27: 1121-1130.
11. Murthy CT, Bhattacharya S. Cryogenic Grinding of Black pepper. J Food Eng. 2008; 85(1): 18-28.
12. Nakatani N, Inatani R, Ohta H, *et al*. Chemical Constituents of Peppers (Piper spp.) and Application to Food Preservation: Naturally Occurring Antioxidative Compounds. Env Health Persp. 1986; 67: 135-142.
13. Pino J, Feo GR, Borges P, *et al*. Chemical and Sensory Properties of Black pepper Oil (*Piper nigrum* L.). Mol Nut Food Res. 1990; 34(6): 555-560.
14. Sabina EP, Nasreen A, Vedi M, Rasool M. Analgesic, Antipyretic and Ulcerogenic Effects of Piperine: An Active Ingredient of Pepper. J pharm Sci Res. 2013; 5(10): 203-206.
15. Sapam R, Kalita PP, Sarma MP, Talukdar N and Das H. Screening of Phytochemicals and Determination of Total Phenolic content, Anti-oxidant, and Antimicrobial Activity of Methanolic Extract of *Piper nigrum* Leaves. Indo Am J Pharmaceut Res. 2018; 8(2): 1354-1360.
16. Shamkuwar PB, Shahi SR, Jadhav ST. Evaluation of Anti-diarrheal effect of Black Pepper (*P. nigrum* L). Asian J Plant Sci Res. 2012; 2: 48-53.
17. Srinivasan K. Black pepper and its Pungent Principle-piperine: A Review of Diverse Physiological Effects. Crit Rev Food SciNutr. 2007; 47: 735-748.
18. Sunila ES, Kuttan G.Immunomodulatory and Antitumor Activity of *Piper longum* Linn. and piperine. J Ethnopharmacol. 2004; 90: 339-346. 9819-9998.
19. Butt MS, Imran Pasha, Sultan MT, Randhawa AR, Saeed F. Waqas Ahmed Black Pepper and Health Claims: A Comprehensive Treatise Crit Rev Food SciNutr. 2013; 53(9):875-86. doi: 10.1080/10408398.2011.571799
20. Meghwal M, Goswami TK.*Piper nigrum* and piperine: An update PhytotherRes. 2013; 27(8): 1121-1130. doi: 10.1002/ptr.4972.
21. Srinivasan K.. Black pepper and its Pungent Principle-piperine: A Review of Diverse Physiological Effects Crit Rev Food SciNutr. 2007; 47(8): 735-48. doi: 10.1080/10408390601062054.
22. Savina. A Review on Bioactive Chemical Compounds, Traditional Medicinal uses and Pharmacological Activities of *Piper nigrum* L. seeds: Demand of the time. 2021; 8(6): b847-b857.
23. Ashok kumar K, Murugan M, Dhanya MK. *et al*. Phytochemistry and Therapeutic Potential of Black pepper [*Piper nigrum* (L.)] Essential Oil and Piperine: A Review. ClinPhytosci . 2021;7: 52-54. https://doi.org/10.1186/s40816-021-00292-2
24. Nair KP. Agronomy and Economy of Black pepper and Cardamom. The King and Queen of Spices: Elsevier Press; 2011. p. 380.

25. Damanhouri ZA, Ahmad A. A Review on Therapeutic Potential of *Piper nigrum* L. (Black Pepper): The King of Spices. Med Aromat Plants. 2014; 3: 161-164. doi:https://doi.org/10.4172/2167-0412.1000161
26. Wong CM, Ling JJ. In Vitro Study of Wound Healing Potential in Black Pepper (*Piper nigrum* L.). UK J PharmaceutBiosci. 2014; 2: 05-9.
27. Gülçin I. The Antioxidant and Radical Scavenging Activities of Black pepper (*Piper nigrum*) Seeds. Int J Food SciNutr. 2005; 56: 491-499.
28. Szallasi A. Piperine. Researchers Discover New Flavor in an Ancient Spice. Trends Pharmacol Sci. 2005; 26: 437-439.
29. Srinivasan K. Black pepper and its Pungent Principle-piperine: A Review of Diverse Physiological Effects. Crit Rev Food SciNutr. 2007; 47: 735-748.
30. Taqvi SI, Shah AJ, Gilani AH. Blood Pressure Lowering and Vasomodulator effects of Piperine. J Cardiovasc Pharmacol. 2008; 52: 452-458.
31. Joshi DR, Shrestha AC, N. Adhikari N.A Review on Diversified use of the King of Spices: *Piper nigrum* (Black pepper). J Pharmaceut Sci Res. 9(10): 4089-4101 doi: 10.13040/IJPSR.0975-8232.9(10).4089-4001.
32. Takooree H, Aumeeruddy MZ, Rengasamy KRR, Katharigatta N Venugopala, Jeewon R, Zengin G, Mahomoodally MF. A Systematic Review on Black pepper (*Piper nigrum* L.): from Folk uses to Pharmacological Applications Crit Rev Food Sci Nutr. 2019; 59(sup1): S210-S243. doi: 10.1080/10408398.2019.1565489.

CHAPTER

6

Nutritional Attributes and Therapeutic Importance of Caraway Seeds

ABSTRACT

Strongly aromatic, caraway is a member of the parsley or Umbelliferae family; a large family of plants that also includes commonly known herbs and spices such as dill, anise, fennel, and Caraway (*Carum carvi* L.) contains health benefiting essential oils. These compounds indeed work as powerful antioxidants by removing harmful free radicals from the body and thus protect from cancers, infection, aging and degenerative neurological diseases. Principle health benefiting volatile compounds are flavonoids antioxidants viz. carvone, limonene, carveol, pinene, cumuninic aldehyde, furfural, and thujone. These active principles in the caraway seeds known to have antioxidant, digestive, carminative, and anti-flatulent properties. Also, dietary fibers occurring in caraway bind to the toxins in the food and helps protect the colon mucosa from cancers. Further, dietary fibers bind to bile salts (produced from cholesterol) and decrease their re- absorption in the colon, and thus help in reducing serum LDL cholesterol levels. Caraway spice is an excellent source of minerals like Fe, Cu, Ca, K, Mn, Se, Zn and Mg. The plant's roots can be eaten, but most people use the caraway fruit, which is mistakenly called seed as a result of its size and texture.

Keywords: Carminative, Crptoxanthin, Carvone, Carveol, Emmenagogue, Thujone, IBS

Introduction

Although frequently mistaken for a seed, this small, brown pod is really the dried fruit of the caraway plant (*Carum carvi* L.) belonging to Umbellifarae family. Caraway is a widely cultivated spice native to Europe, Asia and North Africa. It also appears wild in Iceland, Scandinavia, throughout Russia, in Siberia, Persia, the Caucasus and the Himalayas. Caraway grows extensively all over the Europe, North Africa, and Asia Minor regions. It is a biennial, herbaceous plant which blooms once in every two years. Its creamy flowers appear in umbels. The plant grows to about two feet in height and bears small feathery leaves [1-2]. Caraway seeds, having similar in appearance as that of cumin, have a crescent shape, dark brown, with up to five stripes (ribs) running lengthwise on their surface. Studies have shown that caraway oil has antibacterial and larvicidal properties. Caraway has a long history of use as a household remedy especially in the treatment of digestive complaints where its antispasmodic action soothes the digestive tract and its carminative action relieves bloating caused by wind and improves the appetite. It is often added to laxative medicines to prevent griping. The seed is antiseptic, aromatic, anesthetic, anodyne, antianxiety, diuretic, mildly expectorant, fungicidal, muscle relaxant, soporific, tonic, emmenagogue, expectorant, galactogogue and stimulant. It can be chewed raw for the almost immediate relief of indigestion and can also be made into infusions. The seed is also used in the treatment of bronchitis and are an ingredient of cough remedies, especially useful for children and for mothers for increasing breast milk. A tea made from the seeds is a pleasant stomachic and carminative, it has been used to treat flatulent colic [3-4]. The seed is used in Tibetan medicine where it is considered to have an acrid taste and a heating potency. It is used to treat failing vision and loss of appetite. Caraway boasts a wide variety of essential nutrients, several of which are lacking in Western diets. These include Fe, Zn, Ca and fiber. Caraway boasts a rich supply of health-promoting antioxidants, including limonene and carvone. This plant is also referred to as meridian fennel or Persian cumin. The plant's roots can be eaten, but most people use the caraway fruit, which is mistakenly called seed as a result of its size and texture. They are often compared to fennel, and both make a good substitute for the other, although there is an obvious difference in the taste. Fennel is very heavily licorice-flavored, while caraway tends to have more peppery and citrus notes to it [5-6].

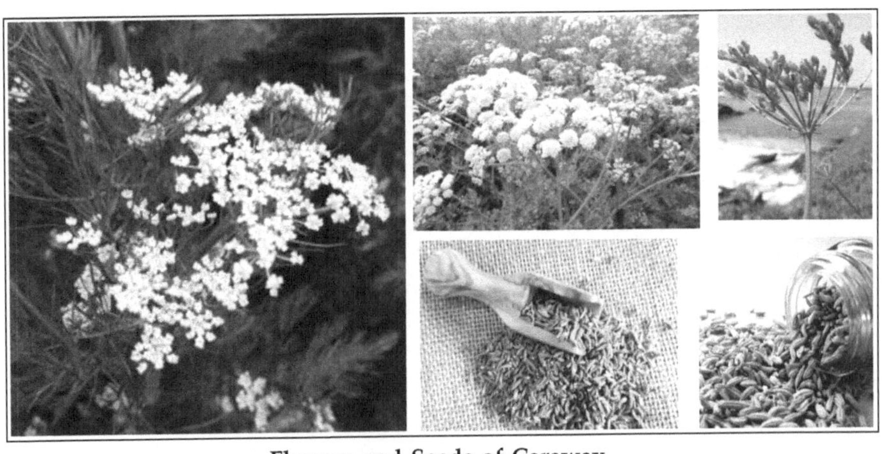

Flowers and Seeds of Caraway

Phytoconstituents

Principle volatile compounds are carvone, limonene, carveol, pinene, cumuninic aldehyde, furfural, and thujone. These active principles in the caraway seeds known to have antioxidant, digestive, carminative, and anti-flatulent properties. Caraway has health benefiting flavonoid antioxidants such as lutein, carotene, cryptoxanthin, and zeaxanthin. Caraway spice is an excellent source of minerals like Fe, Cu, Ca, K, Mn, Se, Zn and Mg.

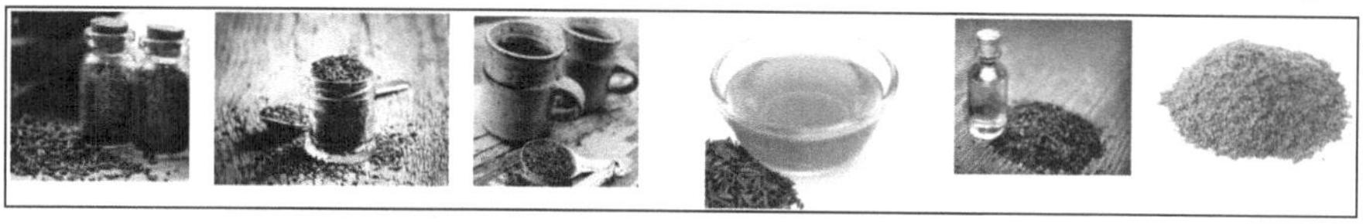

Seed powder, Tea and Oil of Caraway

Limonene	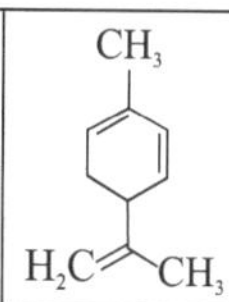
α & β-pinene	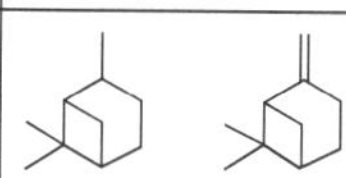
Cumuninic aldehyde	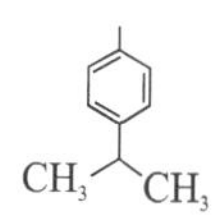
Furfural	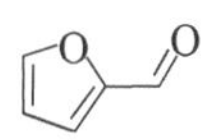
α & β-thujone	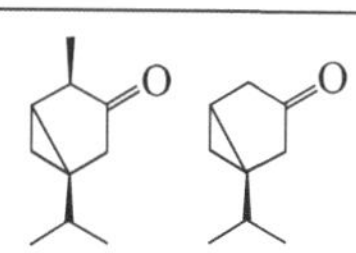

Volatile chemical constituents of Caraway (*Carum carvi* L.)

An essential oil from the seed is used in perfumery, for scenting soap, as a parasiticide etc. The main components of *C. carvi* oil are carvone, limonene, germacrene D, and trans–dihydrocarvone. Gas chromatography (GC) and gas chromatography-mass spectrometry (GC-MS) studies showed the presence of carvone and limonene as the major chemical constituents of the essential oil of *C. carvi*. The herb oil of caraway was found to consist of germacrene D with β-caryophyllene, β-elemene, humulene, germacrene A and B, and two cadinenes. Caraway seeds contained the main components divided into carvone and limonene [4-7].

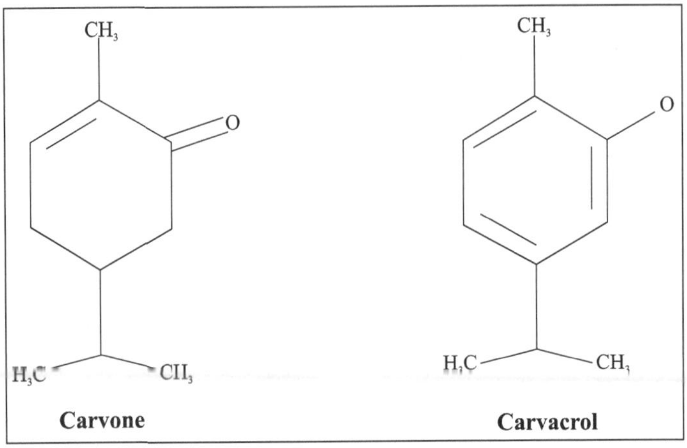

Health Benefits of Caraway Seeds

In addition to their utility as remedial items in the traditional medicines, caraway seeds have their own food value, and indeed, have many health benefiting nutrients, minerals, vitamins and antioxidants. Caraway seeds are a rich source of dietary fiber. 100 g seeds provide 38 g of fiber, 100% of daily recommended intake of fiber. The soluble as well as insoluble dietary fiber increase the bulk of the food and help prevent constipation by speeding up its movement through the gut. Also, dietary fiber binds to the toxins in the food and helps protect the colon mucosa from cancers. Further, dietary fibers bind to bile salts (produced from cholesterol) and decrease their re-absorption in the colon, and thus help in reducing serum LDL cholesterol levels. Caraway contains health benefiting essential oils. These compounds indeed work as powerful antioxidants by removing harmful free radicals from the body and thus protect from cancers, infection, aging and degenerative neurological diseases. Copper present in caraway required for the production of red blood cells [5-8]. Iron required for red blood cell formation. Zinc is a co-factor in many enzymes that regulate growth and development, digestion and nucleic acid synthesis. Potassium is an important component of cell and body fluids that helps regulate heart rate and blood pressure. Manganese used by the body as a co-factor for the powerful antioxidant enzyme, superoxide dismutase. The caraway seeds indeed are the storehouse for many vital vitamins. Vitamin-A, vitamin-E, vitamin-C as well as many B-complex vitamins like thiamin, pyridoxine, riboflavin, and niacin particularly concentrated in the seeds. Caraway water often used as a remedy for flatulence and indigestion in traditional medicines, especially used to relieve colicy pain. It also used in pharmaceuticals as a flavoring agent in mouthwash and gargle preparations. Caraway extraction is used as a rubefacient (to soothe muscle sores), clear the cold, as a remedy for bronchitis and IBS (irritable bowel syndrome) in many traditional medicines [7-10].

Main constituents of Caraway seeds and their nutrition value

Principle	Nutrient Value	Percentage of RDA
Energy	333 Kcal	17%
Carbohydrates	49.90 g	38%
Protein	19.77 g	35%
Total Fat	14.59 g	48%
Cholesterol	0 mg	0%
Dietary Fiber	38 g	100%
Vitamins		
Folates	10 µg	2.5%
Niacin	3.606 mg	23%
Pyridoxine	0.360 mg	28%
Riboflavin	0.379 mg	29%
Thiamin	0.383 mg	32%
Vitamin A	363 IU	12%
Vitamin C	21 mg	35%
Vitamin E	2.5 mg	17%
Electrolytes		
Sodium	17 mg	1%
Potassium	1351 mg	29%
Minerals		
Calcium	689 mg	69%
Copper	0.910 mg	101%
Iron	16.23 mg	203%
Magnesium	258 mg	64.5%
Manganese	1.300 mg	56.5%
Phosphorus	568 mg	81%
Zinc	5.5 mg	50%
Phyto-nutrients		
Carotene-ß	189 µg	–
Crypto-xanthin-ß	58 µg	–
Lutein-zeaxanthin	205 µg	–

Culinary uses

Caraway is a unique spice long used in cooking and herbal medicine. Caraway seeds feature warm, sweet, and slightly peppery aroma when squeezed between index and thumb fingers. They used extensively in European and Mediterranean cooking. To keep their fragrance and flavor intact; caraway seeds roasted gently under low flame and ground just before using them in a recipe. Caraway seed employed widely as a savory spice. It principally added in cooking as a condiment and flavoring base. It features in savory dishes, including cabbage soups, sauerkraut, and salads. Caraway gives a pleasant aroma to bread, cakes, biscuits, and cheese. In France, the seeds offered in a saucer to sprinkle over Munster cheese before eating. Cheddar cheese with caraway seeds is a popular spice mixed, hard cheese in UK. The addition of caraway seeds give this cheddar cheese a savory flavor. Also, along with other spicy items, they are being used to season sausage and other meat preparations. In Central Europe (Poland), caraway-seasoned sausages (*Kielbasa Kminkowa*) are a favorite dish. Caraway seeds have a strong anise-like taste, making them popular in savory dishes, such as sauerkraut and harissa. In modern times, caraway seeds are most often used in baking recipes, from rye bread to pastry toppings and cakes. It's slightly bitter, earthy flavor is reminiscent of licorice, coriander, anise, and fennel. It can be used whole or ground in both sweet and savory dishes, such as breads, pastries, curries, and stews. It's sometimes infused into spirits and liqueurs as well. A tea made from the seeds is a pleasant stomachic and carminative, it has been used to treat flatulent colic [6-10].

Conclusion

Studies have shown that caraway oil has antibacterial and larvicidal properties. Caraway has a long history of use as a household remedy especially in the treatment of digestive complaints where its antispasmodic action soothes the digestive tract and its carminative action relieves bloating caused by wind and improves the appetite. It is often added to laxative medicines to prevent griping. The seed is antiseptic, aromatic, anesthetic, anodyne, antianxiety, diuretic, mildly expectorant, fungicidal, muscle relaxant, soporific, tonic, emmenagogue, expectorant, galactogogue and stimulant. It is used to treat failing vision and loss of appetite. Caraway boasts a wide variety of essential nutrients, several of which are lacking in Western diets. These include Fe, Zn, Ca and fiber.

REFERENCES

1. Antimicrobial Activity of Essential Oil from Seeds of *Carum carvi* and its Composition Begum J, Bhuiyan MNI, Chowdhury JU, Hoque MN, Anwar MN (2008) Banglad J Microbiol 25(2): 85-89.
2. Putievsky E, Ravid U, Dudai N & Katzir I. 1994. A New Cultivar of Caraway (*Carum carvi* L.) and its Essential Oil. J Herbs Spices Med Plants 2(2): 81-84.
3. Toxopeus H & ouwmeester HJ. 1993. Improvement of Caraway Essential Oil and Carvone Production in The Netherlands. Ind CropsProd 1: 295-301.
4. Halva S, Hirvi T, Makinen S & Honkanen E.1986.Yield and Glucosinolates of Mustard Seeds and Volatile Oils of Caraway Seeds and Coriander Fruit. II Yield and Volatile Oils of Caraway Seeds (*Carum carvi*). J Agric Sci Finland 58: 163-167.
5. Iacobellis NS, Cantore PL, Capasso F & Senatore F. 2005. Antibacterial Activity of Cuminumcyminum L. and *Carum carvi* L. Essential Oils. J Agric Food Chem. 53(1): 57-61.

6. Foster S & Duke JA. 1990. A Field Guide to Medicinal Plants: Easternand Central North America. Houghton Mifflin Co, Boston.
7. Coffey T. 1993.The History and Folklore of North American Wild Flowers. Facts on File, New York.13.Tsarong TJ. 1994.
8. Tewari M Mathela CS. 2003. Compositions of the Essential Oils from Seeds of *Carum carvi*Linn. and Carumbulbocastanum Koch. Indian Perfumer. 47: 347-349.
9. Arganosa GC, Sosulski FW & Slinkard AE. 1998. Seed yields and Essential Oils of Annual and Biennial Caraway (*Carum carvi* L.) Grown in Western Canada. J Herbs Spices Med Plants. 6(1): 9-17.
10. Wichtmann EM, Biskup SE (1987) Composition of the Essential Oils from Caraway Herb and Root. FlavFragr J 2(2): 83-89.

CHAPTER 7

Prominent usage of Cardamom [*Elettaria cardamomum* L. (Maton)] for uplifting Invigorating Healthcare

ABSTRACT

Cardamom is one of the most significant, valuable spices in the world. It consists of the small, highly aromatic pods or seed capsules of a perennial plant of the ginger family. Cardamom is a highly valued herbal spice that is used as a culinary spice in Asian cuisines because of its intrinsic flavoring capacity. Moreover, when used as a home remedy it helps cure various ailments like indigestion, nausea, lightheadedness, etc. Cardamom has various chemical compounds that include pinene, pinene, sabinene, myrcene, phellandrene, limonene, cineole, terpinene, cymene, terpinolene, linalool, linalyl acetate, terpinen-4-oil, terpineol, terpineol acetate, citronellol, nerol, geraniol, methyl eugenol and trans-nerolidol. It is useful for curing dental diseases and urinary tract infections such as cystitis, nephritis, and gonorrhea. Cardamom possesses aphrodisiac properties and is also used as a cure for impotence, erectile dysfunction, and premature ejaculation. It possesses antiseptic, aphrodisiac, carminative, digestive, diuretic, stimulant, stomachic, tonic and anti-spasmodic.

Keywords: Cineole, Linalool, Aphrodisiac, Carmative, Geraniol.

Introduction

The cardamom [*Elettaria cardamomum* L. (Maton)] belonging to family Zingiberaceae contains tiny, brown aromatic seeds and is one of the most important spices. *Elettaria cardamomum*, commonly known as green or true cardamom, is an herbaceous, perennial plant in the ginger family, native to southern India. It is the most common of the species whose seeds are used as a spice called cardamom. It is cultivated widely in tropical regions and reportedly naturalized in Réunion, Indochina, and Costa Rica. It is also known as "Queen of Spices" in India and "Hel" in Iran, Saudi Arabia, Kuwait, United Arab Emirates, Iraq, because of its very pleasant aroma and taste. This aromatic spice is straw-green to bright-green in color with small, black seeds inside a pod. The fibrous, oval pod has about 8 to 16 seeds [1-3]. There is another variety of this herb, that is, Black Cardamom (*Cardamomum amomum*) which is mostly found in Asia and Australia. Cardamom is the third most expensive spice in the world. The seeds have a sweet aroma and slightly pungent taste. Its essential oil is obtained by steam distillation of cardamom seeds. The oil and left over resin is used in processed foods, liqueurs and perfumes.

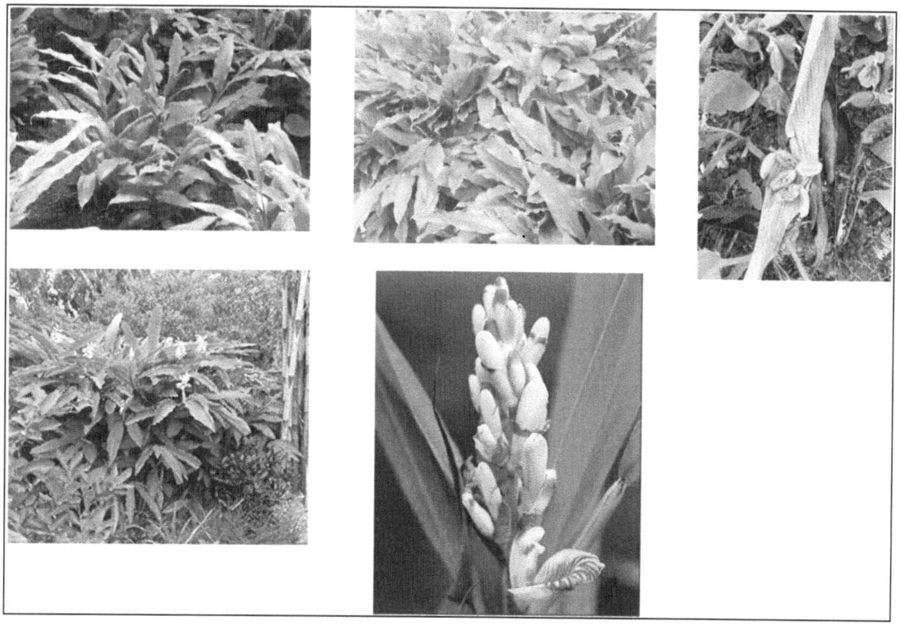

Cardamom plant, leaves, Inflorescence

Cardamom is found in the form of a small pod with black seeds inside. Both the seeds and the pod give a pleasant aroma and flavor. Therefore, they are used as flavoring agents in Indian cuisine. Its use is just not just limited to hot and spicy dishes; the seeds are also added to desserts and beverages to complement the sweet flavor. Cardamom tea is a very famous beverage, along with ginger tea, in India. In India, cardamom was traditionally considered as an herb and was one of the ingredients in Ayurveda and traditional Chinese medicine. It was believed to be a remedy for teeth and gum infections, throat problems, congestion of the lungs, pulmonary tuberculosis, inflammation of the eyelids, gastrointestinal disorders, disintegrating kidneys, and gallbladder stones, and was also used as an antidote for poisons and venoms [4-5]. Cardamom is packed with antioxidants. There are two kinds of cardamoms, green and black. Black cardamoms help in curing colds and cough and certain respiratory problems. It imparts warmth to the body. Due to its strong aroma, it helps in activating our taste and sensory elements and thus, aid digestion. The floral and sweet aroma of cardamoms makes it a natural breath freshener. A major component of cardamom oil called cineole is known for its antimicrobial properties that promote oral hygiene and it also fights bacteria that cause bad breath. Cardamom is known to increase the blood circulation in your body and especially to your lungs and so, is often used as a natural remedy for respiratory disorders. It maintains vitality and keeps your energy levels up. Black cardamom is often touted as an effective remedy for treating high blood sugar levels. Cardamom is rich in manganese which helps in controlling blood sugar levels [6-7].

Nutritional profile of Cardamom

Principle	Nutrient Value	Percentage of RDA
Energy	311 Kcal	15.5%
Carbohydrates	68.47 g	52.5%
Protein	10.76 g	19%
Total Fat	6.7 g	23%
Cholesterol	0 mg	0%
Dietary Fiber	28 g	70%
Vitamins		
Niacin	1.102 mg	7%
Pyridoxine	0.230 mg	18%
Riboflavin	0.182 mg	14%
Thiamin	0.198 mg	16.5%
Vitamin A	0 IU	0%
Vitamin C	21 mg	35%
Electrolytes		
Sodium	18 mg	1%
Potassium	1119 mg	24%
Minerals		
Calcium	383 mg	38%
Copper	0.383 mg	42.5%
Iron	13.97 mg	175%
Magnesium	229 mg	57%
Manganese	28 mg	1217%
Phosphorus	178 mg	25%
Zinc	7.47 mg	68%

Chemical constituents in Cardamom

Cardamom contains essential volatile oil which is made up of monoterpene constituents, such as 1,8-cineole, α-pinene, α-terpineol, linalool, linalyl acetate, and nerolidol and the ester constituent α-terpinyl acetate which exhibit vascular relaxant, anti-inflammatory, analgesic, antimicrobial, antioxidant and antispasmodic properties. The major active component of cardamom oil is a potent antiseptic that is known to kill bacteria producing bad breath and other infections. Cardamom contains flavonoids, terpenoids, anthocyanins, alkaloids, and other phenolic constituents that are responsible for reducing fat storage, cardiovascular, pulmonary, kidney and lung associated disorders and improves insulin function in the body [3-7].

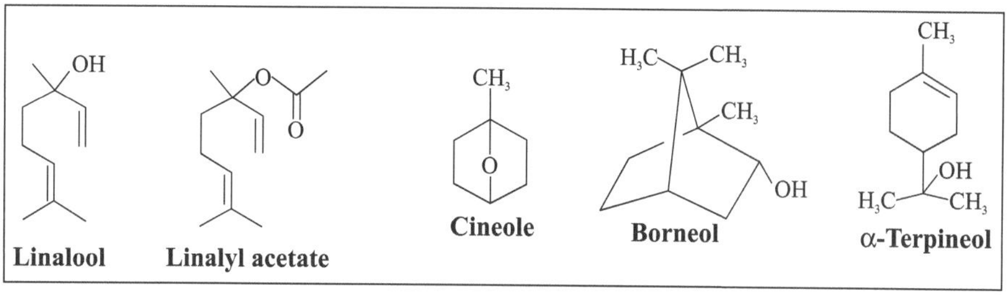

Major Chemical constituents occurring in cardamom

Cardamom benefits

Cardamom boosts energy metabolism and helps the body burn more fat efficiently. Inhaling the sweet and soothing aroma of cardamom essential oil may help in treating sleep issues such as insomnia, restlessness, and anxiety. According to Ayurveda, cardamom is an important spice which is *tridoshic* which means that helps in balancing all the three *doshas* - Vatta, Pitta and Kapha in our body. It has significant warming properties that are soothing for your body. It is also believed in Ayurveda that the excess build-up of *'ama'*, a sticky substance that blocks normal circulation and lowers energy levels, leads to various diseases. Cardamom helps in preventing its accumulation and thus, reduces its negative impact. Since cardamom gives out a sweet flavor, it was traditionally believed to possess aphrodisiac properties. Not only is cardamom regarded as an aphrodisiac, but it is also believed to possess the cure for impotence and premature ejaculation. In Ayurveda, cardamom has been used as a remedy for urinary tract diseases and infections such as cystitis, nephritis, and gonorrhea. There are several remedies prescribed in folk medicine and one of the most popular among them is startling a person who is hiccupping. This may or may not work most of the time [5-7]. However, cardamom is another very effective remedy. Cardamom pods and seeds can be chewed as a breath freshener. The flavors and aroma found in cardamom are due to the presence of essential oil. It is no wonder that the essential oil of cardamom is being used as a popular ingredient in chewing gum. Cardamom contains a high amount of flavonoids contents especially quercetin which improves anxiety-like behavior and depression. Cardamom benefits are due to essential oil, sterol, phenolic acids and lipids which show relaxation of muscles and reduce the volume of gastric ulcer thus prove gastroprotective effect. The presence of phenolic compounds like flavonoids, terpenoids, and tannins (1,8-cineole) in the cardamom show wonderful effects by delayed the severity of seizures. Cardamom increases the production of a good enzyme (superoxide dismutase and ascorbic acid), restores endogenous antioxidants, preserve histopathology and ultrastructure of the myocardium. In simple words, it improves cardiac function thus delay the initiation, progression, and development of myocardial ischemic injury. Cardamom helps improve digestive health, aids in diabetes treatment and helps you cope with depression. The spice also stimulates metabolism, given its antioxidant and anti-inflammatory properties. Cardamom is also known to stimulate the secretion of bile acid in the stomach, further aiding in digestion. The spice also prevents other gastrointestinal ailments like acid reflux, heartburn, diarrhea, etc. Its antioxidant properties can promote heart health. Cardamom also contains fiber, the nutrient that can help lower cholesterol levels and enhance heart health. The spice also can lower blood pressure levels – and this benefits the heart. Cardamom has diuretic properties that can benefit cases of hypertension and epilepsy. These diuretic properties of cardamom also aid in detoxification. Cardamom can indeed help people cope with depression. Cardamom plays a role in fighting asthma symptoms like wheezing, coughing, shortness of breath, and tightness in the chest. The spice makes breathing easier by enhancing blood circulation within the lungs. It also fights related inflammation by soothing the mucus membranes. In accordance with another report green cardamom can be used to treat asthma, bronchitis, and numerous other respiratory issues. Cardamom is extremely rich in manganese – a mineral that can lower the risk of diabetes [3-8]. Cardamom possesses antimicrobial properties that enhance oral health. The pungent taste of cardamom even stimulates the salivary flow – and this can help prevent dental caries. Cardamom can also work well in treating bad breath. One study emphasizes on the use of cardamom for treating a lack of appetite. Even cardamom oil can be used as an appetite stimulant. Cardamom can also aid in the treatment of histoplasmosis – a condition in which one of the symptoms is a lack of appetite. Cardamom is a proven aphrodisiac. The spice is rich in a compound called cineole, and just a small pinch of cardamom powder can release nerve stimulants and fuel your passions. Some reports say that cardamom can also treat impotence. Cardamom has muscle-relaxing properties, and these can help relieve hiccups [8-11].

Cardamom use in Cosmetics

Cardamom is often used in cosmetics to impart fragrance. Due to its distinct spicy, sweet scent, both cardamom and cardamom oil are used in perfumes, soaps, body washes, powders, and other cosmetics. Oriental style perfumes and other scented products often use cardamom as an ingredient in addition to other essential oils. Cardamom can be used in skin care products for antiseptic and anti-inflammatory purposes to calm and soothe the skin, thanks to its therapeutic effects. When added to perfumes, it can stimulate the senses. Facial soaps use cardamom to impart a warming sensation to the skin. These cosmetics using cardamom for therapeutic reasons are known as aromatherapy products. The strong scent of cardamom can ward off unpleasant odors. This makes it a great addition to cosmetic products, such as toners, that serve a specific function but smell unappealing due to the inclusion of certain ingredients. Cardamom is added to these products to mask the unpleasant scent while retaining the benefit of the cosmetic. Cardamom essential oil is often added to cosmetics that are applied to the lips (such as lip balms) to impart the taste of the oil and make the lips smooth. The antibacterial properties of the spice even treat scalp infections, if any. This is a given. Improved scalp health most often means stronger and better-looking hair. The spice strengthens your hair roots and offers shine. The spice helps treat skin allergies and improves skin complexion. It can also be used as a tool to cleanse the skin. One of the benefits of cardamom is that it imparts in making fair skin. Cardamom essential oil helps in removing blemishes, thus giving a fairer complexion. The skin benefits of cardamom can be attributed to its antibacterial and antioxidant properties. Cardamom contains vitamin C, which is a powerful antioxidant. It improves blood circulation throughout the body. Also, the many layers of phytonutrients in the spice can improve blood circulation – which invariably enhances skin health [9-13].

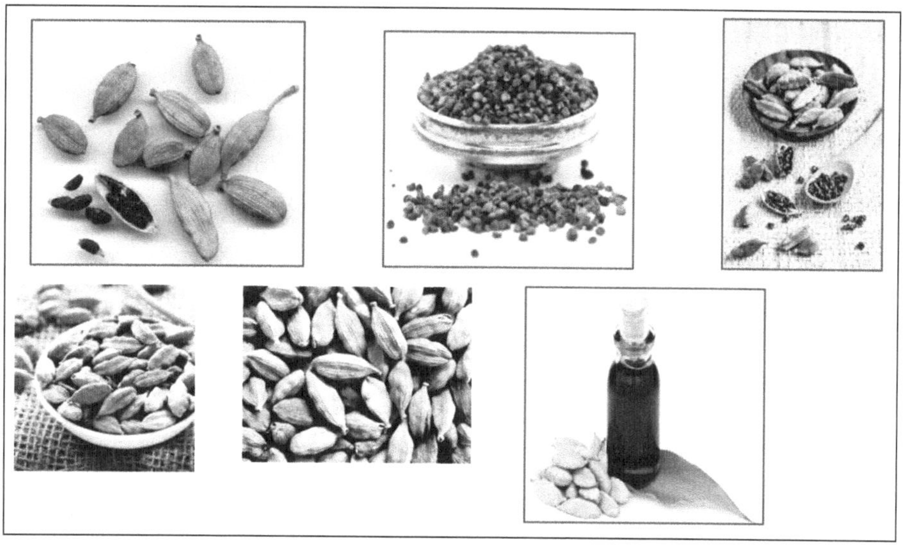

Green and dried Cardamom, Seeds and Oil

Usage of Cardamom products

Cardamom finds use as products in different forms; cardamom seeds, cardamom powder, cardamom oil, cardamom oleoresin, encapsulated cardamom flavor, etc which is used to flavor sweets, baked goods, and hot beverages such as tea and coffee. Cardamom benefits are gastroprotective, treat Seizures, lowers cholesterol and many more. Cardamom oil is used internally for indigestion, nausea, vomiting and pulmonary disease with copious phlegm. Cardamom oil is used for memory enhancement. It is used to flavor coffee, baked goods, curries and pickles, milk desserts and mulled wine. It is also used for perfumery, beverages, cosmetics and a blend of potpourris. Cardamom is used in perfumery blend for manufacturing of men's perfume. It is especially used in the preparation of Curve Cologies, Eau De Toilette spray for men [4, 6, 7-8].

Conclusion

Cardamom has digestive, antispasmodic, carminative, anti-inflammatory, anti-microbial, aphrodisiac and diuretic properties. It boosts digestion and stops nausea, vomiting. Plus, the herb aids in eliminating belching and flatulence. Some other health benefits of cardamom include relief from stomach pain, colon spasms and menstrual cramps. Besides, application of cardamom oil cures teeth and gum infections. Its pleasing fragrance removes bad breath (Halitosis). Furthermore, the herb works as a mild circulatory stimulant. This warm spice improves blood circulation to the lungs. Plus, it can help lower blood pressure, especially in case of primary hypertension. The therapeutic herb also promotes urination and aids in detoxification of the body. Cardamom benefits the immune system as well. In addition, studies show that it has antioxidant properties that can increase the levels of glutathione. It is also believed to have antitumor qualities. Cardamom essential oil has a balsamic aroma and expectorant qualities. Thus, when used in aromatherapy, it helps break up mucus and congestion in sinuses and lungs. It is also beneficial for those suffering from asthma or bronchitis. It has a soothing effect on muscles, nervous system and gives mental clarity. It is high in phytochemical cineole, which is a central nervous stimulant. Further, the herb's diaphoretic properties are useful in increasing perspiration.

REFERENCES

1. Jebur MH, IlhamA. Bnuyan, Amean A. Yasri, Kadhim Hindi NKK.Antimicrobial Effect of Seed Extracts, Leaves and Crude oil of Cardamom (*Elettaria cardamomum*) against different types of BacteriainHilla City, Iraq. World J Pharmaceut Res. 2014; 3(3).123-126.
2. Kaushik P, Goyal P, Chauhan A, Chauhan G. In Vitro Evaluation of Antibacterial Potential of Dry Fruit Extracts of *Elettaria cardamomum* Maton (Chhoti Elaichi). Iranian J Pharnaceut Res.2010; (3): 287-292.

3. Abbas. D. Matter Maliki MA. Isolation and Identification of Phenolic Compounds from *Elettaria cardamomum* Seeds and Study of their Medicinal Activity Against Pathogenic Bacteria of Prostate Gland; J Missan Res 2011; 8: 121-28.
4. Amma K P, Rani M P, Sasidharan I, Nisha VN P. Chemical Composition, Flavonoidphenolic contents and Radical Scavenging activity of four major Varieties of Cardamom.Int J Biol Med Res. 2010; 1(3): 123-129.
5. Savan EK, Küçükbay FZ. Essential Oil Composition of *Elettaria cardamomum* Maton. J ApplBiol Sci. 2013; 7 (3): 42-45.
6. Krishnamurthy KH. Elaa or Cardamom (*Elettaria cardamomum* or repens); J New Approaches Med Health. 2010; 18: 234-240.
7. Mohammed Ali, Shahnaz S. Husain, Analysis of Volatile Oil of The Fruits of *Elettaria cardamomum* (L.) Matonand its Antimicrobial Activity: World Journal of Pharmacy and Pharmaceutical Sciences, 2014; 3: 235-238.
8. Jazila EM, Mount assif D, Amarouch H. Antimicrobial activity of *Elettaria cardamomum*: Toxicity, Biochemical and Histological Studies. Int J Drug Formulat Res Food Chem. 2007; 104: 236-239.
9. Noshad M, Behbahan BA. Identification of Chemical Compounds, Antioxidant Activity and Antimicrobial Effect of *Elettaria cardamomum* Essential Oil on a Number of Pathogenic Qom Univ Med Sci J. 2019; 13(2): 57-56.
10. Abraham P. The cardamom in India. Kachroo P. (ed.) Farm. Bull. (New Series). ICAR, New Delhi (1965) 37: 1-46.
11. Agaoglu S, Dostbil N, Alemdar S. Antimicrobial effect of Seed extracts of Cardamom (*Elettaria cardamomum* Maton). YYU Vet. Fak.Derg. (2005) 16: 99-101.
12. Miyazawa M, Kameoka H. Composition of the Essential Oil and Non-volatile Oil from Cardamom Seeds. Japan. Oil Chem Soc. (Yukagaku). 1975; 24: 22-26.

CHAPTER 8

Enormously Beneficial Chia Seeds in Modern Food Regimen

ABSTRACT

Chia seed is a potential source of antioxidants with the presence of chlorogenic acid, caffeic acid, myricetin, quercetin, and kaempferol which are believed to have cardiac, hepatic protective effects, anti-ageing and anti-carcinogenic characteristics. Chia seed possesses higher proportion of α-linolenic acid makes chia the superb source of ω-3 fatty acid (~65 % of the oil content). It is also a great source of dietary fiber with higher concentration of beneficial unsaturated fatty acids, gluten free protein, vitamin, minerals and phenolic compounds. Therapeutic effects of chia in the control of diabetes, dyslipidaemia, hypertension, as anti-inflammatory, antioxidant, anti-blood clotting, laxative, antidepressant, antianxiety, analgesic, vision and immune improver is scientifically established. This comprehensive review paper describes the huge nutritional and therapeutic potential of chia seed to make it the part of an average diet for better healthcare.

Keywords: ω-3 fatty acids, , Laxative, Anti-inflammatory, α-linolenic acid, Chlorogenic acid, Kaempferol, Widdrol.

Introduction

Chia seeds are tiny black and white seeds from the *Salvia hispanica L.* plant that are also a member of the mint family (Labiatae). Chia seeds were originally grown in Central and South America, and were considered a major food crop in Mexico and Guatemala. The word chia is derived from a Spanish word chian which means oily, it is oilseed, with a power house of ω-3 fatty acids, superior quality protein, higher extent of dietary fiber, vitamins, minerals and wide range of polyphenolic antioxidants which safeguard the seeds from chemical and microbial breakdown. Chia can grow up to 1m tall and has opposite arranged leaves. Chia flowers are small flower (3-4 mm) with small corollas and fused flower parts. The seed color varies from black, grey, and black spotted to white, and the shape is oval with size ranging from 1 to 2 mm [1-2]. Prominently, grown for its seeds, *Salvia hispanica* also produces white or purple flowers. Recently, chia has regained its popularity by becoming one of the main oil sources that contains high levels of PUFA.

Chia, which used to be the major food crop of the indigenous peoples of Mexico and Guatemala, is now widely cultivated and commercialized for its (omega) ω-3 alpha-linolenic acid (ALA) content and antioxidant properties. Today, its cultivation is not only limited to the Americas but is also extended to other areas such as Australia and Southeast Asia. Chia sprouts are used in salads, chia seed is used in beverages and cereals based foods and it can be consumed in raw form. Traditionally seeds have been used as a food, in a wide range of folk medicines, primary cosmetics and a part of religious rituals in pre-Columbian societies. The diets in pre-Columbian regimes were as nutritious as today. The chia seed is widely used in many countries since thousands of years due to its massive nutritional and therapeutic potential [3-5]. Existence of chia as an integral part of the pre-Columbian diet had made their diets even superior to today's diet which is also admitted by the modern science. The massive nutritional and therapeutic potential of chia offers a great future perspective for pharmaceutical sector. In present times, there exists a cumulative consideration and dispersal of the seeds of the plant for the advantages and uses in cookery. The seeds are known as the very rich foundation of nutrients, first of all, the polyunsaturated omega-3 fatty acids which secure your health from inflammation, advance the reasoning presentation and decrease the level of cholesterol. Additionally, sugars founded fibers which exist at high attentiveness level, are linked with decreasing inflammation, dropping cholesterol and adaptable bowel functions which eventually lead to healthy life. This appraisal recapitulates the present in-formation on the photochemistry and pharmacological characteristics of the seeds of chia plant [5-7].

The chia's main fats are α-linolenic acid (ALA) and linoleic acid (LA), with a smaller numbers of (saturated fatty acids), oil (omega-9), and stearic (saturated) acids. The most popular lipids are a ±-linolenic acid. ALA and LA are the two only essential fatty acids which individuals have to put into their diet, as they cannot be synthesized by their bodies. For chia, ALA, fatty acids are ~60%, LA is about 20%. ALA is a source of many benefits, as well as the correlation of cardiovascular and neurological health, to the long-chain Omega-3 fatty acids DHA and Eicosatetraenoic (EPA). In addition, chia seeds are also used in the preparation of cake for example as healthy supplements with oil, and can be used in beverages, cereal and salads [8-9]. Chia seeds in bread products at a value of no more than 5 per cent, including breakfast, cookies, fruit juices and yogurt, have already been permitted in the European Committee. The seeds of chia contain high fiber content (18-30 g/100g). It has been reported that their use can encourage proper intestinal functioning, reduce the level of blood cholesterol and glucose due to the use of chia seed.

Such fatty acids are responsible for the effective functioning of the vision, cardiovascular diseases, cancer, autoimmune and inflammatory diseases, and also for prevention. These fatty acids are not only nutritionally important for health, but also helpful to people with heart disease, and diabetes [10-11].

Phytoconstituents and Nutritional Attributes

The seed contains ω-3 α-linolenic acid (ω-*3ALA*) and ω-6 linoleic acid (ω-6*LA*). Both (PUFAs) Polyunsaturated fatty acids are essential fatty acids required by the human body for good health, and they cannot be artificially synthesized. The protein, fat, carbohydrate, dietary fiber, ash and dry matter contents of chia seeds ranged from 15 to 25%, 30-33%, 41%, 18-30%, 4-5% and 90-93% with a wide range of polyphenols, respectively. The protein content of chia seed grown in different habitats ranged from 18.8% to 21.5%, the variation in protein content was probably be due to agronomic, climatic and soil conditions. In another study regarding the nutritional characterization of chia seed; medicinal characteristics of chia seed reported that seed exhibited 20% protein, 25% fiber and 34% oil. The high fiber content of chia seed as health perspective, fiber increases stool volume, prevent from diverticulosis and cancer [12-14]. Chia is considered as a safe food with no potentially harmful effects and widely used in baked goods, nutritional supplements, cereal bars, cookies, bread, snacks etc. Chia seed contains appreciable amount of fiber, which can absorb up 15x water the weight of seed. The presence of higher extents of fiber help in diabetes mellitus by slowing down the digestion process and release of glucose, it also improves the peristaltic movement of intestine and reducing plasma cholesterol. The biological value of chia is superior to cereals and higher content of calcium, magnesium and potassium than milk. It is revealed from the studies that chia seed had a higher concentration of phytosterols which have and cancer and cardio-protective effect with antimicrobial activities.

Recently, it is established that mucilage of chia seed can be utilized as a functional coating with improved functional properties. The leaves of chia contain an essential oil that contains β-caryophyllene, globulol, γ-muroleno, β-pinene, α-humoleno, germacren-B, and widdrol [15-18].

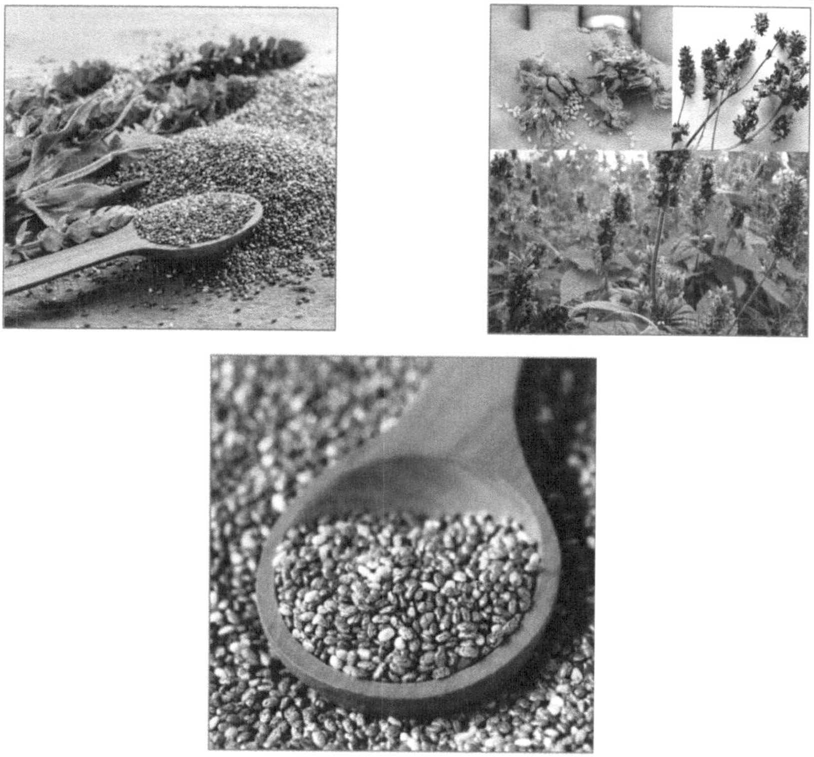

These compounds are believed to have strong repellent characteristics to a wide range of insects. Two tablespoons of this super-seed contain around 140 calories, 4 grams of protein, 11 grams of fiber, 7 grams of unsaturated fat (omega-3 fatty acids) and contain over 18% of your RDA for calcium. They're also a good source of trace minerals like copper and zinc. They contain all nine essential amino acids necessary as the building blocks for protein in the body [19-23]. Not only are chia seeds high in calcium, but they are also loaded with manganese and phosphorous, two crucial minerals involved in bone health. Chia seeds also help us get full, faster, due to their high tryptophan content, also helping to regulate appetite, sleep, and improve our mood.

ω-3ALA (18:3)	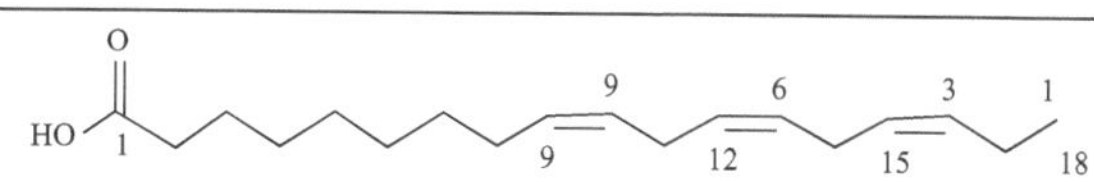
ω-6LA (18:2)	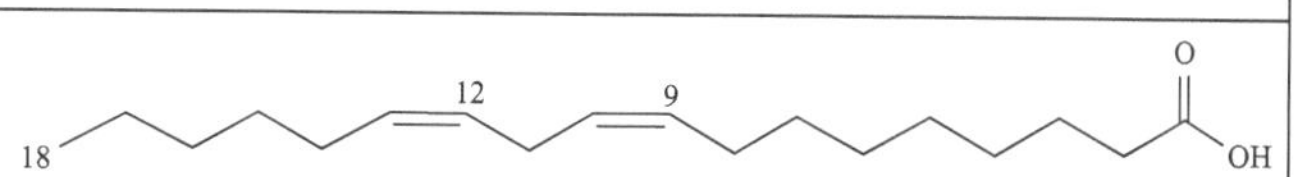

(Contd...)

Myricetin	
Quercetin	
Kaempferol	
Caffeic acid	
Chhlorogenic acid	
β-caryophyllene	
Globulol	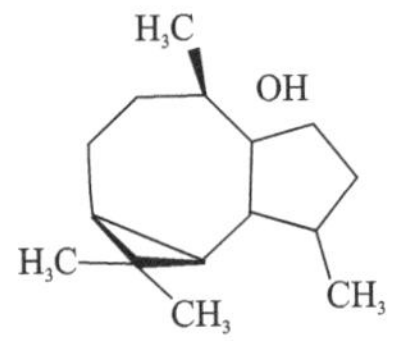
β-pinene	
Germacren-B	
Widdrol	

Chemical structure of phytoconstituents occurring in Chia Seed and leaf

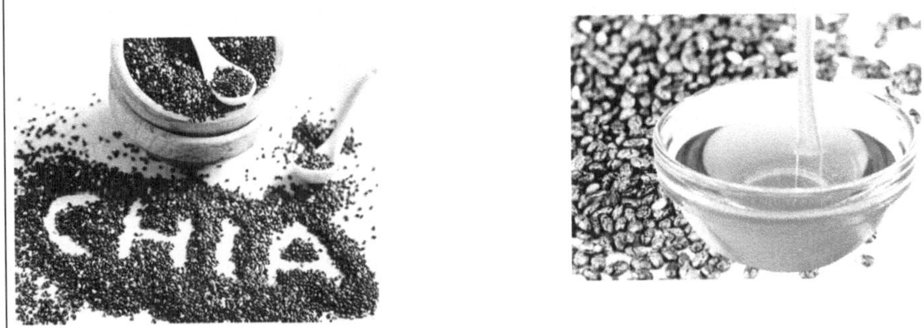

Culinary uses

The European Commission approved the use of chia seed (<5%) in bread products. Other than bread, the food industry of various countries around the world including US, Canada, Chile, Australia, New Zealand, and Mexico has widely used chia seeds or its oil for different applications such as breakfast cereals, bars, cookie snacks, fruit juices, cake, and yoghurt. At present, chia seed is used as a healthy oil supplement and is commonly consumed as salad from chia sprout, in beverages, cereals, and salad dressing from the seed, or it is eaten raw. Biscuits, pasta, cereal bars, snacks and yoghurt and cake are usually supplemented with chia seed. Chia is one of the few medicinal plants that produce essential oil in a great concentration, which is used for the preparation of omega-3 capsules.

Conclusion

Seed from *Salvia hispanica* L. or more commonly known as chia is a traditional food in central and southern America. Currently, it is widely consumed for various health benefits especially in maintaining healthy serum lipid level. This effect is contributed by the presence of phenolic acid and omega 3/6 oil in the chia seed. Isolated polyphenolics from chia seed arechlorogenic acid, caffeic acid, myricetin, quercetin and kaempferol. Quercetin, chlorogenic acid, caffeic acid are believed to have anti-carcinogenic, antihypertensive, neuron protective effects. It is already well established that chia does not have anti-allergic, anti-nutritional and toxic effect on human health. Although the presence of active ingredients in chia seed warrants its health benefits, however, the safety and efficacy of this medicinal food or natural product need to be validated by scientific research.

REFERENCES

1. Cahill JP, Provance MC (2002) Genetics of Qualitative Traits in Domesticated Chia (*Salvia hispanica* L.) J Heredity 93(1): 52-55.
2. Reales A, Rivera D, Palazón JA, Obón C (2004) Numerical Taxonomy Study of Salvia sect. Salvia (Labiatae) Bot J Linn Soc145(3): 353-371.
3. Ullah R, Nadeem M, Khalique A, Imran M, Mehmood S, Javid A, Hussain J (2015) Nutritional and Therapeutic Perspectives of Chia (*Salvia hispanica* L.): A Review.J Food SciTechnol 2016 Apr; 53(4): 1750-1758. doi: 10.1007/s13197-015-1967-0
4. Ali NM, Yeap SK, Ho WY, Beh BK, Tan SW, Tan SG (2012) The Promising Future of Chia, *Salvia hispanica* L. J Biomed Biotechnol 171956. doi: 10.1155/2012/171956
5. Bresson JL, Flynn A, Heinonen M *et al.* (2009) Opinion on the Safety of Chia Seeds (*Salvia hispanica L.*) and Ground whole Chia Seeds as a Food Ingredient. *The Eur Food Safety Auth J* 996: 1-26.
6. Peiretti PG, Gai F (2009) Fatty Acid and Nutritive Quality of Chia (*Salvia hispanica* L.) Seeds and Plant during Growth. Ani Feed SciTechnol1 48(2-4): 267-275.
7. Ixtaina VY, Nolasco SM, Tomás MC (2008) Physical Properties of Chia (*Salvia hispanica* L.) seeds. Indus Crops Prod 28(3): 286-293.

8. Ayerza H R, Coates W (2011) Protein Content, Oil Content and Fatty Acid Profiles as Potential Criteria to Determine the Origin of Commercially Grown Chia (*Salvia hispanica L.*) *Indus Crops Prod* 34(2): 1366-1371.
9. Ayerza H R (1995) Oil Content and Fatty Acid Composition of Chia (*Salvia hispanica L.*) from Five Northwestern Locations in Argentina. *J Am Oil Chemists' Soc* 72(9): 1079-1081.
10. Vedtofte MS, Jakobsen MU, Lauritzen L *et al.* (2011) Dietary Alpha Linoleic Acid, Linoleic Acid and n-3 long-chain PUFA and Risk of Ischemic Heart Disease. The American Journal of Clinical Nutrition. 2011; 94:1097-1103.
11. Ixtaina VY, Nolasco SM, Tomàs MC (2012) Oxidative Stability of Chia (*Salvia hispanica* L.) Seed Oil: Effect of Antioxidants and Storage Conditions. J Am Oil Chemists' Soc 89: 1077-1090.
12. Capitani MI, Spotorno V, Nolasco SM, Tomás MC (2012) Physicochemical and Functional Characterization of by-products from Chia (*Salvia hispanica* L.) Seeds of Argentina. LWT—Food Sci Technol 45(1): 94-102.
13. Ixtaina VY, Mattea F, Cardarelli DA, Mattea MA, Nolasco SM, Tomás MC (2011) Supercritical Carbon dioxide Extraction and Characterization of Argentinean Chia Seed Oil. J Am Oil Chemists' Soc 88(2): 289-298.
14. Uribe JAR, Perez JIN, Kauil HC, Rubio GR, Alcocer CG (2011) Extraction of Oil from Chia Seeds with Supercritical CO_2. JSupercrit Fluids. 56(2): 174-178.
15. Ixtaina VY, Vega A, Nolasco SM, *et al.* (2010) Supercritical Carbon dioxide Extraction of Oil from Mexican Chia Seed (*Salvia hispanica* L.): Characterization and Process Optimization. J Supercrit Fluids 55(1): 192-199.
16. Borneo R, Aguirre A, León AE. Chia (*Salvia hispanica* L) gel can be used as Egg or Oil Replacer in Cake Formulations. Journal of the American Dietetic Association. 2010; 110(6): 946-949.
17. Olivos-Lugo BL, Valdivia-López MÁ, Tecante A (2010) Thermal and Physicochemical Properties and Nutritional Value of the Protein Fraction of Mexican Chia Seed (*Salvia hispanica* L.) Food SciTechnolInt 16(1): 89-96.
18. Illian TG, Casey JC, Bishop PA. Omega 3 Chia Seed Loading as a means of Carbohydrate Loading. J Strength Conditioning Res 2011; 25(1): 61-65.
19. Ayerza R, Coates W (2007) Seed yield, Oil Content and Fatty Acid Composition of Three Botanical Sources of ω-3 Fatty Acid Planted in the Yungas Ecosystem of Tropical Argentina. Trop Sci 47(4): 183-187.
20. Coates W, Ayerza R (1996) Production Potential of Chia in Northwestern Argentina. Indust Crops Prod 5(3): 229-233.
21. Baughman WF, Jamieson GS (1992) Chia Seed Oil. Oil Fat Indust 6(9): 15-17.
22. Basuni AM, Arafat SM, Hikal DM (2021) Chia (*Salvia hispanica* L.) Seed Oil Rich in Omega-3 Fatty Acid: A Healthy Alternative for Milk Fat in Ice Milk. Food Nut Sci 12: 479-493.
23. Food and Nutrition Sciences, 2021, 12, 479-493 Food and Nutrition Sciences, 2021, 12, 479-493.
24. The Chia Company. Request for Scientific Evaluation of Substantial Equivalence Application for the Approval of Chia Seeds (*Salvia hispanica* L.) from the Chia Company for use in Bread. Food Law Consultants, 2010, http://www.food.gov.uk/multimedia/pdfs/thechiacompany.pdf.

CHAPTER 9

Swarm of a Comprehensive and Conversant Review on Phytopharmacological and Traditional uses of *Cassia*

ABSTRACT

Cinnamomum cassia is a tropical aromatic evergreen tree of the Lauraceae family, commonly used in traditional Chinese medicine. It is also a traditional spice, widely used around the world. *Cinnamon cassia* primarily contains vital oils and other derivatives, such as cinnamaldehyde, cinnamic acid, and cinnamate. In addition to being an antioxidant, anti-inflammatory, antidiabetic, antimicrobial, anticancer, lipid-lowering, and cardiovascular-disease-lowering compound, cinnamon has also been reported to have activities against neurological disorders, such as Parkinson's and Alzheimer 's diseases. 166 chemicals have been separated and identified from *C. cassia*. The main constituents of *C. cassia* are terpenoids, phenylpropanoids, glycosides, etc. Modern studies have confirmed that *C. cassia* has a wide range of pharmacological effects, including antitumour, anti-inflammatory and analgesic, anti-diabetic and anti-obesity, antibacterial and antiviral, cardiovascular protective, cytoprotective, neuroprotective, immunoregulatory effects, anti-tyrosinase activity and other effects. This paper summarizes the achievements of modern research on C. cassia, including the traditional uses, phytochemistry, pharmacology and toxicology.

Keywords: Cinnamic acid, Anti-diabetic, Terpinoids, Glycosides, Antiinflamatorry.

Introduction

Cassia [*Cinnamomum cassia* L.) Presl] (also known as *Cinnamomum arromaticum*, Chinese cinnamon or Chinese cassia) belongs to Laurel (Lauraceae) family of plant kingdom. It is harvested from the bark of its tree and is used as a flavouring agent in various Asian cuisines. Common cultivating countries are India, China, Uganda, Vietnam, Bangladesh and Pakistan. The herb is intensely aromatic and has a sweet taste with a tinge of bitterness. The herb is also used in different forms of traditional medicine. Recently, various studies have reported the medicinal use of this herb in different diseased conditions such as diabetes mellitus, peptic ulcer diseases, and various cancers. From the bark of its young branches, cinnamon is obtained, which is widely used all around the world for its fragrance and spicy flavor. It can be used not only as a daily condiment, but also as a raw material for medical products, and has high economic value. Cassia is distributed in China, India, Vietnam, Indonesia and other countries; In China, the producing areas are mainly concentrated in Guangxi, Guangdong, Fujian and Hainan provinces. Cinnamomi cortex is the bark of *C. cassia*, which is often used as a seasoning and spices in the West. For instance, in America, Cinnamomi cortex is used as a food supplements, as a coumarin source of.[1 1] In Asia, Cinnamomi cortex is usually used as a drug.Cinnamomi cortex is a common traditional Chinese medicine in China. Currently, a lot of studies have been done on the pharmacological and phytochemical of *C. cassia*, and more than 166 chemicals have been separated and identified from *C. cassia*. More and more studies have confirmed that *C. cassia* has a wide range of pharmacological effects, including antitumour, anti-inflammatory and analgesic, anti-diabetic and anti-obesity, antibacterial and antiviral, cardiovascular protective, cytoprotective, neuroprotective, immunoregulatory effects, anti-tyrosinase activity and other effects. Cinnamaldehyde derivatives and cinnamic acid, such as 22 hydroxycinnamaldehyde (HCA) were isolated from the bark C. cassia. Mostly bark and leaves of Cinnamon cassia Blumeare used in medicine. [3-6]

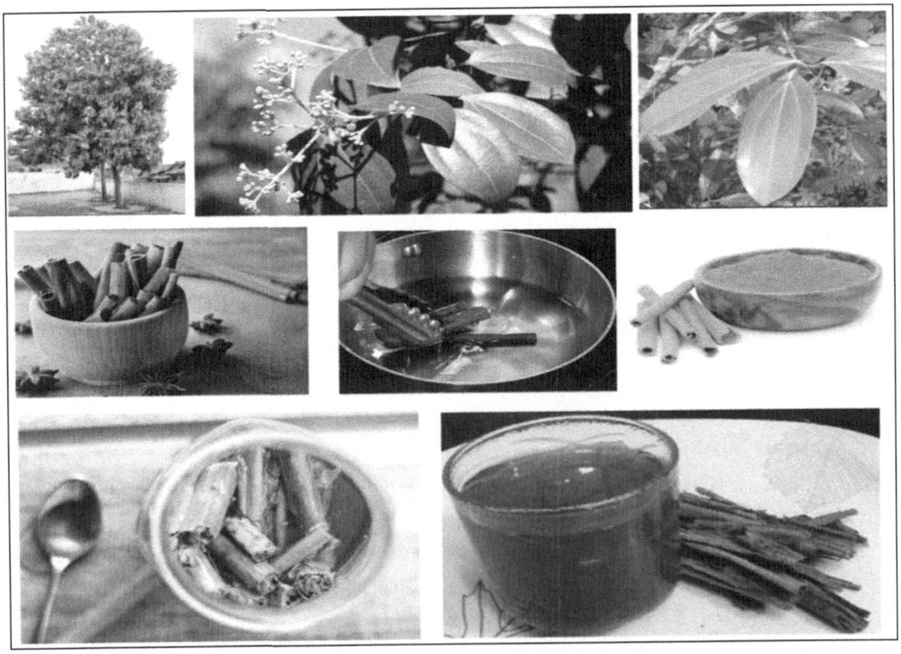

C. cassia bark, cassia tea, cassia waterand cassia with honey

Phytopharmaceutical attributes

There have been a lot of studies about the phytochemistry of *C. cassia*, and 166 components have been separated and identified from the plant. Among them, terpenoids are the most abundant phytochemicals in *C. cassia*, and phenylpropanoids are the bioactive components, among which cinnamaldehyde is considered as the representative component of this plant. In addition to the chemical components found in the bark, the chemical components of other parts of *C. cassia*, including leaves and twigs, were also reported. Terpenoids are the main compounds in essential oil of *C. cassia*. Plant essential oils have a lot of important biological functions and physiological activities. Essential oils with strong antibacterial, antiviral, antitumor and anti-inflammatory effects are the main characteristic components of the Lauraceae. The terpenoids in cassia oil are monoterpenes, diterpenes and sesquiterpenes. So far, 12 monoterpenes have been found in C. cassia. Among them, *endo*-borneol (1) and (–)-α-terpineol (2) were isolated from essential oil of twigs of *C. cassia*. Moreover, 1-terpineol (3) and *cis*-β-terpineol (4) were isolated from essential oil of leaves of *C. cassia*. Other compounds also isolated and identified from the bark, leaves and twigs of *C. cassia*, include α-terpineol (5), β-bisabolene (6), α-bisabolol (7), linalool (8), camphene (9), β-pinene (10), camphor (11) and geranyl acetate (12). Diterpenoids are also important active constituents found in *C. cassia*. To date, 25 diterpenoids have been reported in this plant. These compounds are potentially effective natural immuno modulators in the treatment of autoimmune diseases, tumorigenesis, and chronic inflammatory diseases. The diterpenoids isolated from the barks of *C. cassia* include cinnzeylanol (13), anhydrocinnzeylanol (14), cinnzeylanone (15), 2,3-dehydro- anhydrocinnzeylanine (16), 1-acetylcinncassiol A (17), anhydrocinnzeylanine (18), 18*S*-cinncassiol A 19-*O*-β-D-glucopyranoside (19), 18*R*-cinncassiol A 19- *O*-β-D-glucopyranoside (20), 18-hydroxycinnzeylanine (21), cinncassiol A (22), cinncassiol B (23), cinncassiol C (24), cinncassiol D (25), cinncassiol E (26), cinncassiol F (27), cinncassiol G (28), 16-*O*-β-D-glucopyranosyl-19- deoxycinncassiol G (29), cinnacasol (30), perseanol (31), cinncassiol D1 (32), D1 glucoside (33), D2 glucoside (34), D3 glucoside (35), D4 glucoside (36), 18-hydroxyperseanol (37). Sesquiterpenoids are another class of bioactive constituents found in *C. cassia*. Twenty seven sesquiterpenoids, including curcumene (38), δ-cadinene (39), espatulenol (40), caryophyllene oxide (41), *trans*-caryophyllene (42), germacrene D (43), caryophyllene (44), α-cubebene (45), (–)-isoledene (46), α-bulnesene (47), patchouli alcohol (48), α-copaene (49) [35], α-muurolene (50), α-cadinol (51), copaene (52), isoledene (53), 1-(1,5-dimethyl-4-hexenyl)-4-methylbenzene (54), cedrene (55), α-calacorene (56), cinnamoid A (57), cinnamoid B (58), cinnamoid C (59), cinnamoid D (60), cinnamoid E (61), (–)-15-hydroxy-tmuurolol (62), 15-hydroxy-α-cadinol (63) and *ent*-

4β,10α-dihydroxyaromadendrane (64) are reported from this plant. Phenylpropanoids are the main bioactive components of *C. cassia*. Cinnamaldehyde (65) and *cis*-2-methoxycinnamic acid (66) were isolated from essential oil of bark of *C. cassia* (EOBC), their contents being 42.37% and 43.06%, respectively. In addition, coniferaldehyde (63), *o*-methoxycinnamaldehyde (68), 2-methoxycinnamaldehyde (69), 22 -methoxycinnamaldehyde (70), cinnamylalcohol (71), *cis*-cinnamaldehyde (72), *trans*-cinnamaldehyde (73), ethyl cinnamate (74), eugenol (75), cinnamyl acetate (76), 2-hydroxycinnamic acid (77), 2-hydroxycinnamaldehyde (78), 4-methoxycinnamaldehyde (79), and cinnamic acid (80) were isolated from different parts of *C. cassia*.So far, three glycosides have been isolated from the twigs of *C. cassia*, including cinnacasolide A (81), cinnacasolide B (82) and cinnacasolide C (83), two glycosides isolated from the twigs and leaves of *C. cassia* include cinnacasside A (84) and cinnacasside C (85). Furthermore, 19 glycosides had been isolated from the barks of *C. cassia*, including cinnacasside B (86), cinnacasside F (87), cinnacasside G (88), cinnacassoside D (89), cinnacassoside A (90), cinnacassoside B (91), cinnacassoside C (92), 3,4,5-trimethoxyphenol-β-D–apiofuranosyl (1→6)-β-D-glucopyranoside (93), 3-trimethoxy-4-hydroxyphenol- β -D–apiofuranosyl(1 → 6)- β - D - glucopyranoside (94), 3,4-dimethoxy-phenol-β-D–apiofuranosyl (1→6)-β-D-glucopyranoside (95), (–)-lyoniresinol 3α-*O*-β-D-gluco- pyranoside (96), methyl 2-phenylpropanoate-2-*O*-β-D-apiofuranosyl-(1→6)-*O*-β-D–gluco-pyranoside (97), cinnacasolide E (98), 3,4,5-trimethoxyphenol- β - D - apiofuranosyl-(1→6)-*O*-β-D-glucopyranoside (99), samwiside (100), phenol-β-D-apiofuranosyl-(1→6)-*O*-β-D-glucopyranoside (101), (6*R*,7*R*,8*R*)-7a-[(β-D-glucopyranosyl)oxy]lyoniresinol (102), (6 *S* ,7 *R* ,8*R*)-7a-[(β - D -gluco-pyranosyl)oxy]lyoniresinol (103), (6*R*,7*S*,8*S*)-7a-[(β-D-glucopyranosyl)-oxy]lyoniresinol (104). In recent years, lignanoids have been found in *C. cassia*, and 26 lignanoids have been isolated from it. Cinncassin E (105) was found from the bark of *C. cassia*. Meanwhile, the lignanoids isolated from the twigs of *C. cassia* include cinncassin D (106), picrasmalignan A (107), (+)-leptolepisol C (108), (–)-(7*R*,8*S*,72 *R*,82 *S*)-syringaresinol (109), (+)-isolariciresinol (110), (–)-secroisolariciresinol (111), (+)-*erythro*-(7*R*,8*S*)-guaiacylglycerol-8-vanillin ether (112), (+)-*threo*-(7*S*,8*S*)-guaiacylglycerol-β-coniferyl aldehyde ether (113), (+)-*erythro*-(7*S*,8*R*)-guaiacylglycerol-β-coniferyl aldehyde ether (114), (–)-*erythro*-(7*R*,8*S*)-guaiacylglycerol-β-*O*-42 - sinapoyl ether (115), (–)-*erythro*-(7*S*,8*R*)-syringylglycerol-8-*O*-42 -(sinapoyl alcohol) ether (116), (7*S*, 8*R*)-lawsonicin (117), 52 -methoxylariciresinol (118), (+)-(72 *R*,8*R*,82 *R*)-5,52 -dimethoxylariciresinol (119), (+)-(72 *S*,8*R*,82 *R*)-5,52 -dimethoxylariciresinol (120). The lignanoids isolated from the leaves of *C. cassia* include cinnacassin F (121), cinnacassin G (122), cinnacassin H (123), cinnacassin I (124), cinnacassin J (125), cinnacassin K (126), cinnacassin L (127), cinnacassin M (128), cinnacassin N (129) and cinnacassin O (130). Cinnamomulactone (131), has been isolated from the twigs of *C. cassia*. Later,

5*R*-methyl-3-heptatriacontyl-2(5*H*)-furanone (132), cinncassin A2 (133), cinncassin A3 (134), cinncassin A4 (135), cinncassin A5 (136), cinncassin A6 (137), cinncassin A7 (138) and cinncassin A (139) were found from the twigs of *C. cassia*. In addition to these major compounds mentioned above, some other chemical compounds are found from *C. cassia*, including benzyl benzoate (140), 2-hydroxybenzaldehyde (141), 3-phenylpropanol (142), 2, 2, 4, 6, 6-pentamethylheptane (143), 2, 5, 9-trimethyldecane (144), 2-ethyl-5-propylphenol (145), 3,4-dimethoxyphenethyl alcohol (146), 2,5-dimethylundecane (147), benzaldehyde (148), phenylethyl alcohol (149), 2-methoxyphenylacetone (150) [35], benzenepropanal (151), acetophenone (152), 1,3-dimethylbenzene (153), styrene (154), 2,2,4-trimethyl-1,3-pentanediol (155), decanal (156), 2,6,10-trimethyldodecane (157), epicatechin-(4β→8)-epicatechin-(4β→8)-epicatechin (158), rosavin (159), coumarin (160), dihydromelilotoside (161), methyl dihydromelilotoside (162), evofolin B (163), cinnamomoside A (164), cinncassin C (165) and cinncassin B (166). [5-10]

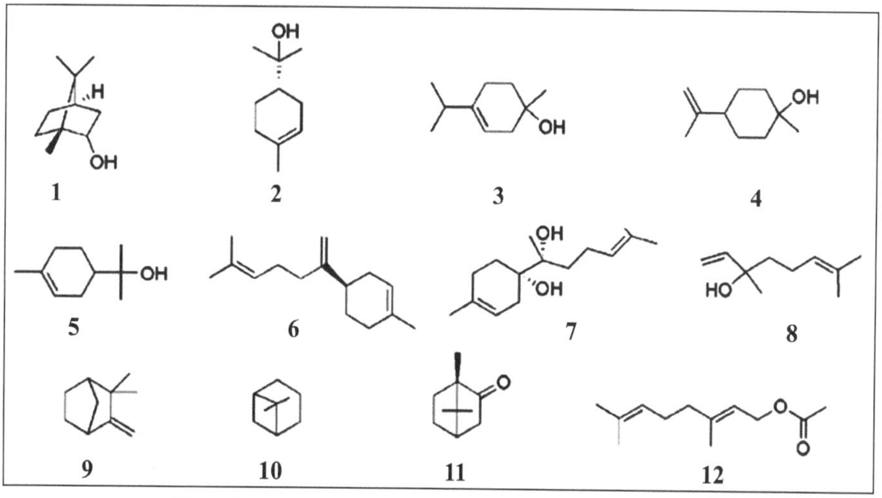

Chemical structures of monoterpenes in *C. cassia*

Chinese cinnamon which is the type of cinnamon sold in the US. and Canada. The fragrance is described as spicy, woodsy, warm, and earthy. However, cinnamon cassia has a sweeter smell and contains more coumarin (a naturally occurring blood thinner). Cinnamon cassia oil is used in Cliganic's cinnamon essential oil which can be made from either the bark or the leaves of the cinnamon plant. Cinnamon bark oil has higher levels of cinnamaldehyde. Because the scent comes from this chemical, cinnamon bark essential oil has a stronger scent than cinnamon leaf essential oil. Also, cinnamon bark oil can be very irritating to the skin, which means it must be diluted before use. Cinnamon leaf oil contains higher levels of eugenol. Besides having a milder aroma, cinnamon leaf oil usually costs less and is not as irritating to the skin.[8-18]

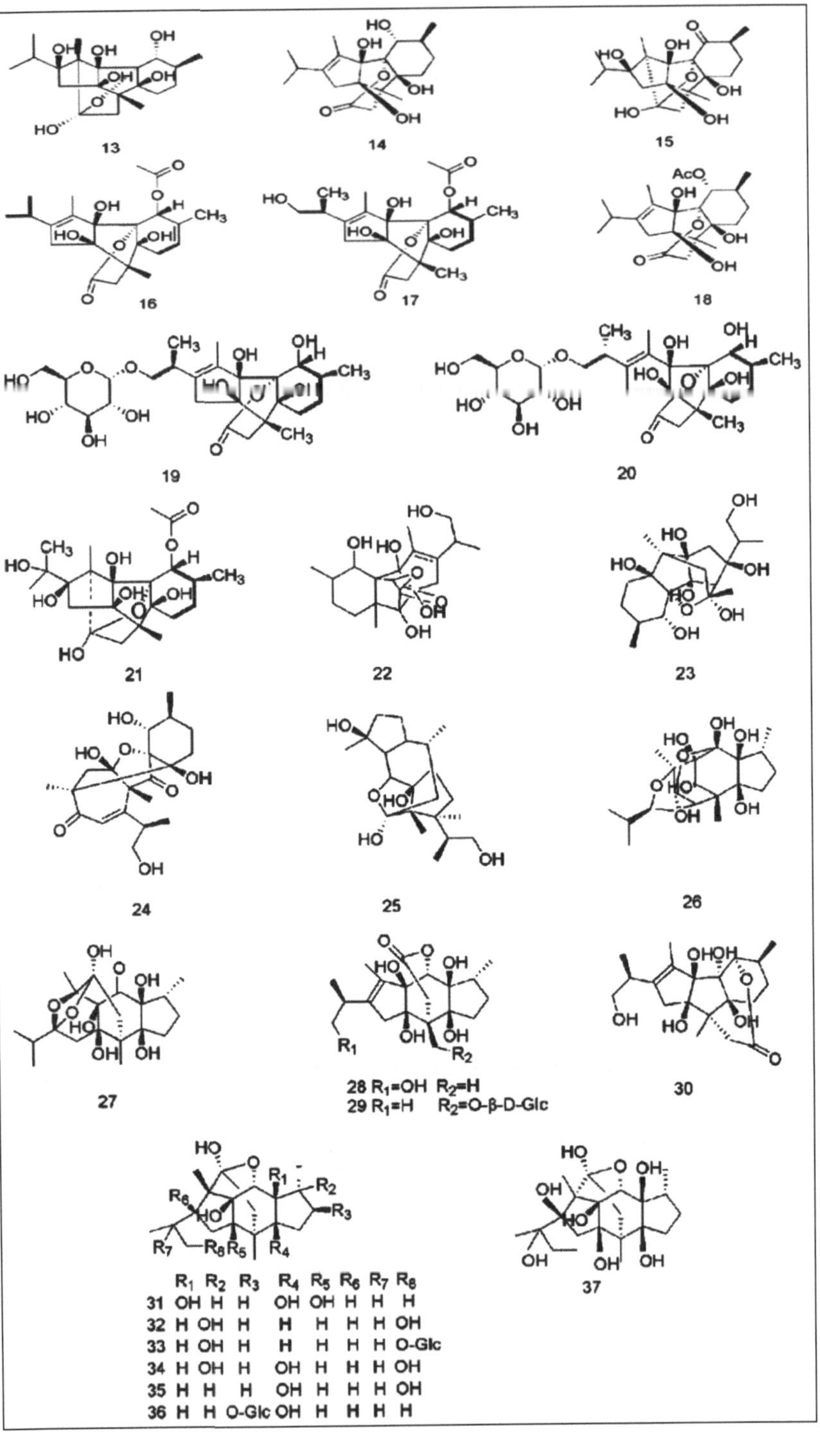

Chemical structures of the diterpenoids in *C. cassia*

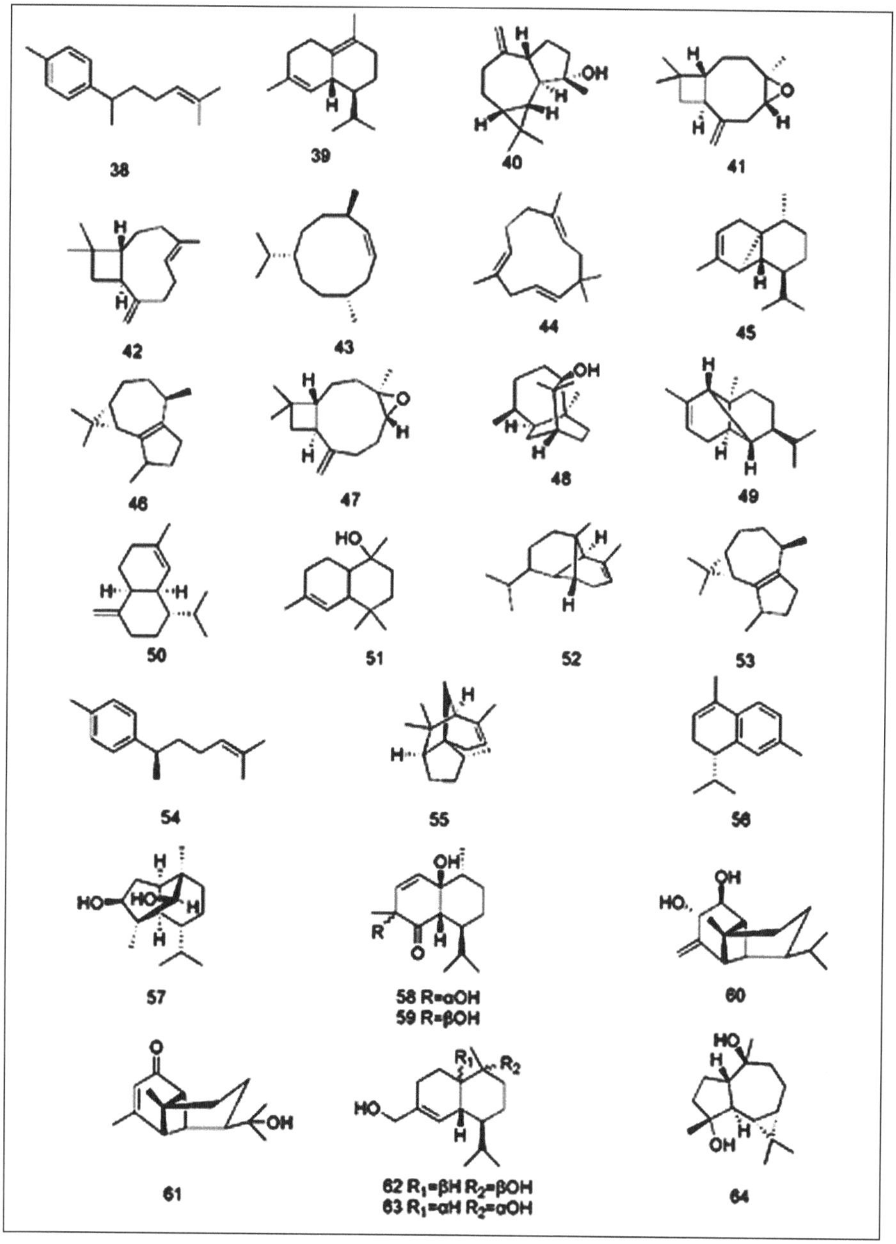

Chemical structures of the sesquiterpenoids in *C. cassia*

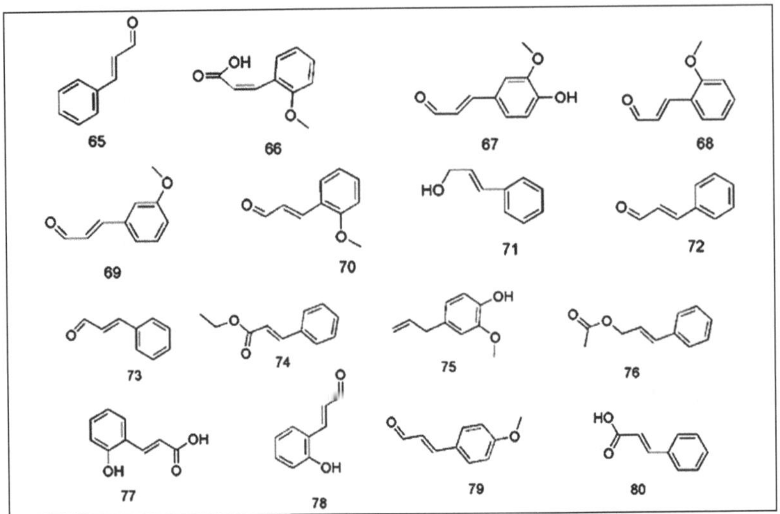

Chemical structures of phenylpropanoids in *C. cassia*

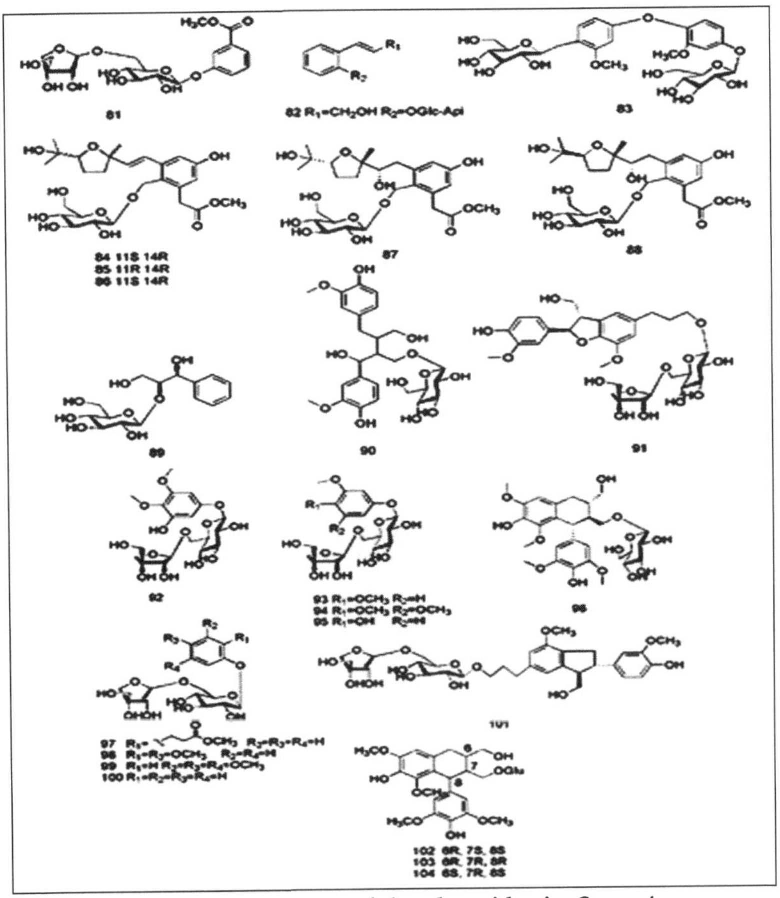

Chemical structures of the glycosides in *C. cassia*

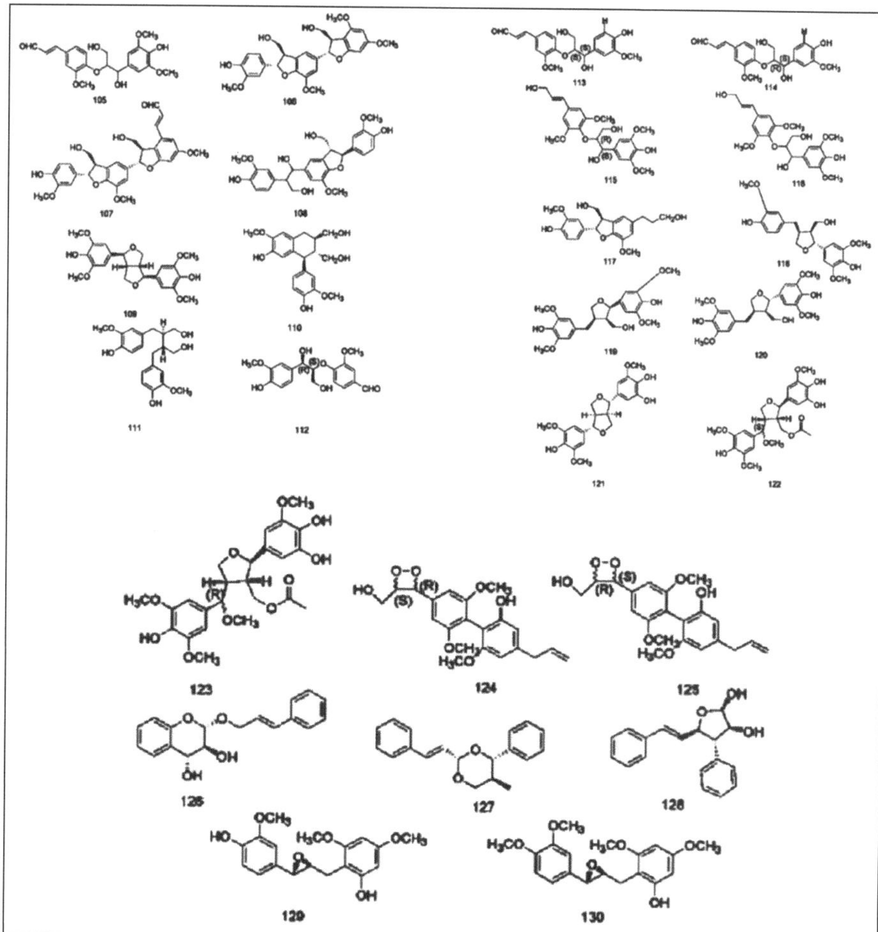

Chemical structures of the lignans in *C. cassia*

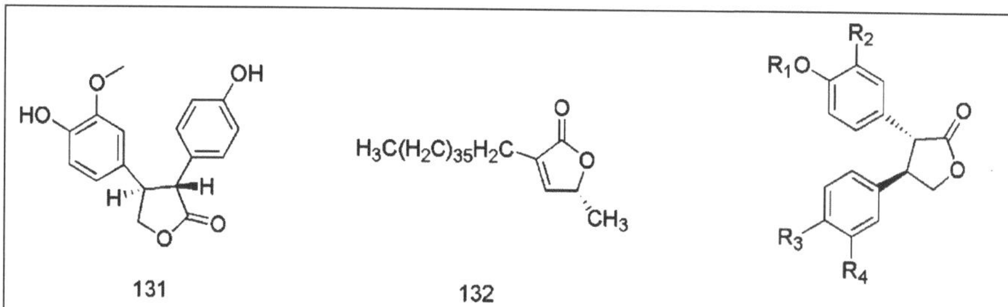

	R_1	R_2	R_3	R_4
133	CH_3	H	OH	OH
134	CH_3	H	OH	OCH_3
135	H	OCH_3	OH	OH
136	CH_3	H	OCH_2O	OCH_2O
137	H	H	OCH_2O	OCH_2O
138	H	OCH_3	OCH_2O	OCH_2O
139	H	OCH_3	OH	OCH_3

Chemical structures of the lactones in *C. cassia*

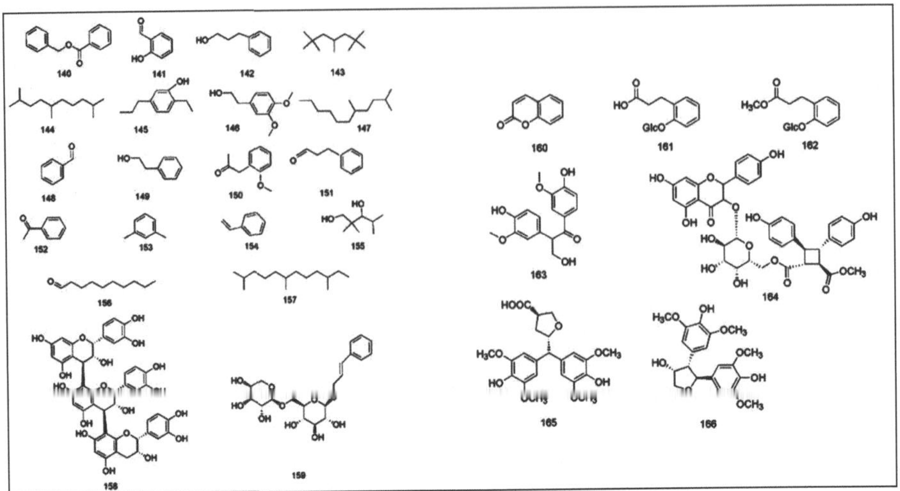

Chemical structures of other compounds found in *C. cassia*

Conclusion

Modern studies have confirmed that *C. cassia* has a wide range of pharmacological activities, including anti-tumor effects, anti-inflammatory and analgesic effects, anti-diabetic and anti-obesity effects, antibacterial and antiviral effects, for which it has been used in the clinic in many countries. Moreover, *C. cassia* has the same origin as a medicine and food which is often used as a condiment in our daily life. Nevertheless, there is still a lack of sufficient research about the alimentotherapy, health products, toxicity and side effects of *C. cassia*. Therefore, more investigations need to be done in *C. cassia* in the future.Firstly, there is a lack of systematic toxicity and side effects studies of the extracts or compounds isolated from *C. cassia*. Essential oils are the main constituents of *C. cassia*, which has been reported to irritate the skin and possibly cause allergies, and the antibacterial effect of essential oil is applied in food and cosmetics. In addition, as a plant with the same origin as medicine and food, people will also eat *C. cassia* for a long time, therefore, in-depth investigations on its toxicity and side effects are a guarantee for the safe use of this plant. Secondly, with the attention humans attach to health preservation, alimentotherapy and health care products are being more and more widely used, thus, there is great space for the development of valuable *C. cassia* health products.

REFERENCES

1. Zhang C, Fan L, Fan S, Jiaqi Wang, Luo T, Tang Y, Chen Z, Yu L. *Cinnamomum cassia* Presl: A Review of its Traditional Uses, Phytochemistry, Pharmacology and Toxicology. Molecules. 2019; 25; 24(19): 3473-3476. doi: 10.3390/molecules24193473
2. Pannee C, Chandhanee I, Wacharee L. Anti-inflammatory effects of Essential Oil from the Leaves of *Cinnamomum cassia* and cinnamaldehyde on lipopolysaccharide-stimulated J774A.1 cells. J. Adv Pharm Technol Res. 2014; 5: 164-170.

3. Xiong YK, Liu XL, Mu ZJ, Yuan E. Sun MS, You QT, Liu ZY. Differences of Chemical Constituents of Volatile Oil from Cinnamomum before and after Drying and Comparison of Anti-Drug Resistant Bacteria Activities. Res Explor Lab. 2018; 37: 56-59.
4. Li YQ, Kong DX, Wu H. Analysis and Evaluation of Essential Oil Components of Cinnamon Barks using GC-MS and FTIR Spectroscopy. Ind Crop Prod. 2013; 41: 269-278.
5. Yan YM, Fang P, Yang MT, Li N, Lu Q, Cheng YX. Anti-diabetic Nephropathy Compounds from *Cinnamomum cassia*. JEthnopharmacol. 2015; 165: 141-147.
6. Pham VC, Nguyen TTA, Vu TO, Gao TQ, Min BS, Kim JA. Five New Diterpenoids from the Barks of *Cinnamomum cassia* (L.) JPresl. PhytochemLett. 2019; 32: 23-28.
7. Zeng JF, Xue, Y.B.; Shu, P.H.; Qian, H.Q.; Sa, R.J.; Xiang, M.; Li, X.N.; Luo, ZW, Yao GM Zhang, YH. Diterpenoids with Immunosuppressive Activities from *Cinnamomum cassia*. Nat Prod. 2014; 77: 1948-1954.
8. Liu X, Fu J, Yao XJ, Yang J, Liu L, Xie TG, Jiang PC, Jiang ZH. Zhu GY. Phenolic Constituents Isolated from the Twigs of *Cinnamomum cassia* and their Potential Neuroprotective Effects. J Nat Prod. 2018; 81: 1333-1342.
9. Zeng JF, Zhu HC, Lu JW. Hu LZ, Song JC, Zhang YH. Two new geranylphenylacetate glycosides from the Barks of *Cinnamomum cassia*. Nat Prod Res. 2017; 31: 1812-1818.
10. Zhang, Y. 1 case of Allergic Reaction caused by Processing Cinnamon. China J. Chin. Mater. Med. 2002, 6, 480-486.
11. Zaidi AF, Aziz M, Muhammad JS, Kadowaki M. Review: Diverse Pharmacological Properties of *Cinnamomum cassia*: A Review. Pak J Pharmaceut Sci. 2015; 28(4): 1433-1438.
12. Rao PV, Gan SH. Cinnamon: A Multifaceted Medicinal Plant. Evid Based Complement Alternat Med. 2014; 2014: 642942. doi: 10.1155/2014/642942
13. Ooi LS, Li Y, Kam SL, Wang H, Wong EY, Ooi VE. Antibacterial Activities of Cinnamon Oil and Cinnamaldehyde from the Chinese Medicinal Herb *Cinnamomum cassia* Blume. Am J Chin Med. 2006; 34: 511-522.
14. Giordani R, Regli P, Kaloustian J, Portugal H. Potentiation of Antifungal Activity of Amphotericin B by Essential oil from *Cinnamomum cassia*. Phytother Res. 2006; 20: 58-61.
15. Park IK, Lee HS, Lee SG, Park JD, Ahn YJ. Insecticidal and Fumigant activities of *Cinnamomum cassia* Bark-derived Materials against Mechorisursulus (Coleoptera: Attelabidae). J Agri Food Chem. 2000; 48: 2528-2531.
16. Bansode VJ. A Review on Pharmacological Activities of *Cinnamomum cassia* Blume. Int J Green Pharm. 2012; 6: 102-108.
17. Shinjyo N, Waddell G, Green J.A Tale of Two Cinnamons: A Comparative review of the Clinical Evidence of *Cinnamomum verum* and *C. cassia* as Diabetes Interventions.J Herbal Med. 2020: 21, 100342.
18. Lee JH, Park DH, Lee S, *et al.* Potential and beneficial effects of *Cinnamomum cassia* on gastritis and safety: Literature review and analysis of standard extract. ApplBiolChem. 2921; 64: 95098. https://doi.org/10.1186/s13765-021-00661-y

CHAPTER 10

Multifaceted *Cinnamomum Zeylanicum* Blume Its Phytopharmacotherapeutic Traditional Applications

ABSTRACT

Cinnamomum zeylanicum, popularly known as cinnamon or ceylon cinnamon are recognized for its sweet flavour and aroma and used as an important spice in India in almost every delicious dishes. The spice has gained more importance due to its well uses as remedy for the treatment of various types of disorders in the Ayurvedic and folklore system of medicine in India from the era of "Charakasamhita". The herb is used for the treatment of dyspeptic conditions, flatulence, loss of appetite, abdominal pain with diarrhoea, inflammation of the eye, leukorrhoea, vaginitis, rheumatism, neuralgia, wounds, and toothache. The oil isolated from the different parts of the plant containing cinnamaldehyde and eugenol as major constituents are considered as active principle of cinnamon. Cinnamon bark essential oil has been used for thousands of years in Ayurvedic medicine to soothe aching joints and numb pain. It is still used for similar purposes in India, presumably because of its anti inflammatory property. It typically contains a very high amount of cinnamaldehyde and a small amount of eugenol, among many other aromatic compounds which have been studied for their antibacterial, antifungal, anti diabetic, anti inflammatory and anticancer activities, among others. In this review paper traditional uses, phytopharmacological aspects and biosynthetic pathway of major chemical constituents in various parts of the plant has been discussed precisely.

Keywords: Euginol, Cinnamaldehyde, Leukorhhoea, Neuralgia, Gastroenterological ailments.

Introduction

Cinnamomam zeylanicum Blume (CZ) a.k.a. Ceylon cinnamon or 'true cinnamon' is indigenous to Sri Lanka and southern parts of India (Family: Lauraceae) popularly known as cinnamon is a reputed spice used in foods and pharmaceuticals since antiquity. *Cinnamomum zeylanicum* is cultivated in south India. But it originates from the island of Sri Lanka, south east of India. Cinnamon spice is obtained by drying the central part of the bark and is marketed as quills or powder. The production of cinnamon is mostly limited to the wettest low land areas of South East Asia. The tree grows to a height of 7-10 meters its wild state and has deeply veined ovate leaves that are dark green underneath, both bark and leaves are aromatic. [1-3]It has small yellowish –white flowers with a disagreeable odour and bears dark purple berries. Several medicinal properties have been attributed to cinnamon. It is carminative, astringent, stimulant; it stops vomiting, relieves flatulence and is useful in treating diarrhea. Recent studies revealed that the extracts of cinnamon were found to have anti-oxidant activity. The essential oil of cinnamon fruit stalk possesses potent antioxidant activity. They also studied the antioxidant activity of cinnamon fruits and the phenolic and flavonoid compounds isolated from them. This paper aims to systematically review the scientific literature and provide a comprehensive summary on the potential medicinal benefits of CZ. In traditional medicine Cinnamon is considered a remedy for respirator y, digestive and gynaecological ailments. *In-vitro* and *in-vivo* studies.In addition to its culinary uses, in native Ayurvedic medicine Cinnamon is considered a remedy for respiratory, digestive and gynaecological ailments. Almost every part of the cinnamon tree including the bark, leaves, flowers, fruits and roots, has some medicinal or culinary use. [4-6]

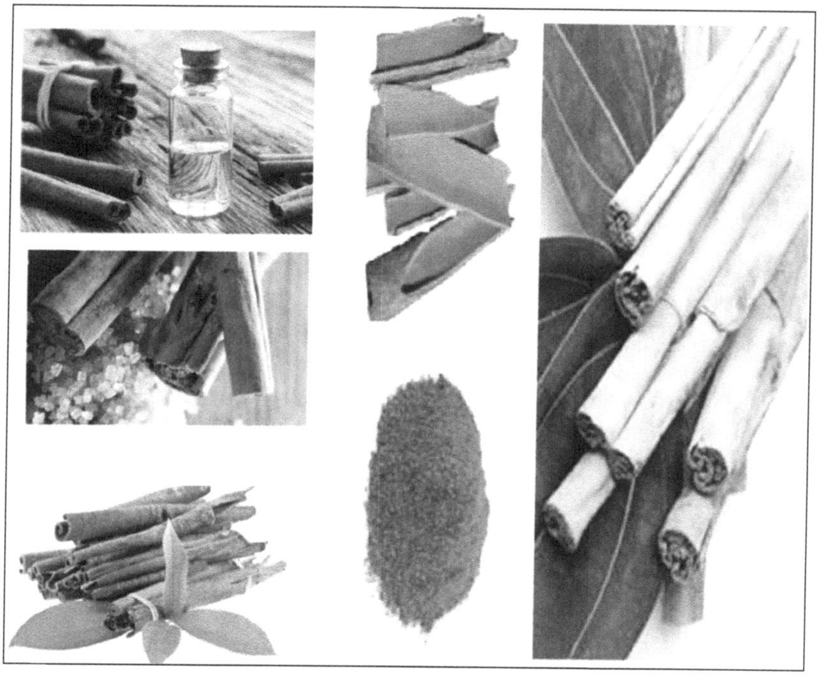

Cinnamon Bark, Powder, oil and sugar

Chemical constituents and Pharmacological attributes

The different parts of the plant possess the same array of hydrocarbons in varying proportions, with primary constituents such as; cinnamaldehyde (bark), eugenol (leaf) and camphor (root). Thus cinnamon offers an array of different oils with diverse characteristics, each of which determines its' value to the different industries. For example the root which has camphor as the main constitute, has minimal commercial value unlike the leaf and bark. It is this chemical diversity that is likely to be the reason for the wide-variety of medicinal benefits observed with cinnamon. Three of the main components of the essential oils obtained from the bark of CZ are trans-cinnamaldehyde, eugenol, and linalool, which represent 82.5% of the total composition. Trans-cinnamaldehyde, accounts for approximately 49.9-62.8% of the total amount of bark oil. Cinnamaldehyde and eugenol are also the major components of CZ extracts.Though both fruits and flowers as well as the fruit stalk oils contain (E)-cinnamyl acetate as the main component, the obvious choice for the raw material to prepare this compound will be the fruit of cinnamon, because cinnamon fruits will be available in large quantities compared to the flowers. [5-14]

Phenyl propanoids found in cinnamon bark, leaf, fruit and flower oils

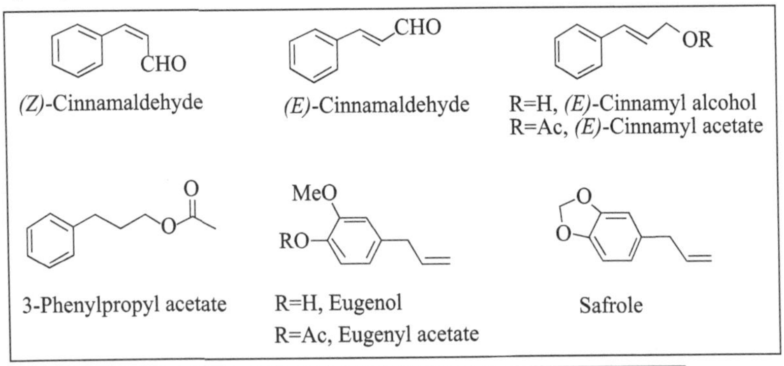

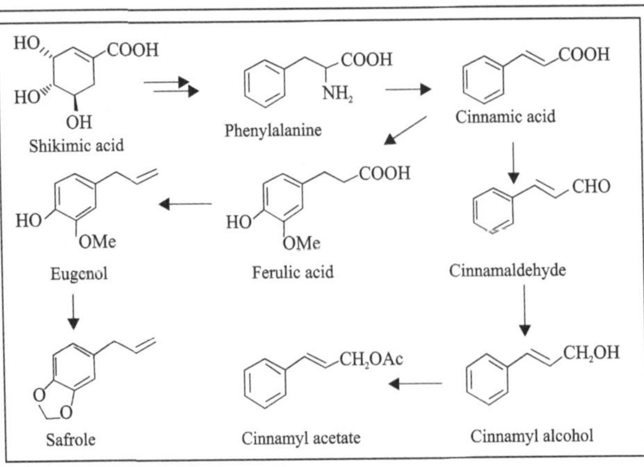

Biosynthetic pathway for the formulation of phenyl propanoids in *C. zeylanicum*

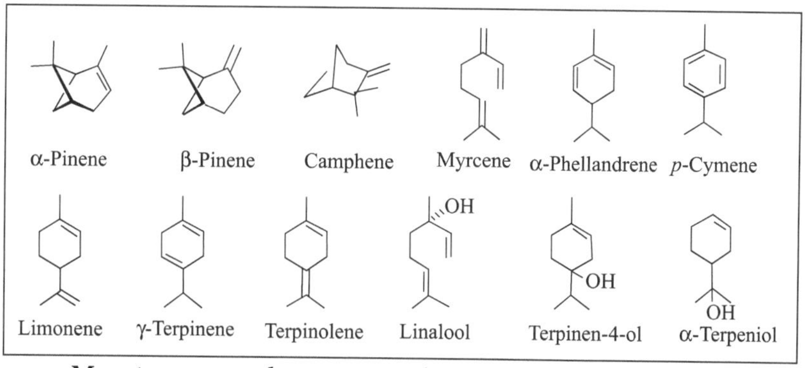

Monoterpenes and oxygenerated monoterpenes found in the oils of bark, leaf, fruit, flower, fruit stalk and bud of *C. zeylancium*

Monoterpenes and oxygenated monoterpenes occurring in the oils of bark, leafm fruit, flower stalk and bud of *C. zeylanicum*

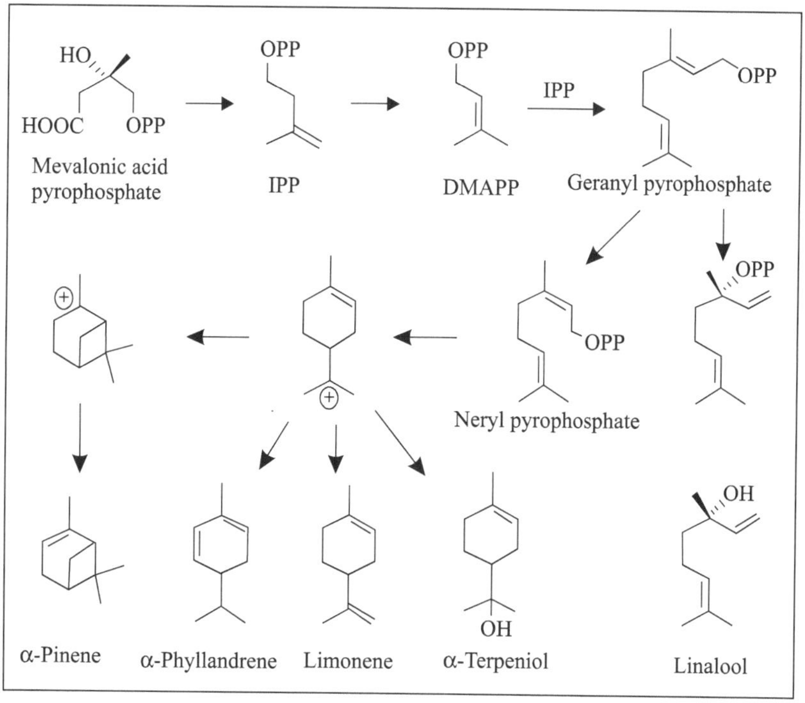

Biosynthesis of nonterpenes in cinnamon

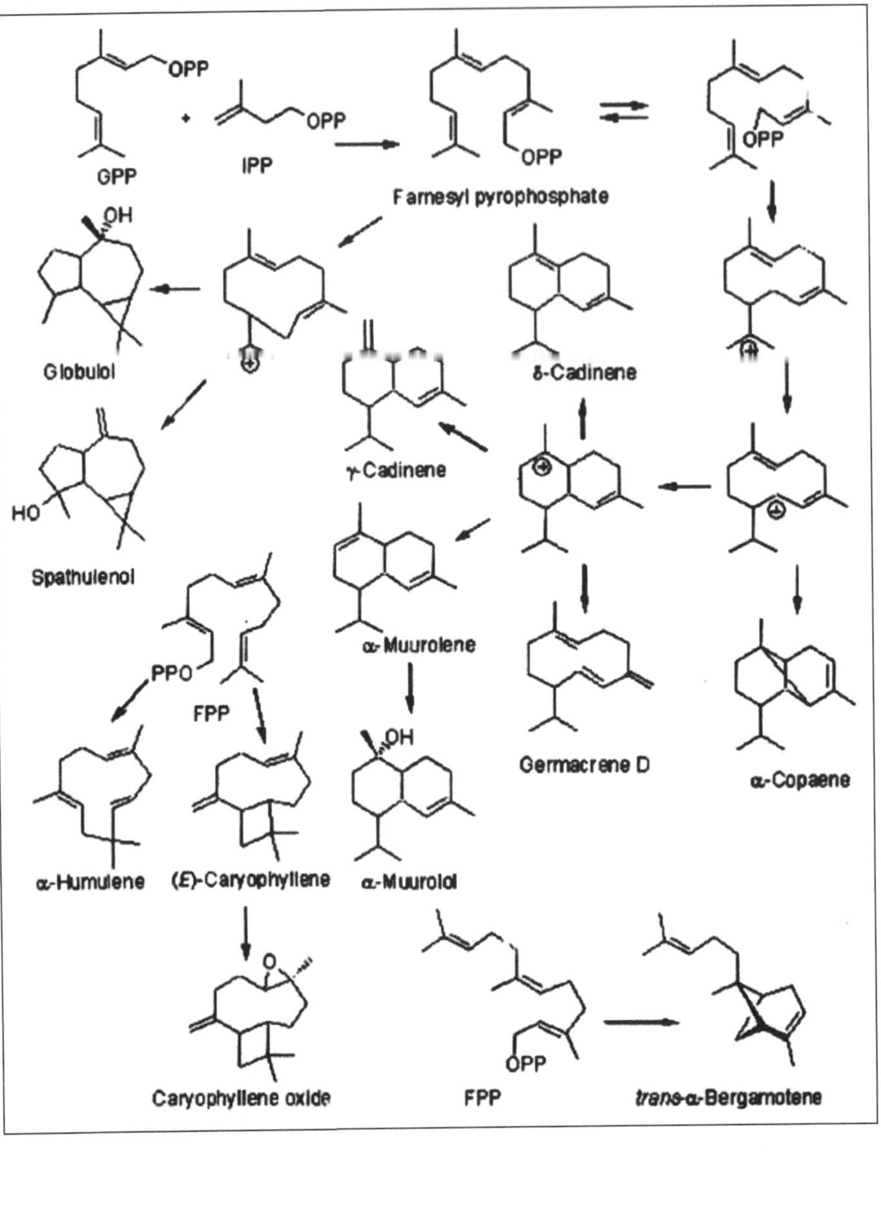

Biosynthetic pathways for the formation of sequesterpenoids in *C. zeylanicum*

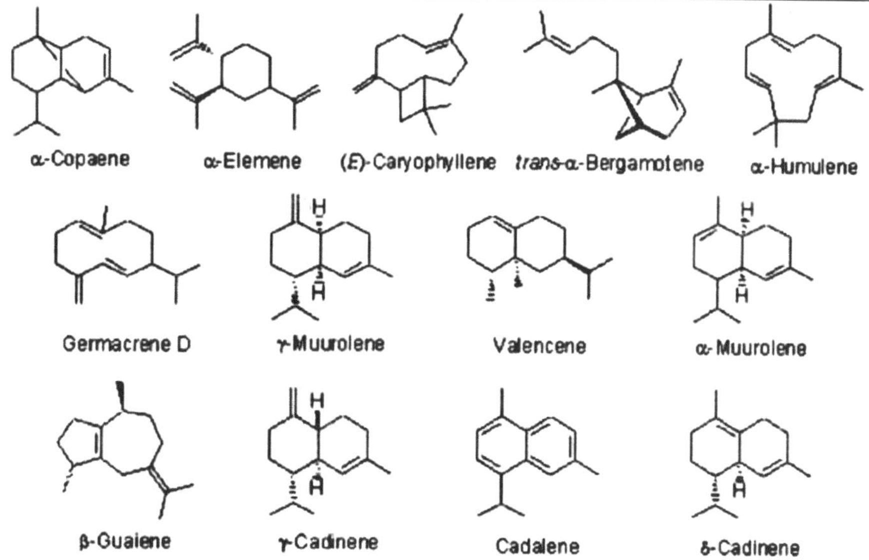

Major sesquiterpenes of the volatile oils of different parts of *C.zeylanicum*

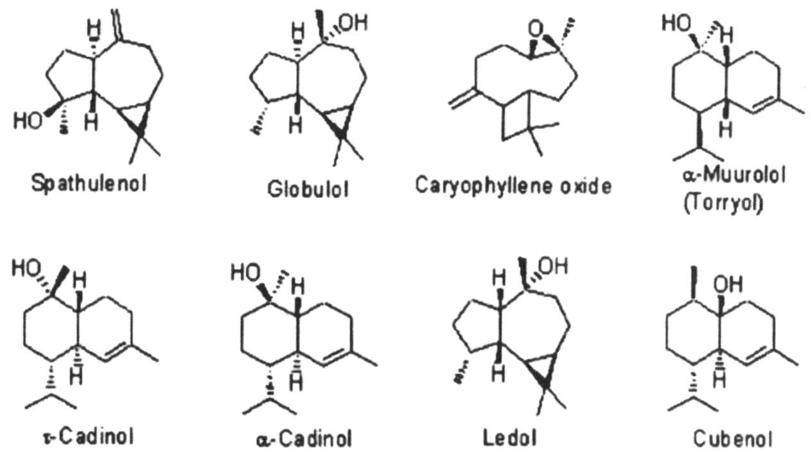

Oxygenated sequiterpinoids in *C. zeylanicum* volatile oils

The volatile oils obtained from the bark, leaf, and root barks vary significantly in chemical composition, which suggests that they might vary in their pharmacological effects as well. In Ayurvedic system, cinnamon (inner bark of shoots) is used in medicine preparation as flu-preventive, indigestion and flatulence control, bark is used in mouth washes. *Cinnamomum zeylanicum* is also used for the treatment of dyspeptic conditions such as mild spastic conditions of the gastrointestinal tract, fullness, and loss of appetite. It is also used to treat abdominal pain with diarrhoea, and pain associated with amenorrhoea and dysmenorrhoea. Folk uses of cinnamon are found in the treatment of impotence, frigidity, dyspnoea, inflammation of the eye, leukorrhoea, vaginitis, rheumatisneuralgia, wounds, toothache and diabetes. *Cinnamomum-zeylanicum* is used as a minor constituent of Unani formulation "JowarishJalinoos" which is used in gastroenterological complaints and it is also used for the preparation of Ayurvedic Drug "Vyaghri Haritaki. "In ancient Egypt cinnamon was used for beverage flavouring, as well as to treat illnesses. Moreover, it has been frequently used in savoury cuisines, Persian sweets soups and pickles. In conventional Chinese medicine,cinnamon has been used as a potential neuroprotective agent, as well as a potent medicine for the control and treatment of type 2 diabetes mellitus. 6 *Cinnamomum* species are commercially valuable source of camphor, cinnamaldehyde and safrol oil in the world. This review presents a summary of *Cinnamomum* species from the Indian Himalaya, Nepal, and Bhutan, focusing on their phytopharmacological attributes. [15-18]Cinnamon leaf essential oil offers numerous benefits. One of the key advantages is that it has antibacterial qualities. Cinnamon leaf Essential Oil is known for its strong antioxidant content and a variety of skin and hair benefits. It is believed to be relaxing to the skin when used topically in a cosmetic blend. It helps to cleanse and tone the skin, making it appear taut and energised. It also helps to reduce wrinkles, age spots, and fine lines while also balancing complexions for a more youthful appearance. Cinnamaldehyde and eugenol are the key elements of cinnamon bark spice oil's composition and natural constituents. The leaf oil does, however, contain eugenol, although the cinnamon bark spice does not. Cinnamaldehyde is known to be responsible for Cinnamon's characteristic warming and comforting scent. Exhibit antifungal, anti-bacterial, and anti-microbial properties. Cinnamyl acetate is known to be a fragrance agent. Have the sweet, peppery, balsamic, spicy, and floral scent that is characteristic of Cinnamon. Be commonly used as a fixative in manufactured perfumes. Enhance circulation, thereby allowing the body and hair to receive the required amounts of oxygen, vitamins, and minerals to sustain the health of each.[19-24]

Culinary uses

Cinnamon bark and leaf have been used in Indian and Western cuisine since antiquity. The bark is used in cakes and other baked goods, chocolates, desserts etc. In India, it is an important ingredient of 'garam masala', a spicy powder containing a variety of spices seed in rice preparations and curries. Both cinnamon bark oil and leaf oil are used in processed meat preparations and in bakery foods. [5,8,11]

Conclusion

Cinnamomum zeylanicum Blume is the integral condiment of the kitchen in Asian traditional dishes and medicine in different cultures and systems. It is used as a flavoring agent, carminative, astringent, germicidal, respiratory, digestive, diabetes, hypertension, cancer and gynecological problems. Volatile oils from different parts of cinnamon species viz leaves, bark, fruits, root bark, flowers, and buds have been proven to exhibit antioxidant, antimicrobial, antifungal, anti-inflammatory, lipid-lowering, and immunomodulatory activities. Cinnamon has also been reported to have activities against neurological disorders, such as Parkinson's and Alzheimer 's diseases. Cinnamaldehyde is majorly constituted in its volatile content responsible for several therapeutic and medicinal applications. This review illustrates the pharmacological prospective of cinnamon and its use in daily life.The Plant *Cinnamomum zeylanicun* Blume offers four types of essential oils to the industry. They are the bark oil having (E)-cinnamaldehyde as the main component, the leaf oil with eugenol as the main component, the root bark oil with camphor as the major component and the fruit oil having (E)-cinnamyl acetate as the major component. Cinnamon bark and leaf oils are already in use in perfumery and flavour industries. Oils from other cinnamon parts are yet to be commercialized by the industry. Eugenol and(E)-cinnamaldehyde are widely used in food flavours and in perfumery. Studies on the antioxidant activity of the cinnamon fruit extracts and the compounds isolated from them revealed the value of the unconventional parts of cinnamon, which have not been utilized commercially at present. Hopefully future research will throw light on the possible application of these extracts and essential oils of cinnamon in the preservation of food products and their use as health supplements and nutraceuticals.

REFERENCES

1. Mallavarapu GR, Rao BRR. Chemical Constituents and Uses of *Cinnamomum zeylanicum* Blume. 2007; In Book: Aromatic Plants from Asia their Chemistry and Application in Food and Therapy Edition: 1, Editors: Jitrovetz L, Dung NX, Varshney VK. Publisher: Har Krishan Bhalla & Sons, Dehradun, India.
2. Wijesekera ROB, Jayewardene A, Rajapakse LS. Volatile Constituents of Leaf, Stem and Root Oils of Cinnamon (*Cinnamomum* zeylanicurzl). J Sci Food Agri. 1974; 25: 1211-1220.

3. Senanayake UM, Lee TH, Wills RBH. Volatile constituents of cinnamon (*Cinnamomum zeylanicum*). J Agnc Food Chem. 1978; 26: 822-824.
4. Nath SC, Pathak MG, Baruah A. Benrylbenzoate the major Component of the Leaf and Stem Bark of *Cinnamomum zeylanicum* Blume. J Essent Oil Res. 1996; 8: 327-328.
5. Cheng BQ, Yu XJ. Introduced Ceylone Cinnamon Cultivars and Chemical Components of their Essential Oils. LinchanHauxe Yu Gongye, 1991; I L: 325-332.
6. Cheng, BQ, Yu XJ. Cultivation of Ceylone Cinnamon and Chemical Components of its Essential Oils. Zhongcaoyao, 1993; 1a (3): 134-137.
7. Kaul PN, Bhattacharya AK, Rao, BR. Seasonal Variationin the Composition of the Essential Oil of Cinnamon (*Cinnamomum*zeylanicura Blume) leaves. Indian Perfum. 1996; 40: 36-38.
8. Jirovetz L, Buchbauer G, Ngassoum MB, Eberhardt R. Analysis and Quality Control of the Essential Oil of the Leaves of *Cinnamomum zeylanicum* from Cameroon. Erniihrung. 1998; 22: 443-445.
9. Jirovetz L, Buchbauer G, Ruzicka J, Shafi MP, Rosamma MK. Analysis of *Cinnamomum zeylanicum* Blume Leaf Oil from South India. JEssent. Oil Res. 2001; 13: 442-443. 30.
10. Jayaprakasha GK, Rao LJ, Sakariah KK. Chemical Composition of the Volatile Oil from the Fruits of *Cinnamomum* zeylanicurm Blume. Flavour Fragr. J1997; 12: 331-333.
11. Syamasundar KV, Ramesh S, Chandrasekhara RS. Volatile Constituents of *Cinnamomum* zeylanicura Blume Fruit Oil. Proceedings of Centennial Conference on Spices and Aromatic Plants, Calicut 2000; pp. 284-286.
12. Kaul PN, Bhattachary AK, Rao, BR., Syamasundar, KV, Ramesh S. Volatile Constituents of Essential Oils Isolated from different Parts of Cinnamon (*Cinnamomum zeylanicum* Blume). J Sci Food Agri. 2003; 83: 53-55.
13. Jayaprakasha GK, Jaganmohan Rao, LJ, Sakariah KK. Volatile Constituents from *Cinnamomum zeylanicum* Fruit Stalks and their Antioxidant Activities. J Agri Food Chem. 2003; 51: 4344-4348.
14. Jayaprakasha GK, Rao, JL, Sakaraih, KK.Chemical Composition of the Flower Oil of *Cinnamomum* zeylanicurz Blume. J Agri Food Chem. 2000; 48: 4294-4295.
15. Jayaprakasha GK, Rao, LJ. Sakariah KK. Chemical Composition of the Volatile Oil from *Cinnamomum* zeylanicurz Buds. Z Naturforsch. 2002; 57c: 990-993.
16. Jayaprakasha GK. Kameyam MO, Ono, Yoshida HM, Rao LJ. (2006). Phenolic Constituents in the Fruits of *Cinnamomum zeylanicum* and their Antioxidant Activity. J Agri Food Chem. 2006; 54(I): 672-1679.
17. Jayaprakasha GK, Negi PS, Jena BS, Rao, LJ. Antioxidant and Antimutagenic Activities of *Cinnamomum zeylanicum* Fruit Extracts. J. Food Comp. Analysis. 2007; 20: 330-33.
18. Ranasinghe P, Pigera S, Premakumara GAS, Galappaththy P, Constantine GR, Katulanda P. Medicinal Properties of 'true' Cinnamon (*Cinnamomum zeylanicum*): A Systematic Review. BMC Complement Altern Med. 2013; 13: 275. doi: 10.1186/1472-6882-13-275.
19. Unlu M, Ergene E, Unlu GV, Zeytinoglu HS, Vural N. Composition, Antimicrobial Activity and in vitro Cytotoxicity of Essential Oil from *Cinnamomum zeylanicum* Blume (Lauraceae). Food ChemToxicol. 2010; 48(11): 3274-80. doi: 10.1016/j.fct.2010.09.001
20. Schmidt E, Jirovetz L, Buchbauer G, Gernot A. Stoilova EI, Krastanov A, Albena Stoyanova A, Geissler M. Composition and Antioxidant Activities of the Essential Oil of Cinnamon (*Cinnamomum zeylanicum* Blume) Leaves from Sri Lanka, J Essen Oil Bearing Plants. 2006; 9: 2: 170-182, doi: 10.1080/0972060X.2006.10643490.

21. Raina VK, Srivastava SK. Aggarwal KK, Ramesh S, Kumar S. Essential Oil Composition of *Cinnamomum zeylanicum* Blume Leaves from Little Andaman, India. 2001;16(5): 374-376. https://doi.org/10.1002/ffj.1016.
22. Gogoi R, Sarma N, Loying R, Pandey SK, Begum T, Lal M.A Comparative Analysis of Bark and Leaf Essential Oil and their Chemical Composition, Antioxidant, Anti-inflammator y, Antimicrobial Activities and Genotoxicity of North East Indian *Cinnamomum zeylanicum* Blume. 2021; 11(1): 74-84. doi: 10.2174/2210315509666191119111800
23. HanX, Parker TL. anti inflammatory Activity of Cinnamon (*Cinnamomum-zeylanicum*) Bark Essential Oil in a Human Skin Disease Model. Phytother Res. 2017; 31(7): 1034-1038. doi: 10.1002/ptr.5822
24. Kumar S, Kumari R. *Cinnamomum*: Review Article of Essential Oil Compounds, Ethnobotany, Antifungal and Antibacterialeffects. Open Access J Sci. 2019; 3(1): 13-16.

CHAPTER

11

Multiple Health benefits of Nutritionally enriched Clove

ABSTRACT

Cloves are the sweet-smelling dried flower buds. Eugenol is the main bioactive compound of clove. With regard to the phenolic acids, gallic acid is the compound found in higher concentration. This essential oil mainly comprises eugenol, followed by β-caryophyllene, α-humulene, and eugenyl acetate as the main components. Other minor constituents including methyl amylketone, kaempferol, gallotannic acid, α-humulene, β-humulene, methyl salicylate, crategolic acid, and benzaldehyde are responsible for the characteristic pleasant fragrance of clove. Cloves help reduce inflammation, thereby preventing heart burns and stomach spasms. Anecdotal evidence suggests that chewing cloves have an alkaline and carminative effect on the stomach and gastrointestinal tract, which doesn't allow gas formation. Furthermore, cloves prevent flatulence and bloating.

Keywords: Eugenol, Anti-microbial, Antidiabetic, Clove bud, Clove essential oil.

Introduction

Clove are the aromatic flower buds of a tree in the family Myrtaceae, *Syzygium aromaticum*. The name comes from the Latin word clavus. The name comes from the French "clou" meaning nail. Clove generally are dried flower buds from the clove tree. Clove were important in the earliest spice trade and are believed to be indigenous to the Moluccas, or Spice Islands, of Indonesia. The clove tree is frequently cultivated in coastal areas at maximum altitudes of 200 m above the sea level. The production of flower buds, which is the commercialized part of this tree, starts after 4 years of plantation. Cloves are harvested mainly in Indonesia, India, Madagascar, Zanzibar, and Sri Lanka. [1-2]They have a numbing effect on mouth tissues. The clove tree is an evergreen that grows to a height ranging from 8-12 m, having large leaves and sanguine flowers in numerous groups of terminal clusters. The flower buds are at first of a pale color and gradually become green, after which they enlarge into a bright red, when they are ready for collect. Cloves are harvested when 1.5-2 cm long, and consist of a long calyx, terminating in four spreading sepals, and four unopened petals which form a small ball in the center. [9]are collected in the maturation phase before flowering. Eugenol, the most important composition of Clove oil, has been accepted as food preservatives by China, US European Union, and other countries and regions. Majorly clove is consumed as a spice in Indian home kitchens. This plant contains active constituents that possess anti-fungal, anti-viral, anti-microbial, antidiabetic, anti-platelet, anaesthetic, anti-inflammatory, anti-oxidant, antithrombotic, pain-relieving, and insect repellent properties. This plant serves as the richest source of phenolic compounds such as eugenol, eugenol acetate, and gallic acid which is used in various applications like in agriculture, pharmaceutical, and in various food preservatives.This review includes the main studies reporting the biological activities of clove and eugenol. The antioxidant and antimicrobial activity of clove is higher than many fruits, vegetables and other spices and should deserve special attention Pharmacokinetics and toxicological studies were also mentioned. [3-5]

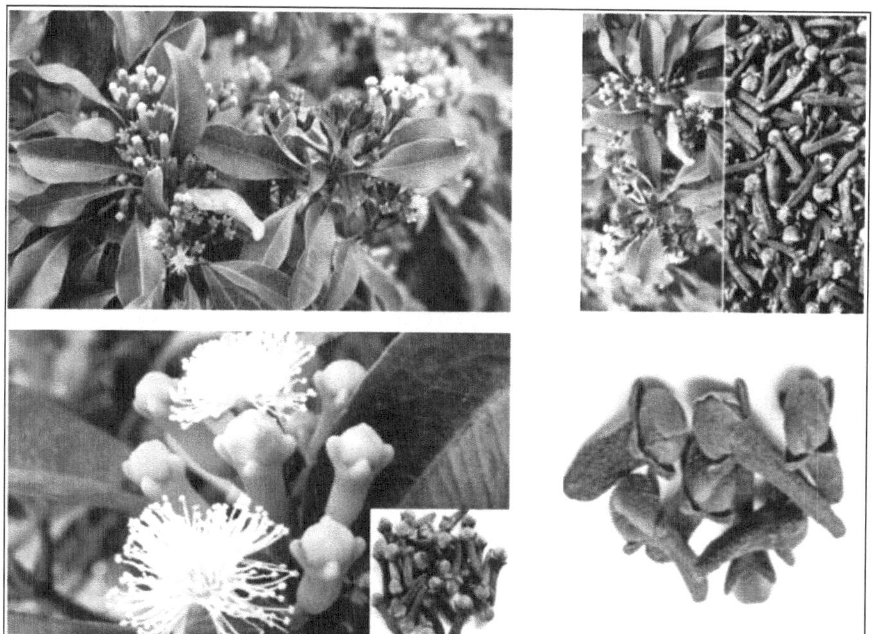

Clove plant, fresh and dried buds

Phytochemicals Constituents of Clove

Clove yields various kinds of volatile oil from leaves, stem, buds and the fruit. Stem oil differs extensively in yield and quality. The main extract of the oil is eugenol. Bud oil contains Eugenol (70-85%), eugenyl acetic acid (15%), and β-caryophyllene (5-12%), which together constitutes 99% of the oil. The constituents of the oil likewise incorporate methyl amyl ketone, methyl salicylate, α and β-humulene, benzaldehyde, β-ylangene, and chavicol. The fragrance of the clove is due to the presence of minor constituents like methyl amyl ketone, methylsalicylate. Stem oil also contains 76.4-84.8% eugenol and 1.5-8.0% eugenyl acetate. Both bud and stem oil contain 7.3-12.4% β- caryophyllene and 1.0-1.4% α- humulene. [6-8]There are 36 compounds extracted from the volatile oil of clove buds. Clove leaves yield 3.0-4.8% basic oil. Clove bud and leaf oil contain different classes of chemical extract, for example, mono terpenes, sesquiterpenes, aldehydes, and ketones. Clove stem contains 6% of oil. The stem oil consists of light yellow fluid containing 80.2% eugenol and 6.6% β-caryophyllene. It contains 2% of oil, which possesses 50-55% eugenol. Non-Volatile Chemical constituents: Few non-volatiles oils have been isolated from clove, which include tannins, sterols, triterpenes, and flavonoids. Tannins: 10-13% of tannins components are present in non-volatile oil among which Eugenin and ellagitannin were separated from the plant. Eugenolglucosidegallate, a chromone C-glycoside, galloyl, and hexahydroxy diphenyl esters of 2, 4, 6- trihydroxy acetophenone- 3-glucopyranoside were extracted from leaves. The two ellagitannins, syzyginin A (1, 2, 3-tri-O-galloyl–4, 6-(S) - tergalloyl- βD-glucoside) and syzyginin B, were also obtained from the clove leaves. Cloves have about 2% of the triterpene and oleanolic acid. Maslinic acid and 2 α-hydroxyoleanolic acids were also extracted from clove buds. Sterols extracted from clove include sitosterol, stigmasterol, and campesterol. Achromone C-glucoside, isobiflorin (5, 7- dihydroxy-2- methoxychromone-8-C-β-D-glucopyranoside), and biflorin were isoated from the ethanolic extract of cloves. The seed of the clove possesses various ailments viz., apigenin 6-C-(β -D-xylopyranosyl-(1→ 2")- β - D galactopyranoside)-7-O-β-D-glucopyranoside and apigenin-6-C-(β-D- xylopyranosyl- (1→2")-β-Dgalactopyranoside)-7-O-β-D-(6-O-p coumaryl glucopyranoside). [5-10]

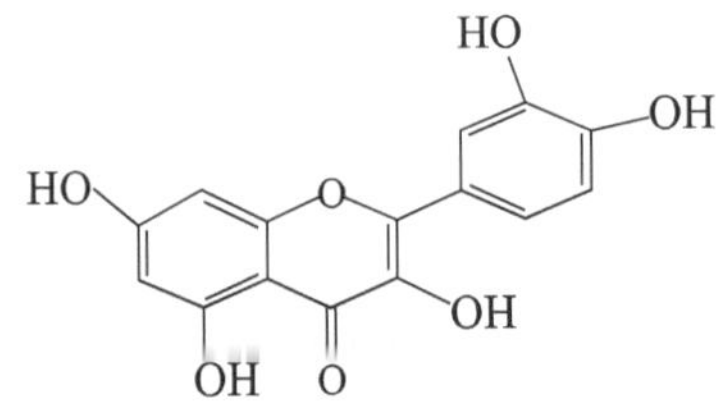

Quercetin

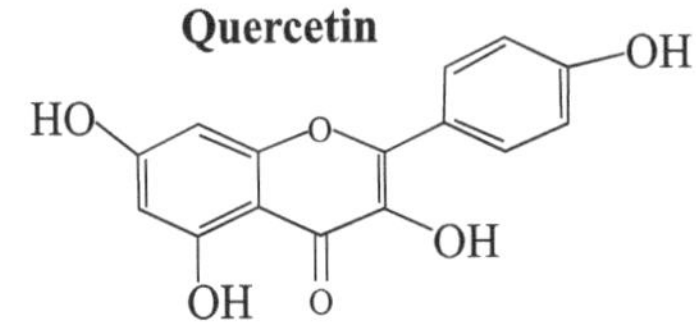

Kaempferol

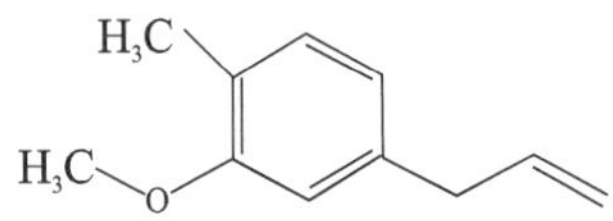

Eugenol

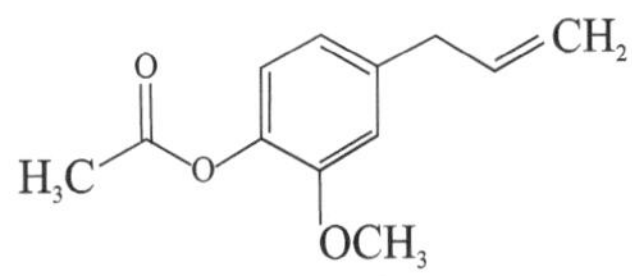

Eugenol acetate

Ethnopharmacological relevance of Clove and its Oil

Clove is known to possess antibacterial properties and is used in various dental creams, tooth pastes, mouth washes, and throat sprays to cleanse bacteria. It is also used to relive pain from sore gums and improves overall dental health. In dentistry, eugenol in combination with zinc oxide is used for provisional filling of cavities. Clove is an anodyne (an agent that soothes or relives pain) for dental emergencies. Cloves are aphrodisiac (an agent for arousing or increasing sexual desire or potency). Clove is used as an anti-inflammatory agent, due to its high content of flavonoids. Aroma therapists use pure clove oil to cure the symptoms of rheumatism and arthritis. Clove is used as a carminative, to increase hydrochloric acid in the stomach and to improve peristalsis. [6-11]Apply the paste of clove powder in honey to treat spots. Paste of clove powder in water promotes faster healing of cut and bite. Cloves can efficiently cure many digestive problems. It is having medicinal qualities to cure flatulence, loose motions, indigestion and nausea. Cloves are useful in relieve the symptoms of diarrhea, gastric irritability and vomiting. Clove and clove oil boost the protected system by purifying the blood and help to fight against various diseases. Clove oil is effective in remedial Athlete's foot and nail fungus. Cloves are good expectorants that promote the free of mucous and secretions in the respiratory passage. The aromatic clove oil, when inhaled can help calm positive respiratory conditions like cold, cough, asthma, bronchitis, and sinusitis. It also helps in clearing the nasal tract. Cloves can successfully prevent the lung cancer as well as the skin cancer. Eugenol helps in minimizing the harmful effects of environmental wastes that can cause cancer of digestive system. Clove oil stimulate blood flow and circulation making it useful for the people having cold extremity. Cloves benefit the diabetic patients by controlling the blood glucose levels. Eugenol is powerful enough for preventing blood clots. Sucking of a clove bud reduce desire for alcohol. Muscular cramps are often relieved, when the oil of clove is applied as a poultice near the affected area. Cloves also help prevent the stop working in retina of the eye, which slows down macular collapse and aids vision in the old age. The underlying mechanism is through the prevention of the breakdown of docosa hexaenoic acid, which preserves vision in elderly people. [11-13] Researchers found that sniffing the spicy aroma of cloves reduces drowsiness, irritability and headaches. One drop of clove oil applied to the roof of the mouth can instantly relieve many headaches. Clove enhances memory retention. It is recommended for relieving brain fog, lethargy and depressive state of mind. Research has shown that clove oil is an effective mosquito repellent. The most prominent use of clove oil in dental care. The germicidal properties of the oil make it very effective for relieve dental pain, tooth ache, sore gums and mouth ulcers. Clove oil contains the composite eugenol, which has been used in dentistry since numerous years. Gargles with diluted clove oil help in easing the throat. The character smell of clove oil helps removing bad breath. As a result, clove oil is added to numerous dental products and medications, including, mouth washes, and tooth pastes. Dentists also mix clove oil with zinc oxide and prepare a white filling material as a temporary alternative to root canal. Clove oil, it's still in dentistry today as antiseptic and pain reliever. According to a 2005 in vivo and in vitro study on immuno suppressed rat, the main compound in clove oil (eugenol) was found to be as effective in treating oral thrush. Clove contain eugenol is the most powerful of these, with antiseptic properties that have been shown to kill the Candida yeast cells. Eugenol is also an immune system stimulant, which means it helps to increase the body's disease fighting powers. Due to its antiseptic properties, clove oil is useful for wound, cuts, scabies, athlete's foot, fungal infections, bruises, prickly heat, scabies etc. It can also be used insect bites and stings. Clove oil is aphrodisiac in nature and hence serves as an outstanding stress reliever. It has a exciting effect on the mind and removes mental collapse and fatigue. When taken internally, in proper amounts, it refreshes the mind. Clove oil also induces the sleeps and is helpful to insomnias patients. It is useful for treating mental problems such as loss of memory, depression and anxiety. Clove oil has a cooling and anti-inflammatory effect, and in this manner clear the nasal passage. This expectorant is useful in various respiratory disorders including coughs, colds, bronchitis, asthma, sinusitis, and tuberculosis. [14-19]

Culinary and other uses

Clove is a valuable kitchen spice which can be used for studding onions, tomatoes, salads, herbal teas, and soups. It is also used to flavor meat products, cookies, chewing gums, spiced fruits, pickles, chocolates, soft drinks, puddings, sandwiches, pastries, and candies. Volatile oil is used to impart essence to perfumes soaps, toothpastes, and pharmaceuticals. In Indonesia, mixture of clove and tobacco in a ratio of 1:2 is used to make a special cigarette "Kretek". Clove possesses antibacterial potential and is used in a variety of mouth washes, dental creams, throat sprays, and tooth pastes to kill pathogens. It is also used to relive sore gums. Mixture of eugenol (major bioactive constituent of clove) and zinc oxide is used for short-term filling of dental cavities. Clove oil has anti-inflammatory properties due to the presence of flavonoids. Pure clove oil is used in aromatherapy of arthritis and rheumatism. Paste of clove powder and honey is used to cure skin conditions. Paste of water and clove powder boosts healing process of bites and cuts. Clove is used to treat various digestive disorders including loose motion, flatulence, nausea, and dyspepsia. Clove oil improves body defense system and help to fight against invading microbes. It is also used to cure Onychomycosis and Athlete's foot disease. Inhalation of clove essential oil soothes various respiratory conditions such as asthma, cold, cough, sinusitis, and bronchitis. Cloves have anticancer potential and are used to cure skin and lung carcinoma. Clove is good for diabetic patients as it controls the blood level of glucose. Eugenol prevents the formation of blood clots. Topical application of clove oil relieves muscular cramps. Cloves also prevent the breakdown in eye's retina, which slows down muscles degeneration and assists vision in the old age. Sniffing of clove aroma reduces lethargy, restlessness, and headaches. Application of one drop of clove oil can soothe headache. Clove improves memory by relieving mental fog, drowsiness, and depression. Clove oil is mosquito repellent. Antioxidant potential of clove is higher than many other medicinal plants. One drop of clove oil is 400 times more potent than blueberries.

Conclusion

Clove (*Syzygium aromaticum*) is one of the most valuable spices that has been used for centuries as food preservative and for many medicinal purposes. This plant represents one of the richest source of phenolic compounds such as eugenol, eugenol acetate and gallic acid and posses great potential for pharmaceutical, cosmetic, food and agricultural applications. Clove is a vital source of phenolic compounds such as flavonoids, hydroxycinamic acids, hydroxybenzoic acids,and hydroxyphenylpropenes. Eugenol is the chief bioactive constituent of clove. Clove consist of acetyl eugenol, beta-caryophyllene and vanillin; crategolic acid; tannins etc. Based on this above information it could be conclude that the clove is a very interesting and important plant which is used for the treatment of various medical conditions because it has various active constituent present in it but most important constituent that is eugenol have various pharmacological activity and for this all miraculous activity of this plant we can confirm that why this plants has been engaged for various centuries. With regard to the phenolic acids, gallic acid is found in higher concentration. Other phenolic acids found in clove are caffeic, ferulic, elagic and salicylic acids. Flavonoids including kaempferol, quercetin and its derivates (glycosilated) are also found in trace amounts. Appreciable amounts of essential oil are present in aerial parts of clove. Good quality clove bud contains volatile oil which mainly comprises of eugenol, eugenyl acetate and beta-caryophyllene.

REFERENCES

1. Yadav M, Yadav P, Sahu S, Yadav V, Gupta SN. Review Literature On Clove 2021; 9(1): 1883-188.
2. Milind P, Deepa K. Clove: A Champion Spice.Int J of Res Ayu Pharm. 2011; 2(1) 47-54.
3. Hu Q, Zhou M, Wei S. Progess on the Antimicrobical Activity Research of Clove Oil and Eugenol in the Food Antisepsis Field. J Food Sci. 2018; 83(6): 13-17.

4. Yadav S, Gupta SK, Bharti D, Yogi B. Syzygium aromaticum (Clove): A Review on Various Phytochemicals and Pharmacological Activates in Medicinal Plant. World J Pharmaceut Res. 2020; 9(11): 13-17.
5. Pulikottil SJ, Nath S. Potential of Clove of Syzgiumaromatium in Development of a Therapeutic Agent for Periodontal Disease: A Review. SADJ 2015:70:108-115.
6. Uddin AM., Shahinuzzaman M, Rana SM, Yaakob Z. Study of Chemical Composition and Medicinal Properties of Volatile Oil from Clove Buds: IntJPharmaceutSciRes. 2017; 8(2): 24-30.
7. Rojas DFC, Fernandes de Souza CR, Oliveira WP. Clove (*Syzygium aromaticum*): A Precious Spice Asian Pac J Trop Biomed. 2014; 4(2): 90-96. doi: 10.1016/S2221-1691(14)60215-X
8. Gülçin I, Elmastas M, Enein HYA. Antioxidant Activity of Clove Oil-A Powerful Antioxidant Source. *Arab J Chem.* 2012; 5(4): 489-499.
9. Hussain S, Rehman R, Mushtaq A, Belaskri PAEZ. Clove: A Review of a Precious Species with Multiple uses Int J CheBiocheSci 11(2017): 129-133.
10. Hussain S, Rahman R, Mushtaq A, Belaskri PAEZ. Deepa MK. Clove: A Championspice. Int J Res Ayurveda Pharm. 2011; 2(1): 47-54.
11. Shan B, Cai YZ, M. Sun MH, Corke H. Antioxidant Capacity of 26 Spice Extracts and Characterization of their Phenolic Constituents. J Agri Food Chem. 2005; 53(20): 7749-7759.
12. Thakur S, Choudhary S, Kumari I, Madhusudan S, Walia B, Kaurav H, Chaudhary G. Clove (*Syzygium aromaticum*) – A Review based upon its Traditional Therapeutic uses.Int J Curr Res. 2021; 13(02): 16368-16375. https://doi.org/10.24941/ijcr.40804.02.2021
13. Nonaka G, Harada M, Nishioka I. Eugenin, a New Ellagitannin from Cloves. Chem Pharmacol Bull. 1980; 28: 685-687.
14. Narayanan CR, Natu AA. Triterpene Acids of Indian Clove Buds. Phytochem. 1974; 13(9): 1999-2000.
15. Brieskorn CH, Munzhuber K, Unger G. Crataegolsaure and Steroid glukosideausblutenknospen von *Syzygium aromaticum.* Phytochem. 1975; 14: 2308-2309.
16. Zhang YW, Chen Y. Isobiflorin, a chromone-C-glucoside from Cloves (Eugenia caryophyllata). Phytochem. 1997; 45: 401-403.
17. Nassar MI. Flavonoid Triglycosides from the Seeds of *Syzygium aromaticum.* Carbohy Res. 2006; 341: 160-163.
18. Cai L, CD Wu. Compounds from *Syzygium aromaticum* Possessing Growth Inhibitory Activity against Oral Pathogens. J Nat Prod. 1996; 59(10): 987-990.
19. Chaieb K, Hajlaoui H, Zmantar T, Nakbi ABK, Rouabhia M, Mahdouani K, Bakhrouf AThe Chemical Composition and Biological Activity of Clove Essential Oil, Eugenia Caryophyllata (*Syzygium aromaticum* L. Myrtaceae): A Short Review Phytother Res. 2007; 21(6): 501-506. doi: 10.1002/ptr.2124.

CHAPTER 12

Study of various Phytopharmacological appraisals of Coriander *(Coriandrum sativum* L.)

ABSTRACT

Coriander (*Coriandrum sativum* L.) is an important seed spice crop grown extensively in India and Indian sub continent for its pleasant herbal aroma and used in traditional Asian cuisine. Apart from its culinary use it has significant medicinal qualities whether used as leaves or intact seeds in ground form. Phytochemical screening of *Coriandrum sativum* showed that it contained essential oil, tannins, terpenoids, reducing sugars, alkaloids, phenolics, flavonoids, fatty acids, sterols and glycosides. It also contained high nutritional values including proteins, oils, carbohydrates, fibers and wide range of minerals, trace elements and vitamins. Various pharmacological activities it possess includes anxiolytic, antidepressant, sedative-hypnotic, anticonvulsant, memory enhancement, improvement of orofacial dyskinesia, neuroprotective, antibacterial, antifungal, anthelmintic, insecticidal, antioxidant, cardiovascular, hypolipidemic, anti-inflammatory, analgesic, antidiabetic, mutagenic, antimutagenic, anticancer, gastrointestinal, deodorizing, dermatological, diuretic, reproductive, hepatoprotective, and detoxification. The current review was designed to give an overview on the phytochemistry and pharmacological attributes of *Coriandrum sativum.*

Keywords: α-tocopherol, Furanocoumarins, Anti-hyperglycemic activity, PUFA, Fatty acids, Phenolics.

Introduction

Coriander (*Coriandrum sativum* L.) being an annual herb is most commonly used for seasoning purpose. It is an upright and short-lived herbaceous plant usually growing 1-2 m. Stems and leaves: The branched stems are hairless (i.e. glabrous), mostly hollow, and have fine lengthwise (i.e. longitudinal) grooves. They are pale green in colour but covered in distinctive purplish or pinkish blotches. The alternately arranged leaves are borne on long hollow leaf stalks (i.e. petioles) that tend to sheath the stem at their bases. They are deeply divided (i.e. bi-pinnatisect), with toothed (serrate) segments, and are ferny in appearance. These leaves (up to 50 cm long and 40 cm wide, but more commonly 12-25 cm long) are hairless (glabrous). The upper leaf surfaces are dark green in colour, while their undersides are a paler green or greyish-green. The stems and leaves give off a strong odour when crushed or damaged. Flowers and Fruit: The white flowers are borne in large numbers in dense flat-topped clusters at the tips of the branches (in terminal compound umbels). [1-4]Individual flowers are small (2-4 mm across), have five in curved petals and five stamens, and are borne on stalks (pedicels) up to 5 cm long. Many (about 15) of these stalks (pedicels) radiate from the same point and form a small cluster of flowers (an umbel), with several (6-20) of these smaller clusters (often called rays) being grouped together into a much larger cluster (a compound umbel) that is subtended by several small leafy bracts (about 5 mm long). Flowering occurs mostly during spring and summer. The fruit turns from green to greyish-brown in colour as it matures and resembles a capsule. It actually consists of two one-seeded structures (mericarps) that readily split apart when the fruit is fully mature. Each of these (seeds), 2-4 mm long, hairless (glabrous), but has five prominent yellowish-coloured ribs. There are many varieties of *Coriandrum sativum* which differ in the fruit size and oil yield. Its plant seeds, leaves and roots are edible, although they have very distinct flavors and uses. Whole plant of coriander mainly fresh leaves and ripe fruits are used for culinary purposes. Coriander leaves have different taste than its seeds, with citrus overtones. Coriander plant is a rich reservoir of micronutrients and nutritional elements which leads us to focus our study on this herb. Coriander is very low in saturated fat however, contains good amount of linoleic acid which is a good source of α-tocopherol and vitamin K. Leaves of plant are rich source of vitamins while seeds are rich in polyphenols and essential oils. Coriander taste is devoted to its essential oil comprising a significant content of linoleic and furano-coumarins (coriandrine and dihydrocoriandrine). [5-8]

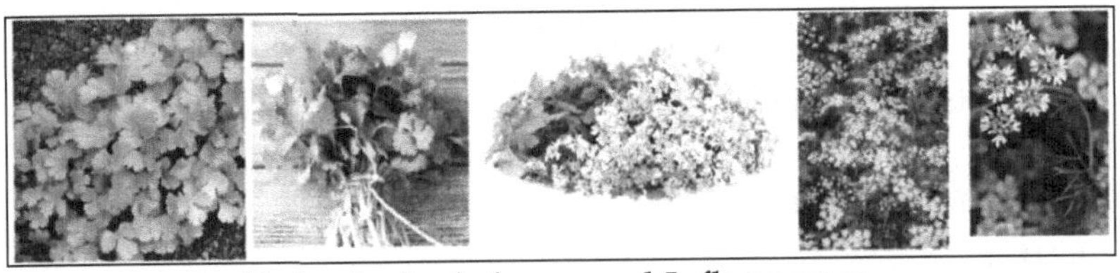

Coriander herb, leaves and Inflorescence

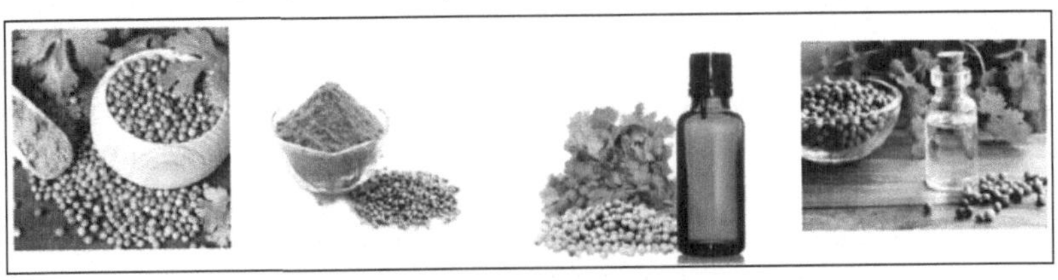

Coriander seeds, powder and essential oil

Coriander is also well known for its antioxidant, anti-diabetic, anti-mutagenic, antianxiety and antimicrobial activity along with analgesic and hormone balancing effect that promotes its use in foods due to numerous health benefits and its protective effect to preserve the food for longer period.The most important constituents of its seeds are the essential oil and fatty oil. It is highly reputed ayurvedic medicinal plant commonly known as "Dhanya" in India. This plant is highly aromatic and has multiple uses in food and in other industries. Plants have played a critical role in maintaining human health and civilizing the quality of human life for thousands of years. It is also used to flavor sausages. All parts of plant are edible, fresh leaves can be used for garnishing and are common ingredient in many foods like chutneys and salads. The green herb is also employed for the preparation of either steam-distilled essential oil or the solvent extracted oleoresin. Fresh juice of coriander is extremely advantageous in curing many deficiencies related to vitamins and iron. One to two teaspoons of its juice, added to refreshing buttermilk, is incredibly beneficial in curing many diseases. Fresh leaves can be eaten as such because of various health benefits however, if it is not harvested freshly seeds mature and ripen in late summer developing delicate aroma which are then used as dried spice. [9-14]

Phytochemical and Nutritional aspects

Coriander is an herb that's commonly used to flavor international dishes. It comes from the *Coriandrum sativum* plant and is related to parsley, carrots, and celery. In the United States, *Coriandrum sativum* seeds are called coriander, while its leaves are called cilantro. In other parts of the world, they're called coriander seeds and coriander leaves. The plant is also known as Chinese parsley. Many people use coriander in dishes like soups and salsas, as well as Indian, Middle Eastern, and Asian meals like curries and masalas. Coriander leaves are often used whole, whereas the seeds are used dried or ground. Coriander nutrition is basically due to its green leaves and dried fruits. Like all other green leafy vegetables, its leaves are a rich source of vitamins, minerals and iron. Its leaves contain high amount of vitamin A (β-carotene) and vitamin C. The green herbs contain vitamin C up to 160 mg/100 g and vitamin A up to 12 mg/100 g. It is very low in saturated fat and cholesterol and a very good source of thiamine, zinc and dietary fiber. Green coriander contains 84% water. Its leaves being good source of β-carotene serve as a precursor of vitamin A. In coriander, β-carotene content, 160 μg/100 g is present whereas total carotenoid content is 1010 μg/100 g. Its foliage is used in various types of foods especially in diets of people facing vitamin A deficiency. Green foliage contains anthocyanin. Anthocyanins are bioactive flavonoid compounds that prevent body from various chronic diseases. Anthocyanin in foliage acts as antioxidants which are very useful in improvement of nutritional value as well as maintenance of health and well being. The characteristic aromatic flavor of its seeds comes from many fatty acids and essential volatile oils. C content of its seeds is nil. Its seeds are considered as an important source of vitamins, minerals and lipids. [15-19]Among minerals, potassium is present in high amount (1267 mg/100 g) followed by calcium (709 mg/100 g), phosphorus (409 mg/100 g), magnesium (330 mg/100 g), sodium (35 mg/100 g), zinc (4.70 mg/100 g). The folate content in coriander seed is 200μg/100 g (fresh weight). Coriander contains high amount of essential oils that are very important for growth and for proper functioning of brain. The main essential fatty acids present in coriander include linoleic and linolenic acids. Linoleic acids belong to PUFA (polyunsaturated fatty acid) group. Dietary supplementation of coriander seed greatly affects the lipid composition of carcass by decreasing saturated fatty acid (SFA) contents (palmitic and stearic acids) and by increasing monounsaturated and polyunsaturated fatty acid (MUFA and PUFA). This plant is a potential source of lipids (rich in petroselinic acid) and an essential oil (high in linalool) isolated from the seeds and the aerial parts. The high content of fats and protein in the fruits make distillation residues suitable for animal feed. Coriander fruits yield 5 to 7% of ash, 13% resin, astringent principle, malic acid and alkaloids. Coriander oil contains coriandrol, jireniol and vebriniol. The functional properties of coriander cannot be under estimated. Besides nutritional benefits, it is well known for its health or medicinal benefits as well as for additional benefits like it acts as antimicrobial agent. The most important and well characterized functional aspect involves antioxidant activity. [20-24]

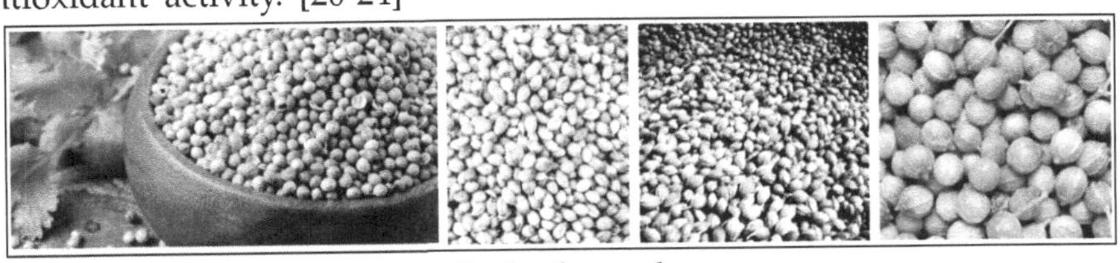

Coriander seeds

For pharmaceutical preparations oil is principally used as a flavoring agent. Coriander can also be used as value added form like other seed spices as volatile oil, curry powder, oleoresin, consumer packed spices, ground spices and organic spices. Essential oil of coriander is used in the flavoring of a number of food products. It is principally used as a flavoring agent in the cocoa, liquor and chocolate industries this may be owing to the nature of chemical composition of coriander essential oil. Like the fruits, it is also employed in medicine as a flavoring or as a carminative agent. It has the advantage of being more stable and of retaining its agreeable odor longer than any other oil of its class. Because coriander oil also has bactericidal and fungicidal properties, it is used as a carminative, stomachic and spasmolytic. It is also used for diarrhea, sub-acid gastritis and dyspepsia of diverse genesis as well as for its stomachic, digestive stimulation and antibilious properties.

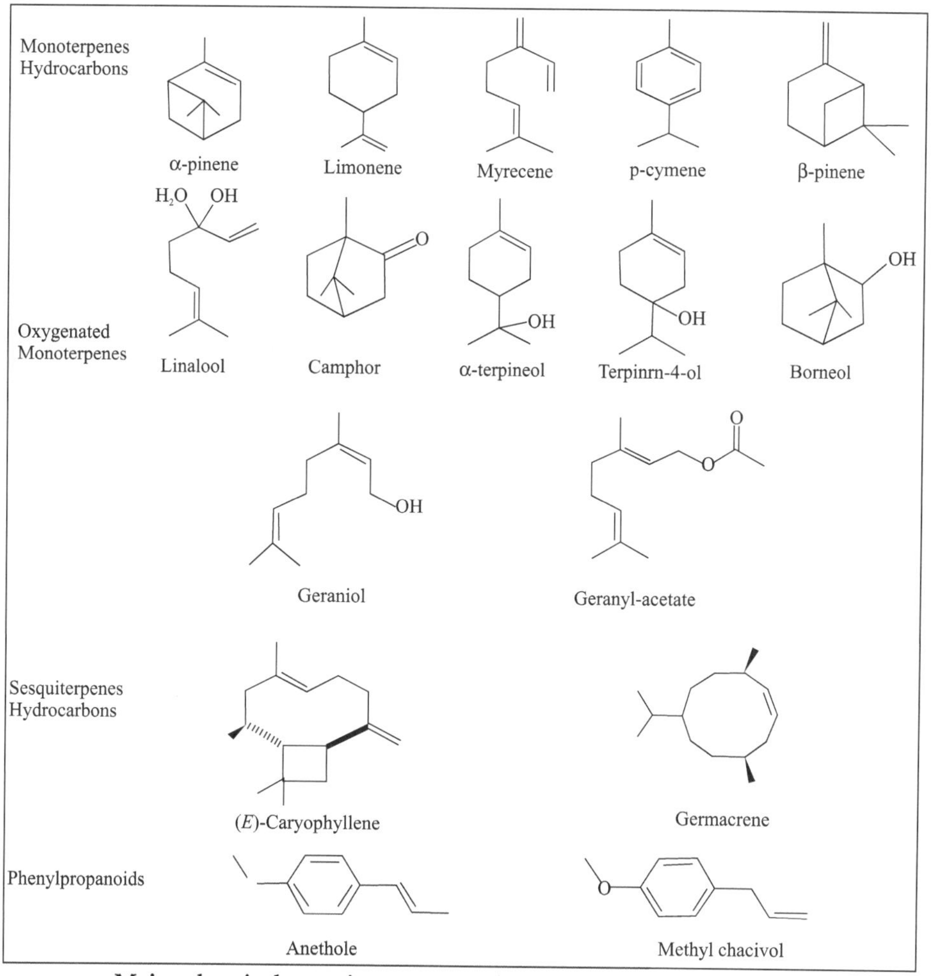

Major chemical constituents occurring in *Coriandrum sativum*L

The different parts of this plant contain linalool, a-pinene, monoterpenes, limpnene, g-terpinene, borneol, p-cymene, camphor, citronellol, geraniol, coriandrin, coriandrons A-E, dihydrocoriandrin, flavonoids and essential oils. [25-28]Linalool is the main volatile compound in coriander seeds; typically constituting morethan 50 percent of total essential oil. The seeds contain on average 18 percent oil (fatty acids/ triglycerides); however, the essential oil content of seeds is approximately 0.84 percent. Beyond essential oil,coriander also contains fatty acid oil which contains oleic, petroselinic and linolenic fattyacids. It forms approximately two-thirds of the oil. Typical compositional analysis of coriander oil is as follows: alcohols: linalool (60-80 percent), geraniol (1.2-4.6 percent), terpinen-4-ol (trace-3%), a-terpineol (0.5%); hydrocarbons: g-terpinene (1-8%), r- cymene (trace-3.5%), limonene (0.5-4%), a-pinene (0.2-8.5%), camphene (trace-1.4%), myrcene (0.2-2%); ketones (7-9%): camphor (0.9-4.9%); esters: geranylacetate (0.1-4.7%), linalyl acetate (0-2.7%). Coriander essential oil were included: Monoterpene hydrocarbons (p-cymene, camphene, Δ-3-carene, limonene (dipentene), myrcene, cis- and trans-ocimene, α-phellandrene, β-phellandrene, α-pinene, β-pinene, sabinene, α-terpinene, γ-terpinene, terpinolene, α-thujene); Monoterpene oxides and Carbonyls (Camphor, 1,8-cineole, linalol oxide, carvone, geranial); Monoterpene alcohols (Borneol, citronellol, geraniol, linalool, nerol, α-terpineol, 4-terpinenol); Monoterpene Esters (Bornyl acetate, geranyl acetate, linalyl acetate, α-terpinyl acetate); Sesquiterpenes (β-Caryophyllene, caryophellene oxide, elemol, nerolidol); Phenols (Anethole, myristicin, thymol); Aliphatic hydrocarbons (Heptadecane, octadecane); Aliphatic alcohols (Decanol, dodecanol); Aliphatic aldehydes (Octanal, nonanal, decanal, undecanal, dodecanal, tridecanal, tetradecanal, 3- octenal, 2-decenal, 5-decenal, 8-methyl-2-nonenal, 8- methyl-5-nonenal, 6-undecenal, 2-dodecenal, 7-dodecenal, 2-tridecenal, 8- tridecenal, 9-tetradecenal, 10-pentadecenal, 3,6-undecadienal, 5,8-tridecadienal and miscellaneous compounds: Acetic acid, α-pdimethyl styrene. [29-34]

Traditional uses

Coriander seeds (Dhaniya) are the aromatic, round, dried seeds (with longitudinal ridges) of coriander plant. The fruits are green in colour and turn brownish yellow colour when they dry out. They are very oily seeds comprising almost 25% of fatty oils. Coriander plant also called dhaniya patta in Hindi is a wonderful herb that resembles parsley and is widely used in cooking all over the world. The seeds are dried and sold in the markets commonly here in India. Coriander seeds have a unique fragrance especially when roasted. At home, we dry roast the coriander seeds to bring out the flavor, grind and then use it in gravies. In home remedies, we mainly make water decoction with it along with other spices like dry ginger and it is popularly called coriander tea all over the world. We use dhaniya also popularly called coriander seeds in English regularly in cooking and also extensively in home remedies as it has amazing health benefits and medicinal uses. It is one of the spices that we regularly keep in our spice box and use it almost in all the dishes. We use both the dried seeds and its ground powder called dhania powder extensively in cooking.In remedies, coriander seeds are used for treating thyroid, aiding weight loss as it regulates digestion and it helps people who are suffering from pcos as it regulates menstrual cycle and treats heavy periods. It reduces high cholesterol and dhania water got by boiling the coriander seeds in water is useful for people suffering from thyroid problems too. It is used for treating hair and skin problems as it has anti bacterial properties and for the same reason it also used for eye care and for treating urinary tract infections too. It is also good for diabetic patients as it reduces blood sugar levels. Coriander seed oil extracted by steam distillation of the seeds also have wonderful medicinal uses.The use of coriander dated back to around 1550 BC, and it was one of the oldest spice crops in the world. Medicinally, it was used as stimulant, aromatic and carminative. The powdered fruit, fluid extract and oil are chiefly used medicinally as flavouring to disguise the taste of active purgatives and correct their griping tendencies. The whole or ground seed (fruit) was an ingredient of pickling spices, also used to flavor various commercial foods, particularly, to prepare some instant soups and dishes, in many cakes, breads and other pastries, alcoholic beverages, frozen dairy desserts, candy, and puddings. The fruit essential oil was a common ingredient in creams, detergents, surfactants, emulsifiers, lotions, and perfumes. However, seeds were applied locally to alleviate swelling and pains. Paste of green coriander were used for headache. Externally, powdered green coriander was used to alleviate burning sensation and pain in diseases like inflammation caused by erysipelas and lymphadenopathy. Decoction of green coriander was used in stomatitis. Nasal drops of green coriander act as a haemostat and thus stop bleeding in epistaxis. Juice or decoction of green coriander was used in conjunctivitis. The seeds were included in many prescriptions as carminative and for the treatment of fever, diarrhoea, vomiting and indigestion. Coriander was used internally as tonics. It was also used for syncope and memory loss. Fresh juice of leaves was used as gargle in sore throat and stomatitis. Paste of leaves were locally applied for swellings and boils and were applied over forehead and temples for headache. [5,9,11-13,32,34]

Conclusion

Coriandrum sativum family Umbelliferae is highly reputed ayurvedic medicinal herb commonly known as the Dhanya. Essential oil, flavonoids, fatty acids, and sterols have been isolated from different parts of C. sativum. The different parts of this plant contain monoterpenes, αpinene, limpnene, γ-terpinene, p-cymene, borneol, citronellol, camphor, geraniol, coriandrin, dihydrocoriandrin, coriandrons A-E, flavonoids and essential oils. Various parts of this plant such as seed, leaves, flower and fruit, possess antioxidant activity, anti-diabetic activity, anti-mutagenic activity, anti-helmintic activity, sedative-hypnotic activity, anticonvulsant activity, diuretic activity, cholesterol lowering activity, protective role against lead toxicity, antifungal activity, anti-feeding activity, anticancer activity, anxiolytic activity, hepatoprotective activity, anti-protozoal activity, antiulcer activity, post-coital anti-fertility activit y, heavy metal detoxification. Various phyto-pharmacological evaluations have been reported in this literature for the important potential of the *Coriandrum sativum*.

REFERENCES

1. Deepa B, Anuradha CV. Antioxidant Potential of *Coriandrum sativum* L. Seed extract Indian J ExpBiol. 2011; 49(1): 30-38.
2. Shahwar MK, Ghorab AHE, Anjum FM, Butt MS, Hussain S, Nadeem M. Characterization of Coriander (*Coriandrum sativum* L.) Seeds and Leaves: Volatile and Non Volatile Extracts. Int J Food Prop. 2012; 15:4, 736-747. doi: 10.1080/10942912.2010.500068
3. Ramadan MFAEAR, Mörsel JT. Oil Composition of Coriander (*Coriandrum sativum* L.) Fruit-seeds. IOSR Jf Pharm. 2016; 6(/37): 17-42.
4. Chung IM, Ahmad A, Kim SJ, Naik PM, Nagella P. Composition of the Essential Oil Constituents from Leaves and Stems of Korean *Coriandrum sativum* and their Immunotoxicity Activity on the Aedesaegypti L. Immunopharmacol Immunotoxicol, 2012; 34(1): 152-156.
5. Bhuiyan NI, Begum J, Sultana M. Chemical Composition of Leaf and Seed Essential Oil of *Coriandrum sativum* L. from Bangladesh. Bangladesh J Pharmacol, 2009; 4: 150-153.
6. Baba K, Xiao YQ, Taniguchi M, Ohishi H, Kozawa M. Isocoumarins from *Coriandrum sativum*. Phytochem. 1991; 30(12): 4143-4146.
7. Melo EA, Filho JM, Guerra NB. Characterization of Antioxidant Compounds in Aqueous Coriander extract (*Coriandrum sativum* L.). Food Sci Technol. 2005; 38(1): 15-19.
8. Harsha SN, Anila Kumar KR. In vitro Free Radical Scavenging and DNA Damage Protective Property of *Coriandrum sativum* L. leaves extract. J Food SciTechnol, 2014; 51(8): 1533-1539.
9. Pathan AR, Kothawade KA, Logade MN. Anxiolytic and Analgesic effect of Seeds of *Coriandrum sativum* Linn. IntJRes Pharm Chem. 2011; 1(4): 1087-1099.
10. Oudah IM, Ali YH. Evaluation of Aqueous and Ethanolic Extraction for Coriander Seeds, Leaves and Stems and Studying their Antibacterial Activity. Iraqi Sci J Nursing. 2010; 23(2): 1-7.
11. Baratta MT, Dorman HJD, Deans SG, Biondi DM, Ruberto G. Chemical Composition, Antimicrobial and Antioxidative Activity of Laurel, Sage, Rosemary, Oregano and Coriander Essential Oils. J Ess Oil Res. 1998; 10: 618-627.
12. Bai VR, Kanimozhi D. Evaluation of Antimicrobial activity of *Coriandrum sativum*. Int JScient Res Rev. 2012; 1(3): 1-10.
13. Reddy LH, Jalli RD, Jose B, Gopu S. Evaluation of Antibacterial and DPPH Radical Scavenging Activities of the Leaf extracts and Essential Oil of *Coriandrum sativum* Linn. World J Pharmaceut Res. 2012; 1(3): 705-716.
14. Silva F, Ferreira S, Queiroz JA, Domingues FC. Coriander (*Coriandrum sativum* L.) Essential Oil: Its Antibacterial Activity and mode of Action Evaluated by Flow Cytometry. J Med Microbiol. 2011; 60 (Pt 10): 1479-1486.
15. M, Faqir Anjum FM, MI, Tehseen S, Ghorab AHE, Sultan JI. Nutritional and Medicinal aspects of Coriander (*Coriandrum sativum* L.) A review May 2013 British Food J.115(5): 743-755. doi: 10.1108/00070701311331526
16. Verma A, Pandeya SN, Sanjay KY, Styawan S. A Review on *Coriandrum sativum* (Linn.) An Ayurvedic Medicinal Herb of Happiness. J Adv Pharm Healthcare Res.1(3): 28-48.
17. Wangensteen H, Samuelsen AB, Malterud KE. Antioxidant Activity in extracts from Coriander. Food Chem. 2004; 88: 293-297.
18. Ullagaddi R, Bondada A Medicinal benefits of Coriander (*Coriandrum sativum* L). J Spatula DD. 2011; 1(1): 51-58.

19. Abidhusen HM, Sawapnil SA, Amit VG. *Coriandrum sativum*: Review of Advances in Psychopharmacology. Afr J Plant Sci. 2012; 3(5): 1233-1239.
20. Darughe F, Barzegar M, Sahari MA. Antioxidant and Antifungal activity of Coriander (*Coriandrum sativum* L.) Essential Oil in Cake. Int Food Res. J. 2012; 19(3): 1253-1260.
21. Ravi R, Prakash M, Bhat KK. Aroma Characterization of Coriander (*Coriandrum sativum* L) Oil Samples. Eur. J. Food Res. Technol. 2007; 225(3-4): 367-374.
22. Sahib NG, Anwar F, Gilani AH, Hamid AA, Saari A, Alkharfy KM. Coriander (*Coriandrum sativum* L.): A Potential source of High-value Components for Functional Foods and Nutraceuticals- A Review. J Phytother Res. 2012; 27(9), doi10.1002/ptr.4897.
23. Silva F, Ferreira S, Queiroz JA, Fernanda CD. Coriander (*Coriandrum sativum* L.) Essential Oil its Antibacterial Activity and mode of action evaluated by Flow Cytometry. J MedMicrobiol. 2011; 60: 1479-1486.
24. Bhat S, Kaushal S, Kaur P, Sharma M. (2014) Coriander (*Coriandrum sativum* L.): Processing, Nutritional and Functional aspects Afr J Plant Sci. 8(1): 25-33. doi:10.5897/AJPS2013.1118
25. Wangensteen H, Samuelsen AB, Malterud KE. Antioxidant Activity in extracts from Coriander. Food Chem. 2004; 88: 293-97.
26. Meloa EA, Filhob JM, Guerrac NB. Characterizations of Antioxidant Compounds in Aqueous Coriander extract (*Coriandrum sativum* L.). Lebensm.-WissU Technol. 2005; 38: 15-19.
27. Matasyoh JC, Maiyo ZC, Ngure RM, Chepkorir R. Chemical Composition and Antimicrobial Activity of the Essential Oil of *Coriandrum sativum*. Food Chem. 2009; 113: 526-529.
28. Eslava JC, Arroyo SG, Pietrini RV. Antimutagenicity of Coriander (*Coriandrum sativum*) Juice on the Mutagenesis Produced by Plant Metabolites of Aromatic Amines. ToxicolLett. 2004; 153: 283-292.
29. Eguale T, Tilahun G, Debella A, Feleke A, Makonnen E. In vitro and in vivo Anthelmintic activity of Crude extracts of *Coriandrum sativum* against Haemonchuscontortus. J Ethnopharmacol. 2007; 110: 428-433.
30. Emamghoreishi M, Heidari-Hamedani G. Sedative-Hypnotic Activity of Extracts and Essential Oil of Coriander Seeds. Iran J Med Sci 2006; 31(1): 22-27.
31. Dhanapakiam P, Joseph JM, Ramaswamy VK: The Cholesterol Lowering Property of Coriander Seeds (*Coriandrum sativum*): Mechanism of Action. J EnvironBiol. 2008; 29(1): 53-56.
32. Ravi R, Prakash K, Keshava B. Aroma Characterization of Coriander (*Coriandrum sativum* L.) Oil samples. Eur Food Res Technol. 2007; 225: 367-374.
33. Momin AH, Acharya SS, Amit V. Gajjar *Coriandrum sativum*-Review of Advances in Phytopharmacology. Int JPharmaceutSci Res. 2012; 3(5): 1233-1239.
34. Saxena SN, Agarwal D. Pharmacognosy and Phytochemistry of Coriander (*Coriandrum sativum* L.) Int J Seed Spices. 2019; 9(1): 1-13.

CHAPTER 13

Miraculous Health benefits of Cumin (*Cuminum cyminum* L.)

ABSTRACT

Cumin is most widely used for culinary and medicinal purposes. It is generally used as a food additive and flavoring agent in many cuisines. Cumin has also been widely used in traditional medicine to treat a variety of diseases, including hypolipidemia, cancer, and diabetes. The literature presents ample evidence for the biological and biomedical activities of cumin, which have generally been ascribed to its content and action of its active constituents, such as terpens, phenols, and flavonoids. The present paper provides an overview of phytochemical profile, biological activities, and ethnomedical and pharmacological uses of Cumin.

Keywords: Cuminaldehyde, Thymol, Pyrazines, Thymoquinon, Insomnia, Bronchitis, Lactation, Anticarcinogenic activity; Hypolipidermia.

Introduction

Cumin (*Cuminum cyminum* L.) is a small annual and herbaceous plant belonging to the Apiaceae family. It is a multipurpose plant species cultivated in the Middle East, India, China, and several Mediterranean countries, including Tunisia. Dubbed as the second most popular spice in the world (next to black pepper), cumin comes from a small flowering herbaceous plant from the Apiaceae or Umbelliferae famil y, which also includes parsley, fennel and hemlock. It is native to Asia, Africa, and Europe, but it is widely used in cooking throughout the world. It is the second most popular spice after black pepper. The plant, which grows about 1 to 2 feet tall, is actually native to the Middle-East Asian region, but is now grown all over the world. The aromatic seeds are the part of the plant that's most widely utilized. These cumin "seeds," which are actually the plant's small dried fruits, look very similar to caraway seeds. They're yellow-brown, oblong-shaped and longitudinally ridged. Today, cumin is a spice that's highly valued in different cuisines. Mexicans, Indians and North Africans love using it to add color and flavor to their dishes. Cumin is also a primary component of curry powder, blended with other herbs and spices. [1-2]Cumin seeds' health benefits mainly come from their phyto-chemicals, which are touted to have carminative, antioxidant and anti-flatulent properties. Cumin is a good source of energy, vitamin A, C, E and B6, thiamine, riboflavin, niacin, antioxidant carotenes lutein, zeaxanthin and minerals like iron, manganese, copper, calcium, magnesium, phosphorous, and potassium. This spice also works as an expectorant that loosens mucus and phlegm in the respiratory tract. One curious characteristic of cumin is that although it's a stimulant, it can also work as a relaxant, making it potentially helpful for alleviating insomnia.[2-4] Research is still ongoing, but animal studies found that cumin may help reduce the risk of hypoglycemia. Cumin may have anticancer properties, as it stimulates the secretion of chemopreventive and detoxifying enzymes from the glands. This study provides scientific support for the anti-stress, antioxidant, and memory-enhancing activities of cumin extract and substantiates that its traditional use as a culinary spice in foods is beneficial and scientific in combating stress and related disorders. Because of its strong aroma, only a small amount of cumin essential oil is used in recipes to provide these with a powerful punch. Cumin essential oil is also attributed to its bactericidal, carminative, digestive, diuretic and antiseptic properties for numerous other benefits. It is also rich in protein and amino acids, carbohydrates, dietary fiber and a reasonable amount of fats & fatty acids. Cumin is known for the benefits it offers, more than its taste or flavor, as it helps in losing weight, improving digestion and immunity, and treating skin disorders, boils, piles, insomnia and respiratory disorders. [5-6]

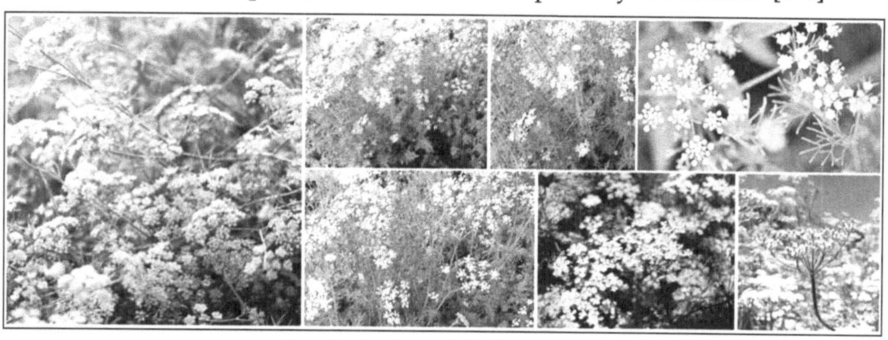

Cumin herb and Inflorescence

Phytochemistry

Phytochemical analysis showed that *Cuminum cyminum* contained: alkaloid, anthraquinone, coumarin, flavonoid, glycoside, protein, resin, saponin, tannin and steroid. Nutrient contents of cumin (in 2 g of seeds) were included: calories 7.50, calories from fat 4.00, calories from saturated fat 0.28, protein (g) 0.36, carbohydrates (g) 0.88, dietary fibre (g) 0.22, total fat (g) 0.44, saturated fat (g) 0.04, monounsaturated fat (g) 0.28, polyunsaturated fat (g) 0.06, water (g) 0.16, Ash (g) 0.16, vitamin A (IU) 25.40, vitamin A (RE) 2.54, α-carotenoid (RE) 2.54, beta carotene (μg) 15.24, thiamin – B1(mg) 0.02, niacin – B3(mg) 0.10, niacin equiv 0.10, vitamin C 0.16, vitamin E alpha equiv 0.02, vitamin E (IU) 0.04, vitamin E (mg) 0.02, folate (μg) 0.20, vitamin K (μg) 0.11, calcium(mg) 18.62, copper(mg) 0.02, iron(mg) 1.32, magnesium (mg) 7.32, manganese (mg) 0.06, phosphorus (mg) 9.98, potassium (mg) 35.76, selenium (μg) 0.10, sodium (mg) 3.36, zinc (mg) 0.10, palmitic acid (g) 0.02, oleic (g) 0.28, linoleic acid (g) 0.06 and omega 6 fatty acids (g) 0.06. Organic acids (aspartic, citric, malic, tartaric, propionic, ascorbic, oxalic, maleic and fumaric acids) were isolated from seeds of *Cuminum cyminum*. Cumin fruits contained 2.5 to 4.5% volatile oil and 10% fixed oil. It appeared that the constituents of *Cuminum cyminum* essential oil were differ according to the area from which the *Cuminum cyminum* samples were taken. The major compounds in the Turkish cumin (*Cuminum cyminum*) seed oil were cuminaldehyde (19.25-27.02%), p-mentha-1,3-dien-7-al (4.29-12.26%), p-mentha-1,4-dien-7-al (24.48-44.91%), γ-terpinene (7.06-14.10%), p-cymene (4.61-12.01%) and β-pinene (2.98-8.90%). Cuminaldehyde, γ-terpinene, o-cymene, limonene and β-pinene were determined to be the major constituents of Syrian *Cuminum cyminum*. The major compounds in cumin essential oil of Egyptian cultivars were cuminaldehyde (35.25%), tetradecene (12.25%), γ-terpenene (12%), β-ocimene (9.72%), p-mentha-2-en-ol (9%), α-terpinyl acetate (5.32%), α-terpinolene (3%), lmonine (0.5%), myrcene (0.2%), β-pinene(0.9%) and α-pinene (0.19%).

Tunisian variety of *Cuminum cyminum* contained cuminlaldehyde (39.48%), gamma-terpinene (15.21%), Ocymene (11.82%), beta-pinene (11.13%), 2-caren-10-al (7.93%), trans-carveol (4.49%) and myrtenal (3.5%) as major components. Analysis of the fruit oil of *Cuminum cyminum* from Delhi showed that the major constituents were transdihydrocarvone (31.11%), γ-terpinene (23.22%), p-cymene (15.8%), α- phellandrene (12.01%) and pmenth-2-en-7-ol (3.48%) and cuminlaldehyde constituted only 0.58%. Analysis of cumin oil samples from four different German regions showed that the major compounds in all samples were monoterpenes beta -pinene, p-cymene, gamma –terpinene, the terpenoid aldehydes, cuminic aldehyde and the isomeric menthadien carboxaldehydes. However, Li and Jiang found that Chinese cumen seed oil contained cuminal (36.31%), cuminic alcohol (16.92%), γ-terpinene (11.14%), safranal (10.87%), p-cymene (9.85%) and β-pinene (7.75%) as major components. Thymol (40.65%), γ-terpinene (24.51%), b-pinene (5.38%), a-pinene (3.47%), camphene (2.31%), terpinene- 4 – ol (2.00%), cuminaldehyde (1.79%), a-thujene (1.45%), a-terpinolene (1.17%), myrcene (1.07%), limonene (1.04%), α-phyllanderene (0.94%), acetoxylinalool (0.57%) and sabinene (0.37%) represented the major components isolated from cumin essential oils from Kurdistan mountain of Iran(91). 20 compounds from the *Cuminum cyminum* (seeds) oil including: α-pinene 2.14, sabinene 1.01, β-pinene 4.89, β-myrcene 1.45, α-terpinene 0.84, p-cymene 1.77, limonene 0.24, g-terpinene 1.07, α-terpinolene 0.08, Camphor 0.12, Terpinen-4-ol 0.04, α-terpineol 2.47, geraniol 0.07, geranyl acetate 4.11, β-caryophyllene 3.44, α-phellandrene 1.09, cuminaldehyde 60.01, thymol 2.04, β-farnesene 3.01 and caryophyllene oxide 6.12. However, 32 compounds from *Cuminum cyminum* oil including: isobutyl isobutyrate 0.8, a-thujene 0.3, a-pinene 29.1, sabinene 0.6, myrcene 0.2, d-3-carene 0.2, p-cymene 0.3, limonene 21.5, 1,8- cineole 17.9, (E)-ocimene 0.1, g -terpinene 0.6, terpinolene 0.3, linalool 10.4, a-campholenal 0.03, transpinocarveole 0.07, d-terpineole 0.09, terpinene-4-ol 0.5, a-terpineole 3.17, trans-carveole 0.4, cis-carveole 0.07, geraniol 1.1, linalyl acetate 4.8, methyl geranate 0.2, a-terpinyl acetate 1.3, neryl acetate 0.09, methyl eugenol 1.6, b-caryophyllene 0.2, a-humulene 0.2, spathulenol 0.07, caryophylleneb epoxide 0.1, humulene epoxide II 0.08 and acetocyclohexane dione-2 0.4(93). 49 components were identified in the essential oil constituents of the *Cuminum cyminum* fruit grown in Delhi, which represented 99.78% of total detected constituents. The essential oil was characterized by the presence of monoterpene (79.61%), sesquiterpene (2.66%), aromatic (16.55%) and aliphatic compounds (0.66%). Among thirty four monoterpenes detected, there were fourteen hydrocarbons (41.28%), twelve alcohols (5.76%), six keto compounds (31.92%), one aldehyde (0.54%) and two esters (0.11%). The predominant monoterpene hydrocarbon was γ-terpinene (23.22%) followed by α-phellandrene (12.01%), α-pinene (1.78%) and α-terpinene (1.24%).

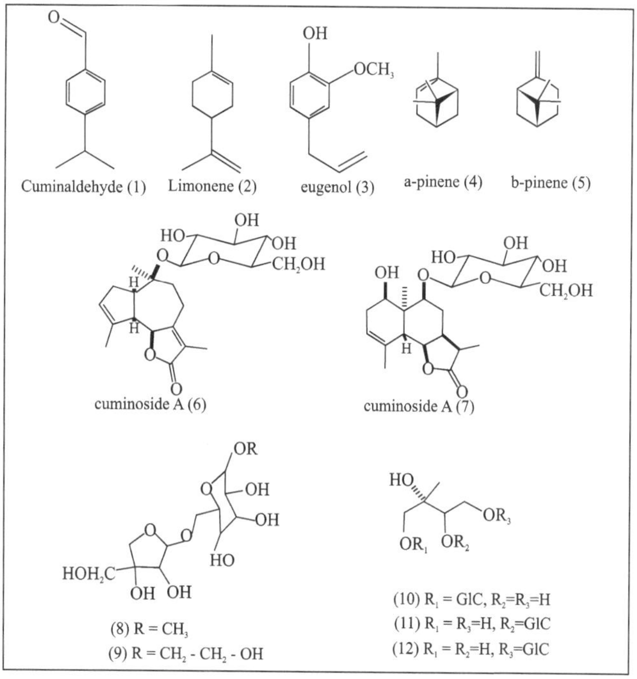

Structure	Name	Formula	Structure	Name	Formula
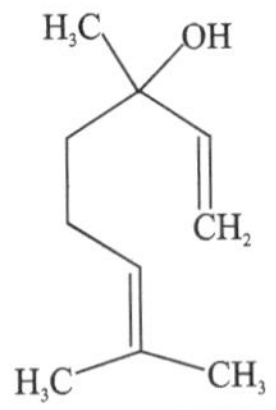	Linalool	$C_{10}H_{18}O$	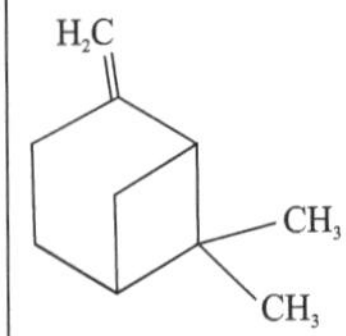	β-Pinene	$C_{10}H_{16}$
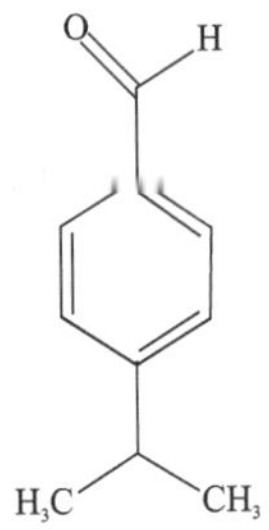	Cuminaldehyde	$C_{10}H_{12}O$	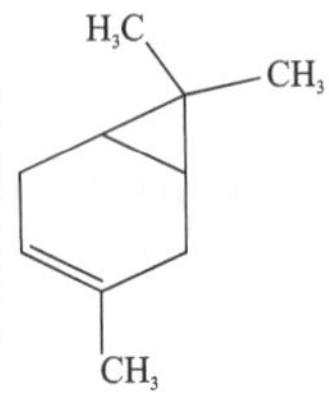	Δ -Carene	$C_{10}H_{16}$
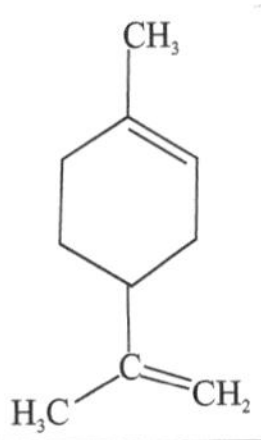	Limonene	$C_{10}H_{16}$	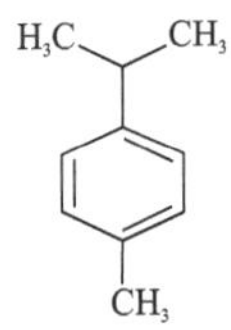	*p*-Cymene	$C_{10}H_{14}$
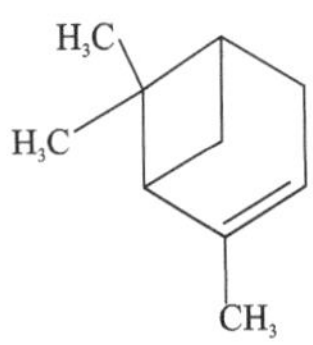	α-pinene	$C_{10}H_{16}$	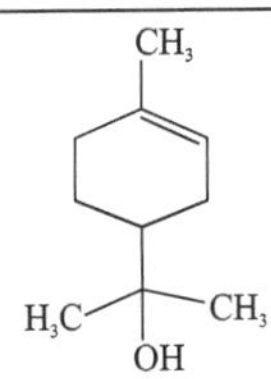	α-Terpineol	$C_{10}H_{18}O$

Among twelve monoterpenic alcohols, p-menth-2-en-7-ol (3.48%) was the major alcoholic constituent and trans-dihydrocarvone (31.11%) was the prominent monoterpenic ketone in the essential oil. The sesquiterpenes identified in the oil were teresantalol (2.62%) and karvaknol (0.04%). The aromatic compounds detected were p-cymene (15.87%), 8a-methyl octahydro-2(1H)- naphthalenone, 2-isopropyl-5-methyl phenol, pcymen-7-ol, o-cymen-5-ol, p-cymen-3-ol, 6-allyl-4,5-dimethoxy-1,3-benzodioxole and 2,a,8,8-tetramethyl decahydrocyclopropanal [d] naphthalene. The aliphatic compounds included 1-(1, 2, 3-trimethyl-2- cyclopenten1-yl) ethanone, 3-isopropyl phenol, 2-methyl-4-isopropyliden-cyclopentan-1-al, 1-methyl-4-iso propyl-3- cyclohexen-1-ol, 2-isopropenyl-5-methyl-hex-4-enal, 4-isopropyl cyclohex-1,3-dien-1-yl) methanol, 4- isopropyl-1-cyclohexen-1-carbaldehyde, hexadecylene oxide and (3,4-dimethyl-2-oxo-cyclopenten-1-yl) acetic acid(88). Analysis of the methanolic extract of the fruits of *Cuminum cyminum* led to the isolation of five terpenic and steroidal constituents, they were characterized as 1,4,5,8-tetrahydroxynaphthyl geranilan-10 -al 1 -oate, lanost 5, 20 (22)-dien-3α-olylndocosanoate, labdan-6α,16,20-triol-16-(10,11 -dihydroxy anthraquinone-2 -oate), stigmast-5-en- 3β-O-D-arabinopyranosyl-2 -benzoate and lanost-5,24-dien-3β-ol 3β-O-D- arabinopyronosyl-2 noctadec-9, 12 -dienoate. The characteristic odour of cumin was attributed to the presence of sminaldehyde, 1, 3-p-menthadien-7al, 1-4-pmenthadien-7-al. 14 free amino acids were also isolated from the seeds. While, flavonoid glycosides isolated from the plant were included apigenin-7-glucoside, luteolin-7-glucoside, luteolin-7-glcuronosyl glucoside, luteolin and apigenin. Total polypheols in cumin were 4.98 ± 0.31. (mg GAE/g DW). Phenols (salicylic acid, gallic acid, cinnamic acid, hydroquinone, resorcinol, P-hydroxybenzoic acid, rutin, coumarine, quercetin) were isolated from seeds of *Cuminum cyminum*. However, *Cuminum cyminum* roots, stems and leaves, and flowers were investigated for their total phenolics, flavonoids, and tannins contents. In all *Cuminum cyminum* organs, total phenolics content ranged from 11.8 to 19.2 mg of gallic acid equivalents per gram of dry weight (mg of GAE/g of DW). Among the polyphenols studied, 13 were identified in roots, 17 in stem and leaves, and 15 in flowers. The major phenolic compound in the roots was quercetin (26%), whereas in the stems and leaves, p-coumaric, rosmarinic, trans-2- dihydrocinnamic acids and resorcinol were predominant. In the flowers, vanillic acid was the main compound (51%). A total of 19 phenolic compounds were successfully identified during the ripening of cumin seeds. Rosmarinic acid was the major phenolic acid for the unripe seeds, while, half ripe and full ripe seeds were dominated by pcoumaric acid. [5-20]

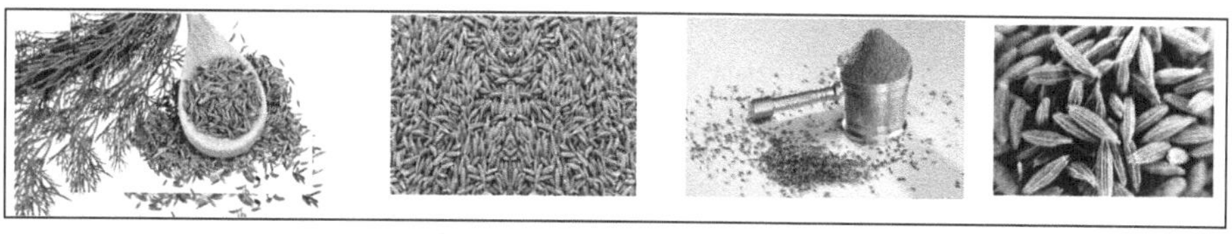

Cumin seeds and powder

Traditional Health Benefits

Cumin is extremely good for digestive problems. The very aroma, which comes from an organic compound called Cuminaldehyde, the main component of its essential oil, activates the salivary glands in our mouth, which facilitates the primary digestion of food. Next is thymol, a compound present in cumin, which stimulates the glands that secrete acids, bile, and enzymes responsible for complete digestion of the food in stomach and intestines. Cumin is also carminative, which means that it relieves you from gas troubles, and thereby, improves digestion and appetite. Due to its essential oils, magnesium, and sodium content, cumin promotes digestion and also gives relief from stomach-aches when taken with hot water. The main cause behind piles (hemorrhoids) is constipation added with infections in the wound in the anal tract, which is also caused by constipation. Cumin because of its dietary fiber content, and carminative, stimulating, antifungal and antimicrobial properties, acts as a natural laxative in powdered form. These characteristics are due to the presence of essential oils comprised mainly of cuminaldehyde and certain pyrazines. [4-6] It is important to note that it is capable to clear up all of the symptoms and causes of hemorrhoids. Although research is still ongoing, early studies report that cumin, among a number of other spices, can have a powerful effect in preventing diabetes by reducing the chances of hypoglycemia. The animals that were tested showed a sharp decline in hypoglycemia when fed cumin seeds in their diet. They also showed a decrease in glucosuria, which is a condition where the urine contains too much glucose, also resulting in hypoglycemia and diabetes. Some of the components of cumin essential oil are hypnotic in nature and have tranquilizing effects, which also help to relieve stress and anxiety that commonly cause insomnia. The presence of caffeine (the stimulating agent), and the richly aromatic essential oils (the disinfectants) make cumin an ideal anti-congestive combination for those suffering from respiratory disorders such as asthma and bronchitis. It acts as an expectorant, meaning that it loosens up the accumulated phlegm and mucus in the respiratory tracts, and makes it easier to eliminate those from the system via sneezing or coughing up and spitting. The common cold is a viral infection which affects our body frequently when our immune system becomes weakened. Again, the essential oils present in cumin act as disinfectants and help fight viral infections which can cause the common cold. Cumin also suppresses the development of coughing in the respiratory system since it dries up the excess mucus. Cumin is rich in iron and has a considerable amount of vitamin C, which is essential for a healthy immune system and keeps infections from forming or becoming worse.Cumin is rich in iron and thus very good for lactating mothers or pregnant women, as well as for women who are undergoing menses. Moreover, cumin is said to help ease and increase secretion of milk in lactating women due to the presence of thymol, which tends to increase the secretions from our glands, including milk, which is a secretion from the mammary glands. Also, cumin is more beneficial if taken with honey. Cumin has a remarkable amount of calcium (> 900 mg/100 grams) which accounts for over 90% of our daily requirement of calcium. This calcium is an important constituent of milk and hence cumin is very good for lactating mothers.As stated above, cumin is very rich in iron (> 66 mg/100 grams) which is more than 5x the daily requirement of iron for an adult. [5-7]So, cumin can be a nutritious additive to the daily diet of anemic people. It can help reduce the symptoms of anemia like fatigue, anxiety, cognitive malfunction, and digestive issues. The amount of iron in cumin leads to an increased hemoglobin production and subsequent prevention of anemia, but the increased blood flow has other benefits as well. When your blood circulation is at its best, adequate amounts of oxygen are able to reach the organs and the brain, leading to an optimal performance of those bodily systems. The Proper amount of oxygen and iron in the brain lead to increased cognitive performance and a decrease in cognitive disorders like Alzheimer's disease and dementia. Almost everyone knows that vitamin-E is good for the maintenance of skin and the prevention of premature aging symptoms. It keeps the skin young and glowing. This vitamin is also present in abundance in cumin. The essential oils present in cumin have disinfectant and antifungal properties. This prevents any microbial and fungal infection from affecting the skin. Not all skin issues are disorders or infections, some of them are simply signs of aging. Vitamin E acts as an antioxidant in this regard and combats the free radicals that attack the skin and result in signs of premature aging like wrinkles, age spots, and sagging skin. This, combined with the antibacterial capacity of cumin, makes for healthy, beautiful skin that lasts far into your old age.Boils are outlets for the removal of toxic substances and foreign matters such as microbes from the body. This means that they are the symptoms which show that a high amount of toxic substances have accumulated in the body. Those who regularly use cumin in food have a significant reduction in the occurrence of boils, rashes, pimples, and other signs of excess toxin content. Components such as cuminaldehyde, thymol, and phosphorus are good detoxifying agents which help in the regular removal of toxins from the body. The healthy way of removing toxins is through the excretory system, not through boils.As discussed above, an abundance of iron, the presence of essential oils, vitamin C, and vitamin A in cumin boosts our immune system in a number of ways. Vitamin C is one of the most powerful antioxidants that we have in our body, and it stimulates the function and activity of white blood cells. [8-11]As an antioxidant, vitamin C fights the detrimental effects of free radicals, which are the dangerous byproducts of cellular metabolism. They are constantly being created in the body, and therefore, must be eliminated. Antioxidants neutralize free radicals that lead to many diseases, including, but not limited to, cardiovascular diseases and cancer. Cumin itself has detoxifying and chemo-preventive properties, and accelerates the secretion of detoxifying and anti-carcinogenic enzymes from the glands, as it also does to other secretions. Furthermore, it has beneficial antioxidants like vitamin C and vitamin A within its chemical makeup, in addition to those essential oils. Besides having countless other benefits, the antioxidants have anti-carcinogenic properties too, and those found in cumin are particularly good for colon cancer prevention. [12-20]

Culinary Uses

Spices play an important role in making a dish more flavorful. Indian cuisine is especially known to have some of the healthiest traditional spices as its main ingredients. Cumin is one such spice that forms an integral part of various dishes in the Indian cuisine.Cumin is traditionally used as a spice in Indian cooking, either as whole seeds or in powdered form. It is a major component in a curry's preparation and other food products. Derived from cumin seeds, this oil is used as a scent in cosmetics including creams, perfumes, and lotions. It is used to add flavor to alcoholic beverages and desserts. Cumin seeds are used to make medicines that help in treating problems like diarrhea, colic, inflammation, bowel and muscle spasms and gas. When ground cumin is mixed with honey and pepper, it works as an aphrodisiac.

Discussion and Conclusion

Besides its culinary uses, this aromatic spice is known for its medicinal properties since ancient times. Being an excellent source of iron, it aids in digestion, boosts the immune system and has anti-carcinogenic properties. Black cumin seeds contain about 100 chemical compounds including vitamins, proteins, carbohydrates, minerals and fatty acids. They are known for their healing qualities. Thus, this spice has a rich history and was particularly favored by the ancient Egyptians, Greeks and Romans. Regular usage of cumin in your food helps in keeping your skin free from boils, rashes, pimples etc. This is because it has components such as Cuminaldehyde, Thymol and phosphorus which are good detoxifying agents. Cumin has a high content of vitamin E which keeps your skin healthy and glowing. Besides, the essential oils, cumin have disinfectant and anti-fungal properties which protect your skin from fungal and microbial infections. Cumin is also a good source of dietary fiber which helps in the cleaning process and removes toxins. Vitamin E present in cumin triggers the anti-ageing processes within the body, thus preventing premature ageing symptoms. It acts as an antioxidant to combat the free radicals that attack the skin and cause signs of ageing like wrinkles, age spots and sagging skin. Oil extract from cumin is a great stimulant, carminative, antioxidant and diuretic. It is often used for massage in aromatherapy and scalp treatments to get rid of dandruff. Cumin helps to lower blood sugar levels and thus helps in maintaining proper blood content levels in the body. This is a great boon for people suffering from Diabetes. Cumin seeds are very rich in iron, which makes it an essential natural health ingredient. Cumin seeds contain Thymoquinone, which reduces inflammatory processes and other mediators that cause asthma. They also act as a bronchodilator. This is achieved by its anti-oxidant characteristics that fight against impurities and free radicals. This helps in making the body's immunity better in combating diseases. Cumin seeds are rich in iron which is necessary for the formation of haemoglobin in the blood. This in turn is required for the transportation of oxygen in the body. Consuming cumin seeds will keep one protected from anaemia. Cumin is healthy for women of all age groups and is known to influence a healthy menstrual cycle. Cumin is helpful in treating colon and breast cancer. The seeds contain thymoquinone, dithymoquinone, thymohydroquinone and thymol which are anti-carcinogenic agents. Cumin is rich in Vitamin C and has anti-fungal properties. These help to cure cold and other respiratory problems. Cumin seeds are also suggested for kidney health. Good metabolism process helps to keep all the other body processes in check. Iron present in cumin helps to properly maintain our metabolic activity.Enzymes present in cumin help to breakdown foods and thus aid in digestion. In traditional medicine, cumin was used to treat hoarseness, jaundice, dyspepsia and diarrhoea. Its seeds were used for stomachic, diuretic, carminative, stimulant, astringent and abortifacient properties. The oil of cumin was used in perfumery and as a seasoning in curry powders, soups, stews, sausages, cheeses, pickles, meats and chutneys. In America, Africa and India the drug is used as an abortive and as an emmenagogue. In Indonesia, it was used in cases of bloody diarrhea and headache (paste is applied to the forehead). It was also taken orally for rheumatic ailments. In India, cumin was used as an abortifacient, for kidney and bladder stones, chronic diarrhea, leprosy and eye disease. In Unani system of medicine, the fruits of *Cuminum cyminum* were used as an astringent, carminative, emmenagogue, for the treatment of corneal opacities, ulcers, boils, styes and to relieve cough and inflammation. Phytochemical analysis showed that *Cuminum cyminum* contained: alkaloid, coumarin, anthraquinone, flavonoid, glycoside, protein, resin, saponin, tannin and steroid. The previous pharmacological studies revealed that *Cuminum cyminum* exerted antimicrobial, insecticidal, anti-inflammatory, analgesic, antioxidant, anticancer, antidiabetic, antiplatelet aggregation, hypotensive, bronchodilatory, immunological, contraceptive, anti-amyloidogenic, anti-osteoporotic, aldose reductase, alpha-glucosidase and tyrosinase inhibitory effects, protective and central nervous effects. This review highlights the chemical constituents and pharmacological effects of Cuminum cyminum.

REFERENCES

1. Nasim R, Lahooti M, Roodbari S, Aein A, Ganjali A. The Effect of Salinity Stress on Germination and Seedling Growth of Cumin (Cuminum Cyminum L.). J Agri Food Technol. 2011; 5 (3): 1-4.
2. Esmaei E; Habashi AA, Ghareyazie B, Ghannadha M, Mohammadie M.A Rapid and Efficient method for Regeneration of Plantlets from Embryo Explants of Cumin (*Cuminum cyminum*). Plant Cell, Tissue and Organ Culture. Netherlands: Kluwer Academic Publishers. 2003; 75: 19-25.
3. Bettaieb I, Bourgou, S, Sriti, J, Msaada K, Limam F, Marzouk B. "Essential Oils and Fatty Acids Composition of Tunisian and Indian Cumin (*Cuminum cyminum* L.) Seeds: A Comparative Study. J Sci Food Agri. 2011; 91 (11): 2100-2107. doi:10.1002/jsfa.4513

Hindi, Kariveppilai in Tamil, Karivepaaku in Tamil or Karivempu in Malayalam. Derived from the Tamil word "Kari" meaning spicy, leaves are mentioned in ancient Tamil scriptures dating back to the 4th century AD for its amazing benefits and culinary significance. *Murraya koenigii*is an unarmed, semi deciduous aromatic shrub or small tree with slender but strong woody stem and branches covered with dark grey bark, leaves are imparipinnate, glabrous, and very strongly aromatic. Leaflets 9-25 or more, short stalked, alternate, gland dotted and strongly aromatic. The stem of *Murraya koenigii*is an aromatic and more or less deciduous shrub or small tree up to 7 meters in height and 14 to 42 cm in diameter. Kadi Patta should also not be mistaken for the plant, *Helichrysum italicum,* as it is unrelated. The main stem is dark green to brownish [1-4]. The bark of the stem can be peeled off longitudinally which exposes the white wood underneath. Flowers are small, white fragrant ebracteate, calyx deeply five cleft, pubescent. Petals five, free, whitish, glabrous and with dotted glands. Fruits occur in close clusters, small ovoid or subglobose, glandular, thin pericarp enclosing one or two seeds having spinach green color. The aromatic leaves are seen in the form of pairs on the branches of the tree. The plant produces small white flowers which can pollinate themselves and it produces small, black, shiny semi-globose fruits with a single large seed. Though the fruits are fleshy and edible, neither the flower nor the fruits are used for culinary purposes [5-6].

Murraya koenigii Spreng belongs to the family of Rutaceae. The plant is distributed and cultivated throughout India. It is found wild from Himalaya's, Uttarakhand, Sikkim to Garhwal, Bengal, Assam, Western Ghats and Travancore - Cochin. Propagation is done by seeds, which germinate freely under partial shade. It is also available in other part of Asian region like in moist forests of 500-1600 m height in Guangdong, S Hainan, S Yunnan (Xishuangbanna), Bhutan, Laos, Nepal, Pakistan, Sri Lanka, Thailand, Vietnamurraya Together with South Indian immigrants, leaves reached Malaysia, South Africa and Réunionisl and outside the Indian sphere of influence, they are rarely found. A scrutiny of literature reveals some notable pharmacological activities of the plant. Carbazole alkaloids which are abundantly present in the leaves, fruits, roots and bark of this plant, have been reported for their antidiabetic, anticancer, antibacterial, anti-nociceptive and antioxidant activities. Besides these activities, the plant is described to have a wide array of therapeutic activities [7-9]. There are three different morphotypes of *Murraya koenigii* possessing different intensity in its flavor. The regular type of *Murraya koenigii* is the fastest growing plant with good looking leaves and with dark green in color. The dwarf type grows as shrub and branches are spread and appears like bushy and the leaves are in light green in color with little taller like regular type and poses its own aroma. The brown type is the most fragrant one, with thick and smallest leaf structure and in dark brown in color. Previous study has been done widely on leave from its stem up to its bark and, thus this review gathers variety of idea from multifarious research which has been done on leave and provides a better cognizance of its therapeutic and non-therapeutic properties. The phytoconstituents isolated so far from the leaves are alkaloids viz., mahanine, koenine, koenigine, koenidine14, girinimbiol, girinimibine, koenimbine, O-methyl murrayamine A, Omethylmahanine, isomahanine, bismahanine, bispyrayafoline16 and other phytoconstituents such as coumaringlycoside viz., scopotin, murrayanine, calcium, phosphorus, iron, thiamine, riboflavin, niacin, vitamin C, carotene and oxalic acid. The essential oil from leaves yielded di-alpha phellandrene, D-sabinene, D-pinene, dipentene, D-terpinol and caryophyllene. It is reported to possess antioxidant, antibacterial, antifungal, larvicidal, anticarcinogenic, hypoglycemic, anti-lipid peroxidative, hypolipidemic, antihypertensive activity. It is also reported to contain 5, 8-dimethylfuranocoumarin, 1- al, 3 [6′, 6′ dimethyl 5-hexene] carbazole and sitosterol [10-14]. Fresh leaves, dried leaf powder, and essential oil are widely used for flavoring soups, curries, fish and meat dishes, eggs dishes, traditional powder blends, seasoning and ready to use other food preparations. The essential oil is also utilized by soap and cosmetic aromatherapy industry. Leaves are boiled with coconut oil till they are reduced to blanked residue which is then used as an excellent hair tonic for retaining natural hair tone and stimulating hair growth. It is traditionally used as a whole or in parts as antiemetics, antidiarrheal, febrifuge, blood purifier, antifungal, depressant, anti-inflammatory, body aches, for kidney pain and vomiting.

Pharmacological Studies

Antibacterial activity-the essential oil from *Murraya koenigii* leaves showed antibacterial effect against *B. subtilis, S.aureus, C. pyogenes, P. vulgaris* and *Pasteurella multocida*. The aim of this review study is to update information about pharmacognostical, Phytochemical and pharmacological studies of *Murraya koenigii*. To evaluate the versatile multi-potential medicinal use of *Murraya koenigii*. Phytochemistry and pharmacology of this plant necessitates a comprehensive review of its prospects as an important therapeutic agent for the management of numerous diseases commonly affecting humans [15-18].

Customary and Contemporary uses

Leaves being popular for their various antioxidant properties and the ability to control diarrhea and several gastrointestinal problems satisfy the current trend to look out for an alternative such as herbal medicines. Barring this they have cancer fighting traits. Several systematic scientific studies are also being conducted regarding the efficacy of whole plant or its parts in different extract forms for the treatment of different diseases. *Murraya koenigii* contains a number of chemical constituents that interact in a complex way to elicit their pharmacodynamic response. A number of active constituents responsible for the medicinal properties have been isolated and characterized. This plant has been reported to have anti-oxidative, cytotoxic, antimicrobial, antibacterial, antiulcer, positive inotropic and cholesterol reducing activities [19-24]. Therefore the present review summarizes the available literature till date on isolation of phytoconstituents, biological activities of the isolated compounds and pharmacological actions of extracts along with the clinical studies. In traditional system of Medicine, it is used as antiemetic, antidiarrheal, dysentery, febrifuge, blood purifier, tonic, stomachic, flavoring agent in curries and chutneys. The oil is used externally for bruises, eruption, in soap and perfume industry. The barks and roots are used externally to cure the bites of the poisonous animals; the green leaves were eaten raw as a cure for dysentery, diarrhea [25-28]. Infusion of roasted leaves were given in order to stop emesis. Furthermore, patta has also have been a used as blood purifier, tonic and cure for stomachache and used as flavoring agents in curries and chutneys. Leaves were also used as calcium source to those having calcium deficiency besides that it also consist Vitamin A, Vitamin B and B_2, Vitamin C and iron. For the treatment of morning sickness, fresh juice of leaves together with lime juice and sugar is given and it is also applicable for vomiting due to indigestion. In the case of stomach upsets, the leaves is grounded to a fine paste and mixed with buttermilk and consumed orally. A paste of leaves is applied on the boils for swift relief, besides that, renal pain can be cured by consuming the root as a juice. The fresh juice of leaves can prevent the progression of cataract. *Murraya koenigii* will retain the black color of the hair or in other words, it will prevent the premature greying of the hair. Karipatta is a valuable plant for its characteristic aroma and medicinal value. *Murraya koenigii* is widely used in Indian cookery from centuries and have a versatile role to play in traditional medicine. The plant is credited with tonic and stomachic properties. Green leaves are eaten raw for cure of dysentery, diarrhoea and vomiting. Leaves and roots are also used traditionally as bitter, anthelmintic, analgesic, curing piles, inflammation, itching and are useful in leucoderma and blood disorders. Packed with a multitude of nutrients like carbohydrate, fiber, calcium, phosphorous, iron, magnesium, zinc, multivitamins and flavonoids, leaves are an arcade of health benefits [29-30]. It is extensively used in the treatment of anemia, diabetes, indigestion, obesity, kidney problems, hair and skin problems. Leaves are an excellent source of fiber. It improves our digestive health and regular bowel movements. It is helpful in treating diarrhea and nausea and also controls the blood glucose levels in the body. Leaves have a high concentration of proteins which are considered to be the building blocks of the body. It is pivotal for the proper growth and development of the body and strengthens our immune system. Calcium is widely known for its significance in improving bone health. Being a powerhouse of calcium, leaves are effective for strengthening the teeth and bones and preventing diseases like osteoporosis and osteomalacia. Being one of the major nutrients in leaves, phosphorus helps in cleansing the kidneys. It maintains a normal heartbeat, reduces painful muscle spasm after exercise and also strengthens the teeth and bones. At the cellular level, phosphorus is used for the growth and repair of cells and tissues.Apart from the minerals and vitamins, leaves are a powerhouse to a number of volatile essential oils like α-pinene, sabinene, β-pinene, α-terpinene etc. These essential oils possess anti-inflammatory, anti-bacterial, anti-diabetic, anti-dysenteric, carminative and digestive properties which are extremely beneficial for the hair, skin and oral health. It is also effective against hyperglycemia, high cholesterol and aids in digestion. The hypoglycemic property of the leaves plays a significant role in alleviating the blood sugar level of the body. The production of insulin from the pancreatic β-cells becomes active on the consumption of leaves [31-33]. It helps in reducing the breakdown of starch into glucose which in turn leads to low blood glucose levels. The deficiency of iron in the body causes anemia. Leaves having a high concentration of iron, is extremely effective in increasing the hemoglobin and red blood cell count of the blood. It acts as a natural blood purifier, improves symptoms of tiredness and fatigue and reduce the chances of getting infections. Leaves being abundant in Vitamin A and β-carotene, play a vital role in improving eyesight and treating eye-related problems. It prevents the cornea from drying up and cloud formation in front of the eyes, thus reducing the chances of Xeropthalmia and night blindness. The leaves have potent anti-bacterial, anti-fungal, anti-inflammatory and antioxidant properties. So, regular consumption of leaves shields our body against various infections and germs. Leaves are considered a boon by people under a weight loss management program. The presence of carbazole alkaloids in the leaves prevents weight gain and reduces the LDL cholesterol (i.e. bad cholesterol) in the blood. It washes out the harmful toxins from the body and burns excess fat. The high content of fiber in the leaves has proven to be beneficial in treating several gastrointestinal troubles. The carminative, digestive, antiemetic and anti-dysenteric properties of leave not only aid in digestion but also prevent constipation, diarrhea, dysentery, piles, nausea, bloating etc. Being a natural stimulant, it enhances the appetite. Recent researches suggest that the presence of phenols and carbazole alkaloids are extremely effective in treating and preventing prostate and colorectal cancers. Leaves have anti-bacterial and anti-microbial properties that are extremely effective in maintaining good oral health [34-37]. The essential oils present in the leaves strengthen the gum and teeth, removes bad odor and protects the teeth and gum from any foreign microbes and infections. Although the humble leaves have a wealth of healthful nutrients including protein, fiber, calcium, vitamins and minerals, and spectacular properties, quite often we tend to throw it away. Here are a few more reasons, why it should probably be a part of the daily dietary regimen and should be consumed alongside the food prepared using it. The abundance of high amounts of an alkaloid called mahanimbinein leaves makes it extremely beneficial for the heart and plays a pivotal role in treating a host of heart ailments. It relaxes the cardiac system, by calming the mind, which is beneficial for patients suffering from arrhythmias and palpitations. Regular intake of leaves imparts heart-healthy properties by strengthening the heart muscles, lowering cholesterol levels in the blood and preventing lipid build-up, which in turn reduces the risk of atherosclerosis, heart attacks, heart blocks, blood clots, etc. Since long back these mighty leaves offer a traditional remedy to increase the functioning of the brain [38-40]. The presence of bioactive components prevents the breakdown of brain chemicals including glutathione reductase (GRD), glutathione peroxidase (GPx), and superoxide dismutase (SOD) that are needed for enhancing the memory. Hence, it helps improve memory capacity, focus, concentration, calmness, alertness of an individual. Being a potent brain tonic and stimulator, people including leaves in their daily diet or consuming other formulations have improved memory, reasoning, problem-solving, and other cognitive abilities and are thus used for treating Alzheimer's and other psychotic conditions like dementia. Imbued with potent anti-bacterial and expectorant properties, leaves are highly significant for quite a few respiratory problems. It helps clear mucus and rheum deposits from the nasal passage and provides relief from chest congestion. The soothing nature of this leaf plays a quintessential role in treating dry, irritated throat. It also serves as a potent remedy for sinus, headache, asthma, bronchitis and pharyngitis [41-43].

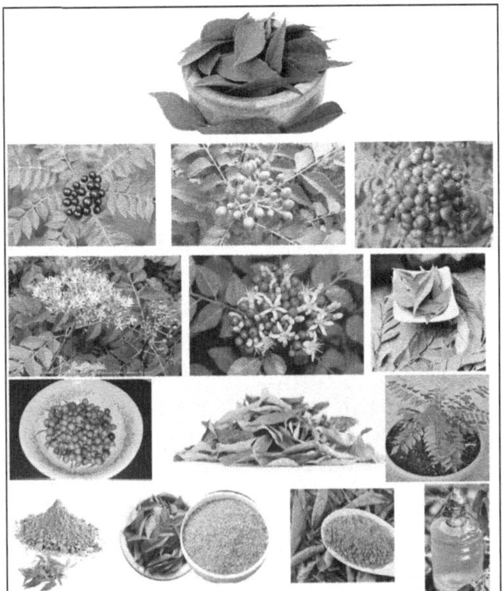

Patta tree, green leaves, dried leaves, inflorescence, fruits and seeds pattapoder, Churn and oil

Chemical constituent (occurring in stem, fruits, leaves, roots & seeds) and Phytopharmacotherapeutics

The fresh leaves of *Murraya koenigii* contain 61.77-66.2% of moisture, 2.1-12.5% of protein, 14.6-18.97% of total sugar, 9.7-13.06% of total ash, 1.35-1.82% of acid insoluble ash, 1.35-1.82% of alcohol soluble extractive and water extractive value ranges between 27.33-33.45%. Solvents used in preparation of the extract are ethyl acetate, ethanol, petroleum ether, water and chloroform and compounds such as alkaloids, flavonoids and sterols have been extracted. In leaves by acetone extract, Koenigine, koenine, koenidine and (-) mahanine were isolated. Form the hexane mahanimbine, isomahanimbine, koenimbidine and murrayacine where isolated. Isomahanimbicine was isolated in the petroleum ether. Seed of *Murraya koenigii* consist of furocoumarin lactone, carbazole alkaloids, glycolipids, Phospholipids and terpinene. It also contains 4.4% of total lipids in which 85.4 % are neutral lipids, 5.1% are glycolipids and 9.5% are phospholipids. 73.9% triacylglycerol, 10.2% free fatty acids and small amounts of diacylglycerols, monoacylglycerols and sterols which are present in neutral lipids. The seeds of *Murraya koenigii*contain terpinene these are as follow terpinene, terpinen-4-ol, linolol, ocimene, limblee, limbolee and simbolee [44-46]. The fruit contain pulp which is having 64.9% of moisture, 16.8% of total soluble solids,[48] 9.76% of total sugar,[54] 9.58% of reducing sugar,0.17% of non-reducing sugar, 13.35% of vitamin C,[56] 2.162% of total ash, 1.97% of protein, 0.082% of phosphorus, 0.811% of potassium (32,2), 0.166% of calcium, 0.216% of magnesium, 0.007% of iron and 0.00057% of tannin. The chemical constituent of matured stem and bark of *Murraya koenigii* are carbazole alkaloids, coumaringalactoside, Carbazole carboxylic acid, glycolipids, Phospholipids etc.The roots of *Murraya koenigii* include many types of bioactive compounds. The extraction of root was done in benzene and petroleum ether [45-55].

Chemical Composition	Structure	Nature	Extracted From
(1)	(2)	(3)	(4)
α-Copaene	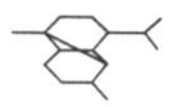	Sesquiterpenoid	Leaves
α-Pinene	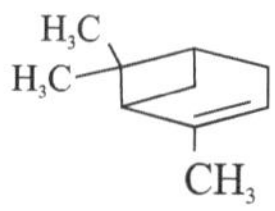	Turpentine	Leaves
α-Humulene	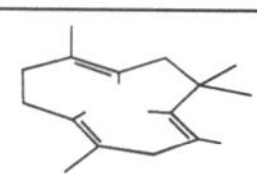	Sesquiterpene	Leaves
Aromadendrene	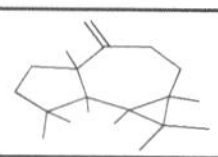	Sesquiterpene	Leaves

(Contd...)

(1)	(2)	(3)	(4)
α-Selinene		Monoterpenoid	Leaves. Stems
β- Elemene		Sesquiterpene	Leaves. Stem
Bismurrayafoline E		Carbazole Alkaloid	Leaves, Stems
Bispyrafoline	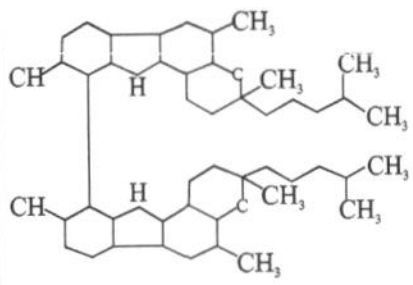	Carbazole Alkaloid	Leaves, Stems
β-Myrcene		Olefinic Natural Organic Hydrocarbon	Leaves, Stems
Bornyl Acetate		Terpene	Leaves, Stems, Roots
Bicyclomahanimbicine		Terpenoid Alkaloids	Leaves, Stems
β-Bisabolene		Sesquiterpene	Leaves
β-Pinene		Terpene	Leaves
β-Caryophyllene	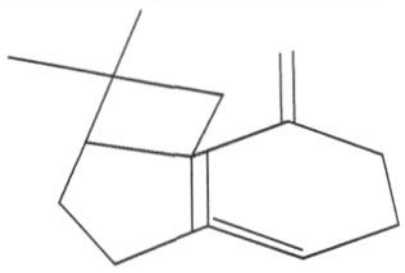	Sesquiterpene	Leaves, Seeds
β-Costol	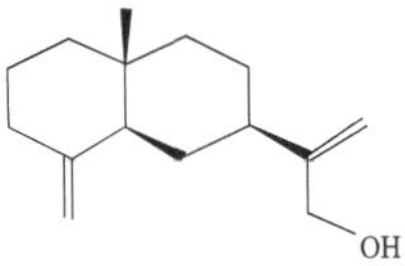		Alcohols
β-Eduesmol	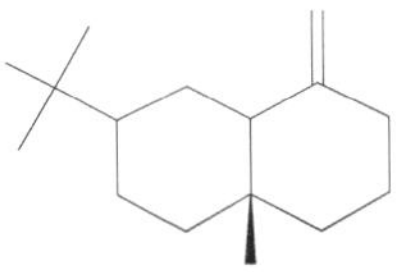	Alcohols	Leaves
β-Phellandrene		Cyclic Monoterpenes	Leaves
Bikoeniquinone		Indole Alkaloid	Roots
Bicyclomahanimbine		Alkaloids	Leaves, Stems, Roots
Butanedioic Acid		Dicarboxylic Acid	Leaves, Stems
Butyl Myristate		Esters	Leaves, Stems
β-Selinene		Sesquiterpenes	Leaves, Stems
Bismahanine	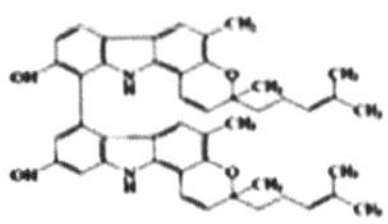	Indole Alkaloid	Leaves, Stems
Bis-3-Hydroxy-3-Methyl Carbazole		Indole Alkaloid	Roots

(Contd...)

(1)	(2)	(3)	(4)
β-Terpineol		Alcohols	Leaves
β- Cadina		Oleoresin	Leaves
Carotene		Terpene	Leaves
Camphene	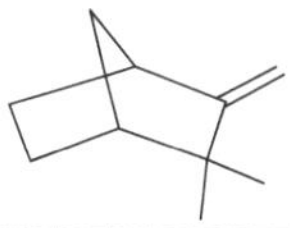	Bicyclic Monoterpene	Leaves
Cis-2-Cyclohexen-1-Ol	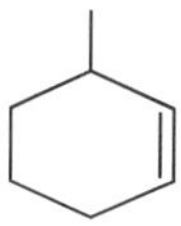	Monoterpenoid Alcohol	Leaves
Chrysanthenyl Acetate	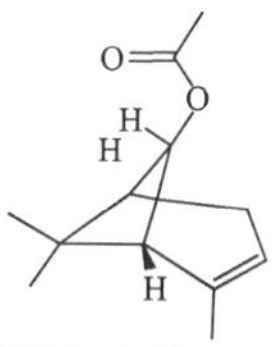	Monoterpene	Leaves, Stem
Cycloheptane	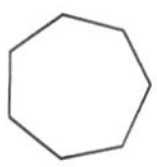	Cycloalkane	Leaves
Citral	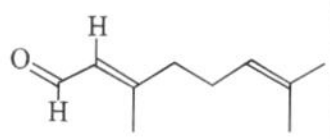	Monoterpenoidal Aldehyde	Leaves, Stems
3-Carene	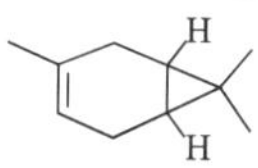	Bicyclic Monoterpene	Leaves, Stems
Cadinene	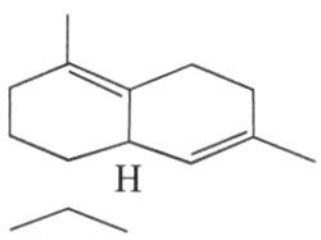	Sesquiterpene	Leaves
Cyclomahanimbine	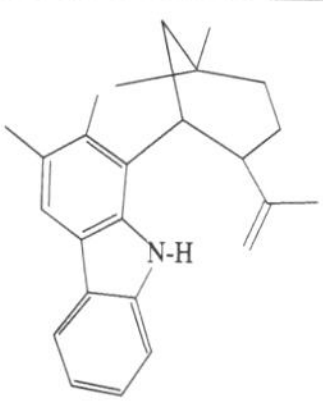	Indole Alkaloid	Leaves
anine	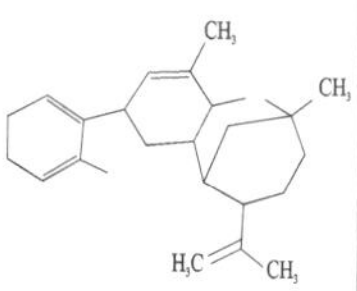	Indole Alkaloid	Stems

(Contd...)

(1)	(2)	(3)	(4)
Δ-Cadinene	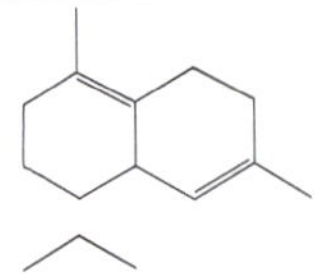	Sesquiterpene	Leaves
Cis-Caryophyllene	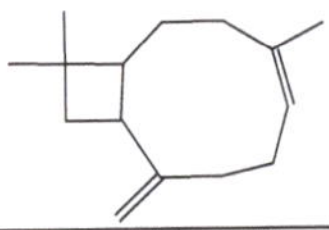	Sesquiterpense	Leaves
CarvoMenthone	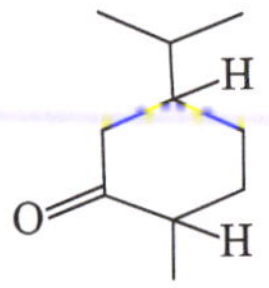	Ketone	Leaves
Cubenol	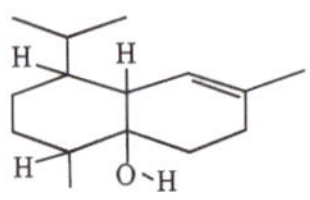	Sesquiterpenes	Leaves, Stems
4-Diene	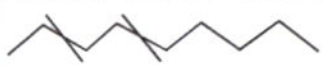	Diolefin	Leaves, Stems
Dipentene	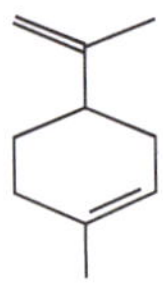	Monoterpene	Leaves
6,7-Dimethoxy 1-Hydroxy Carbazole	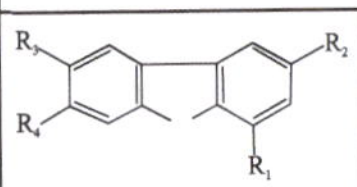	Carbazole Alkaloids	Leaves, Stems, Roots
Dehydro Aromadendrene	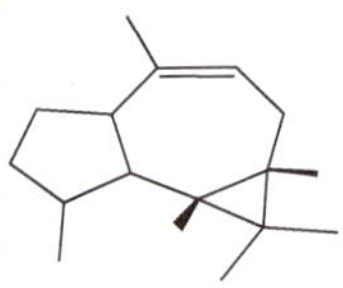	Sesquiterpense	Leaves, Stems, Roots
Euchrestine	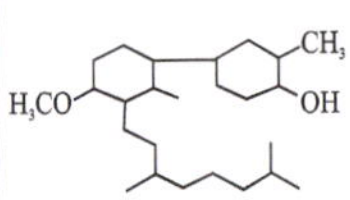	Protein	Leaves
Eustifoline-D	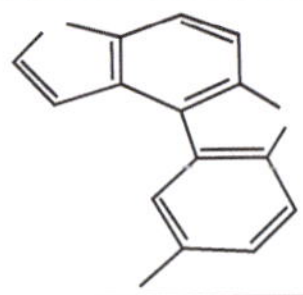	Indole Alkaloid	Roots
Formlycarbozole	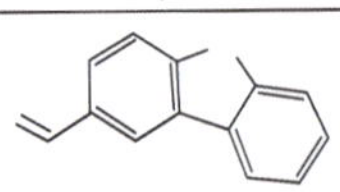	Indole Alkaloid	Roots

(Contd…)

(1)	(2)	(3)	(4)
Frnesols	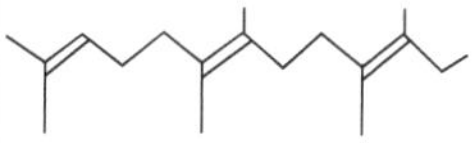	Alcohols	Leaves
Girinimbine	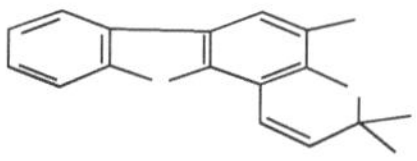	Indole Alkaloid	Leaves, Stems, Roots, Fruits, Seeds
Glycozoline	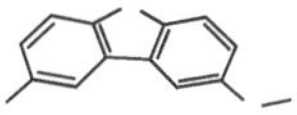	Carbazole Alkaloids	Stems
Gurjunene	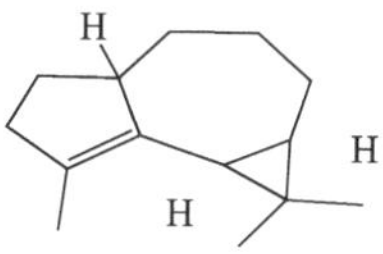	Carbotricyclic Sesquiterpene	Leaves
Girinimbilol	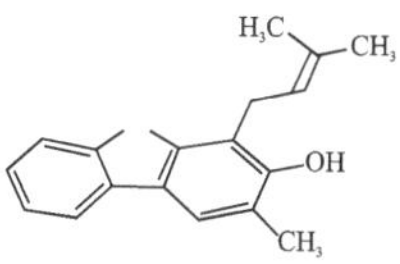	Indole Alkaloid	Leaves, Stems, Roots
Heraclenin	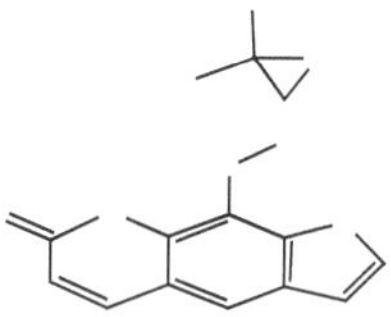	Coumarin	Leaves
1-Hydroxy-3-Methyl Carbazole	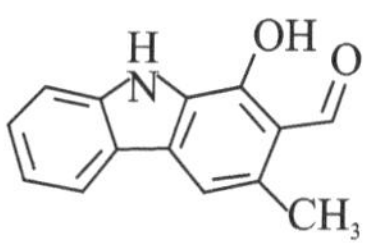	Indole Alkaloid	Stems
Isomahanine	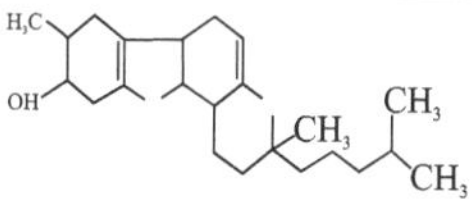	Pyranocarbazole Alkaloids	Leaves
Isomurrayazoline		Carbazole Alkaloid	Leaves, Stems
Isomurrayazolinine		Carbazole Alkaloid	Leaves, Stems
IsoCaryophyllene		Sesquiterpense	Leaves, Stems
Isogirinimbine		Carbazole Alkaloids	Leaves, Stems
Imperatorin		Furocoumarin	Leaves
IsoMenthone	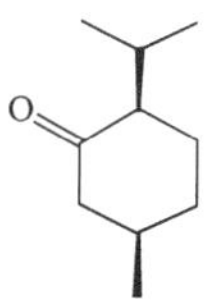	Ketone	Leaves, Stems, Roots

(Contd...)

(1)	(2)	(3)	(4)
Isomahanimbine (+)	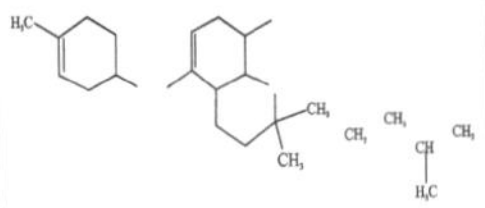	Indole Alkaloid	Leaves, Fruit
Juniper Camphor	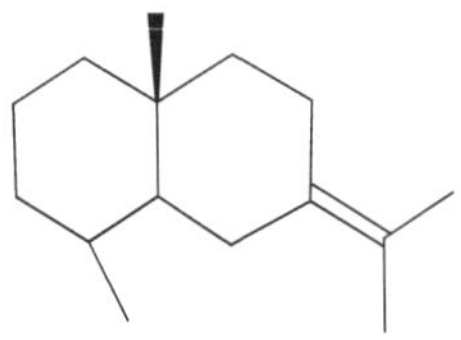	Terpenoid	Leaves
Junipene	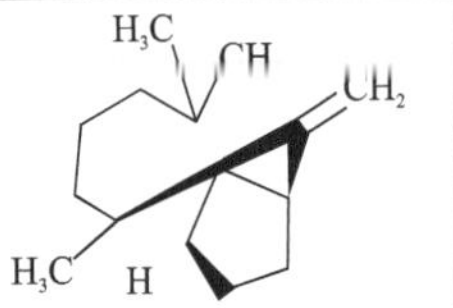	Sesquiterpense	Leaves
Koenimbine	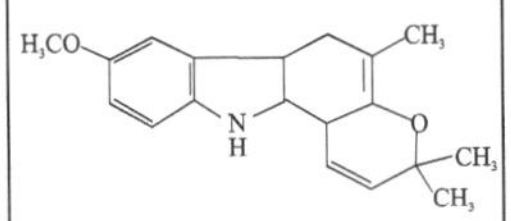	Indole Alkaloid	Leaves, Fruits
Koenoline		Carbazole Alkaloid	Leaves, Seeds
Kurryam		Carbazole Alkaloid	Leaves
Koenimbidine	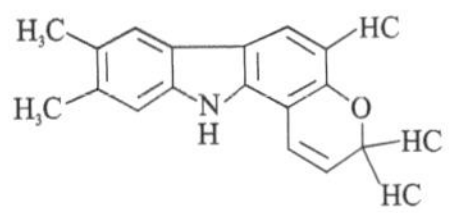	Carbazole Alkaloid	Leaves, Stems
Koenigicine		Carbazole Alkaloid	Leaves, Stems
Koenigine		Indole Alkaloid	Leaves
Koenine		Indole Alkaloid	Leaves
Linalool		Terpene Alcohol	Leaves, Stems, Roots
Lutein	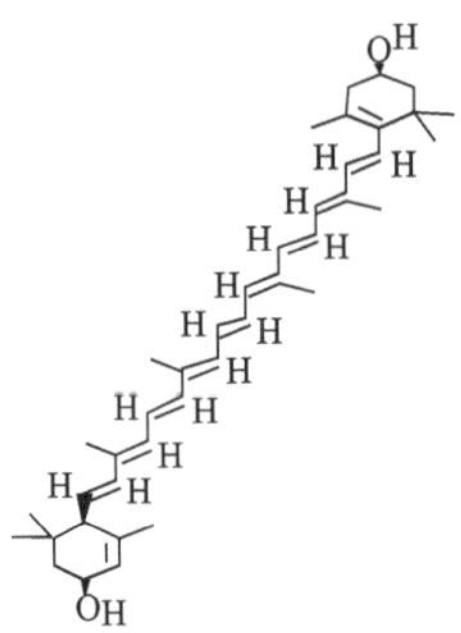	Xanthophyll	Leaves

(Contd...)

(1)	(2)	(3)	(4)
Linalyl Acetate		Acetate Ester	Leaves, Stems
Limonene		Cyclic Terpene	Leaves, Stems
Lavandulyl Acetate		Acetate Ester	Leaves, Stems
Mahanimbinine		Terpenoid Alkaloid	Leaves, Stems
Murrayamine-J		Carbazole Alkaloid	Leaves, Stems
Marmesin-1′-O-Beta-D Galactopyranoside		Coumarin Galactoside	Stems
Murrayamine-M		Carbazole Alkaloid	Leaves, Stems
Murrayamine-G		Carbazole Alkaloid	Leaves, Stems
Murrayazolidine		Pentacyclic Carbazole Alkaloid	Leaves, Stems
Murrayacine		Pyrano-Carbazole Alkaloid	Leaves, Stems
Murrayacinine	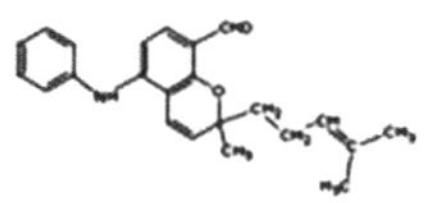	Carbazole Alkaloid	Leaves, Stems
Mahanimboline	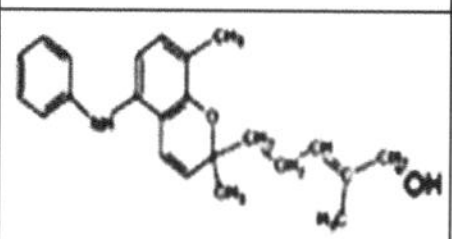	Carbazole Alkaloid	Leaves, Stems
Mukoeic Acid		Carbazole Carboxylic Acid	Leaves, Stems
Mukonine		Carbazole Alkaloid	Leaves, Stems, Roots
3-Methyl Carbazole		Carbazole Alkaloids	Leaves, Stems, Roots
Mahanimbicine		Alkaloids	Leaves, Stems
Mukonidine	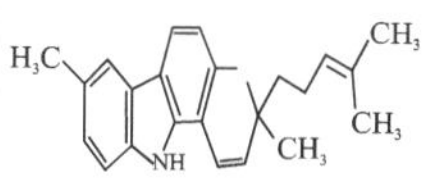	Carbazole Alkaloids	Leaves, Stems
Murrayakoeninol		Alkaloids	Leaves
Mahanimbine		Indole Alkaloid	Roots, Leaves
Mukoline		Carbazole alkaloid	Roots
Murrayanol		Alkaloids	Roots, Leaves, Stems
Murrayazolinine	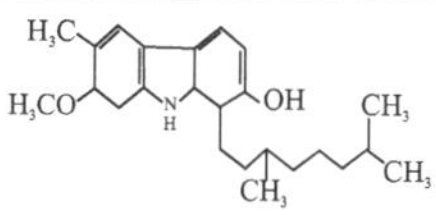	Carbazole Alkaloid	Leaves, Seeds
Murrafoline-I	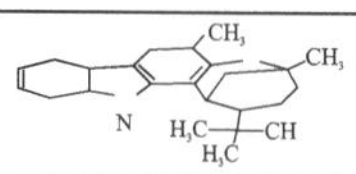	Biscarbazole Alkaloid	Leaves, Stems, Seeds

(Contd...)

(1)	(2)	(3)	(4)
Mukonicine		Carbazole Alkaloid	Fruits, Seeds, Leaves
Murrayacinine		Carbazole Alkaloid	Leaves, Stems
Mukoenine A		Indole Alkaloid	Leaves, Roots
2-Methoxy-3-Methyl		Indole Alkaloid	Leaves, Stems
O-Methyl Murrayanine		Carbazole Alkaloids	Roots, Leaves, Stems
Mukolidine	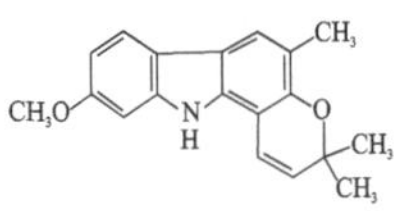	Carbazole Alkaloid	Leaves
Mukonal		Carbazole Alkaloid	Leaves
Murrayazolinol		Carbazole Alkaloid	Leaves
Murrayazoline	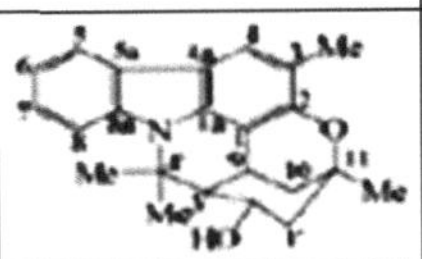	CarbozoleAlkaloid	Leaves
Mahanimbinol	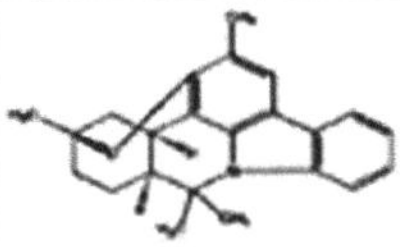	Indole Alkaloid	Stems, Leaves, Roots
Mahanine		Indole Alkaloid	Stems, Leaves, Roots
Murrayanine		CarbazoleAlkaloid	Stems, Leaves
Menthol	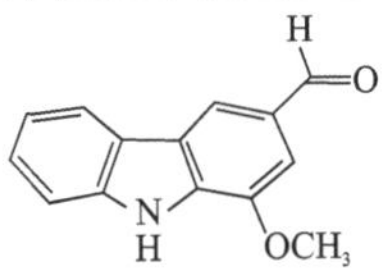	Alcohols	Leaves
Nicotinic Acid	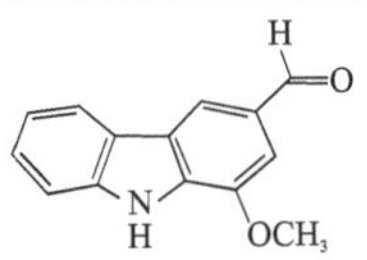	Carboxylic Acid	Stems, Leaves, Roots
2-Naphthalenemethanol	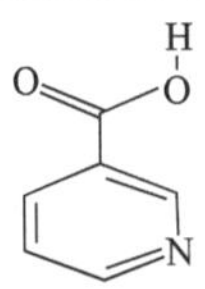	Naphthalenes	Stems, Leaves
Steary Alcohol	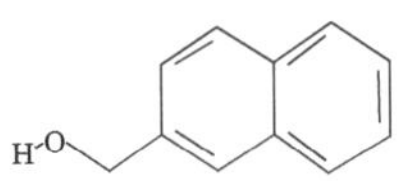	Alcohols	Stems, Leaves, Roots
Stearaldehyde	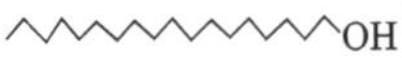	Aldehyde	Stems

(Contd...)

(1)	(2)	(3)	(4)
Sabinene	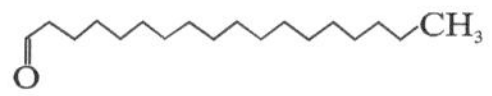	Terpenes	Stems, Leaves
Tocopherol	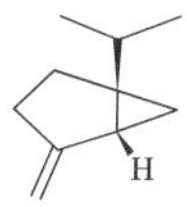	Alcohol	Leaves
α-Terpinene	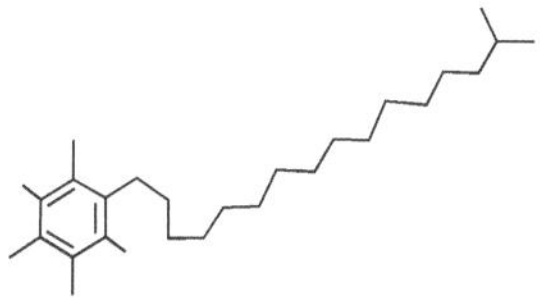	Terpenoids	Leaves, Stems

The leaves having an appearance similar to bay leaves but slightly smaller in size are also termed as Indian bay leaves. The aromatic scent of these leaves is due to the high content of essential volatile oils that get extracted through steam distillation method and this essential oil is used in healing skin disorders. Leaves have a distinct bitter and pungent taste with acidic undertones. The leaves are not only sought after for their aromatic flavor in the foods, but also enhance the health benefits of the meal making it more appealing. The leaves have found its way in many holistic treatments like Ayurveda, Siddha, Unani and traditional Chinese treatments for their medicinal properties in treating diabetes, diarrhea, gastro intestinal disorders etc. The extract from the leaves have an active constituent which is antidiabetic in nature and hence are widely used for the treatment of diabetes. The paste from the dried grounded leaves also have anti-helminthic, anti-fungal and anti-bacterial properties, which are potent against various infections and skin disorders. In the primeval times, the leaf branches have played a significant role in good oral hygiene [56-58]. The thin twigs or branches were used as a datun (i.e. natural brush) for cleaning the teeth, strengthening the teeth and gums and protecting them from harmful bacteria and air borne microbes. These days in modern Ayurvedic treatments the powder of the leaves or the raw leaves is being used as tooth powder for preserving good oral health. Leaves play a pivotal role in the field of weight loss. The leaves when eaten raw or consumed as juice, serves as a detox drink to cleanse body from within, burn fat, reduce bad cholesterol and enhance digestion. Taking leaves regularly is bound to show promising results [59-61].

The fresh leaves or kadipatta are an indispensable part of Indian cuisine and Indian traditional medicines. They are most widely used in southern and west coast Indian cooking, usually fried along with vegetable oil, mustard seeds and chopped onions in the first stage of the preparation. They are also used to make thoran, vada, sambhar, koshimbir, rasam and kadhi. The fresh leaves are valued as seasoning in the cuisines of South and Southeast Asia. In Cambodia, where the leaves are called *sloekkontroap*, the leaves are roasted and used as an ingredient in a soup, *majukrueng*. In Java, the leaves are often stewed to flavour *gulai*. Though available dried, the aroma and flavor is greatly inferior. The oil can be extracted and used to make scented soaps. Sauté leaves in ghee at high heat and then add the ghee and softened leaves to any dish of your liking. Infuse broths with leaves for a fresh flavor. Combine fresh or dried leaves with other spices, such as red chili, turmeric and cumin seeds, to make a flavorful seasoning blend. Top any savory dish with diced or crumbled dried leaves for a pop of flavor. Cook leaves in hot oil and then use the infused oil as a dip or topping for crusty bread. Add leaves to chutneys and sauces or make a leaves churna. [62-64]Toss chopped leaves into savoury baked food recipes like breads and crackers. Leaves pair well with lentils, yoghurt, coconut milk, aromatics such as onions, garlic, and ginger, mustard seeds, chilli peppers, eggplant, pork, and fish. Leaves are edible after they are cooked and do not need to be removed before eating. Kadi Patta add a bright flavor to stews, curries, soups, rice dishes, and dals. The branches of leaves play a significant role in good oral hygiene. The thin twigs or branches are used as a datun. The leaves when eaten raw or consumed as juice, serves as a detox drink to cleanse body from within, burn fat, reduce bad cholesterol and enhance digestion. The chemical constituents present in leaves are carbazole. The leaves are commonly added to dishes to bring about a robust, rich flavour and popularly used in meat dishes, curries, and other traditional Indian recipes. Leaves are used in many holistic treatments like Ayurveda, Siddha, Unani and traditional Chinese treatments for their medicinal properties in treating diabetes, diarrhea, gastrointestinal disorders etc. In Ayurveda, leaves are considered to have anti-diabetic, antioxidant, antimicrobial, anti-inflammatory, anti-carcinogenic, and hepatoprotective. There are different forms of *Murraya koenigii* due to which they are found as the useful plant such as extract, essential oil, or directly used due to the presence of following active constituent bismahanine, murrayanine, murrayafoline-A, bi-koeniquinone-A, bismurrayaquinone, mukoenine-A, mukoenine-B, mukoenine-C, murrastifoline, Murrayazolinol, murrayacine, murrayazolidine, murrayazoline, mahanimbine, girinimbine, koenioline, xynthyletin, koenigine-Quinone A and koenigine-Quinone B for therapeutic purpose by folk people.[64-66]

Benefits of the Hair Oil and Powder

Ayurveda mentions leaves as Giri nimba or Krishna nimba, entitled after Lord Krishna, the God of Protection in several ancient scriptures. The essential oil extracted from the leaves of the leaf tree is widely employed in this traditional holistic healing for the treatment of hair and skin problems, diabetes, eye problem, dental problem, diarrhea etc. The leaves have Tikta (bitter) and Kashaya (astringent) properties. It is blessed with all the trigunas i.e. Laghu (light), Rukhsha (dry) and Tikshna (sharp). It has Ushna Virya (hot potency) and KatuVipaka (pungent metabolic property). It aggravates the Pitta doshas (digestion) and pacifies Vata (air) and Kapha (earth and water) doshas. The richness of antioxidants and nutrients in these leaves work wonders in giving one a lustrous long hair. It treats damaged hair, strengthens the hair roots, prevents hair fall and also treats dandruff. It is also a natural aid for premature greying of hair. The oil acts like a magic potion in giving one a beautiful mane. It rejuvenates hair follicles, stimulates the growth of hair, repairs damaged roots, strengthens the hair, prevents hair fall and premature greying. Since the oil has a pungent smell, addition of an essential oil while applying it to your hair will not only nourishes the hair but also adds a beautiful fragrance to your hair. Leaves being a powerhouse of antioxidants and Vitamin C are extremely beneficial in providing a beautiful healthy skin. It protects the skin from tanning. Boil 30-40 fresh leaves in coconut oil and store for later use. Add few drops of leaf oil to 2-3 drops of jojoba oil and massage your skin regularly, to prevent wrinkles, reduce dark circles and other signs of aging. Addition of few drops of leaf oil to your regular skin care regime can prevent infections associated with pimples, acne and boils. The pure leaf oil having anti-bacterial and anti-inflammatory properties can be used to reduce inflammation and pain from insect bites and bee stings. Add 2 drops of leaf oil in a cup of warm water and gargle to strengthen teeth, prevent teeth and gum infections and acquire a refreshing breath. Massage 2-3 drops of pure leaf oil with few drops of olive oil to reduce swelling and inflammation on various parts of the body and get instant relief. Dry 2-3 bowls of freshly plucked leaves under direct sun. Grind them without water. Sieve the powder to remove any hard particles or impurities and store for later use. Consuming one spoonful of this powder with water daily on empty stomach can cause wonders in naturally treating your diabetes and reducing your blood sugar level. 1 spoon of leaf powder added to the buttermilk can be consumed to get relief from gastro-intestinal troubles. 1 teaspoon of the powder or the decoction of the dry bark consumed with water regularly reduces nausea and vomiting. Powder from the dried roots of the tree is believed to relieve kidney disorders.[56, 59-61, 67-69]

Conclusion

Murraya koenigii was one of the medically beneficial plant which has been used many century ago by our ancestors. In the current globalization era, it is difficult to find a plant in majority of the houses and many diets has been dependent to synthetic agent as taste enhancer against leaves. Thus, the importance of this beneficial plant should be emphasized and the bioactive components of *Murraya koenigii* should be analyzed further and used against the disease that have been developed resistance and synergistic studies should be carried out. The various pharmacological activities of the *Murraya koenigii* plant has been seen such as such as activity on Antidiabetic, cholesterol reducing property, antimicrobial activity, antiulcer activity, Antioxidant property, cytotoxic activity, anti-diarrhoea activity, anti-cancer activity with many other phagocytic activity. The chemical composition of the *Murraya koenigii* consists of essential oil alkaloids and terpenoid. Thus leaves merits further phytochemical, pharmacological and clinical investigations for development of an effective natural plant. Leaves being a staple food crop in India are an extremely essential ingredient found in almost all Indian households. The aromatic flavor and high nutritional benefit make this leaf an amazing spice which can be relished as different cuisines.

REFERENCES

1. Nishan M, Subramanian P. *Murraya koenigii* (leave) - A Review on its Potential. Int J of PharmTech Res. 2015; 7(4): 566-572.
2. Singh S, More PK, Mohan SM. Floral Composition and Taxonomy of Mangroves of Andaman and Nicobar Islands. Ind J Scient Res. 2014; 43(6):1037-1050.
3. Priyanka Gupta P, Alok Nahata A, Vinod K. *et al.* An update on Murayya Koenigii: A Multifunctional Ayurvedic Herb. J Chinese Integra Med. 2012; 9(8): 824-833.
4. Jain V, Momin M, Laddha K. *Murraya koenigii*: An updated Review. Int J Ayur Herbal Med. 2012; 2(4): 607-627.
5. Ajay S, Rahul S, Sumit G, *et al.* Comprehensive Review: *Murraya koenigii*Linn. Asian J Pharm Life Sci. 2011; 1(4): 417-425.
6. Bonde SD, Nemade LS, Patel MR, *et al. Murraya koenigii*(leaf): Ethnobotany, Phytochemistry and Pharmacology - A Review. Int J Pharmaceut Phytopharmacolo Res. 2007; 4(5): 45-54.
7. Khosa RL, Prasad S. Pharmacognostical Studies of Leaf of *Murraya koenigii* and Murrayapaniculata. J Res Indian Med. 1972; 7(3): 78.
8. Khosa RL, Prasad S. Pharmacognosy of Roots of *Murraya koenigii* and Murrayapaniculata. J Res Indian Med. 1974; 9(3): 105.
9. Handral HK, Pandith A, Shruthi SD. A Review on *Murraya koenigii*: Multipotential Medicinal Plant. Asian JPharmaceutClin Res. 2012; 5(4): 5-14.
10. Dineshkumar B, Mitra A, Mahadevappa M. Antidiabetic and Hypolipidemic Effects of Mahanimbine (Carbazole Alkaloid) from *Murraya koenigii*(Rutaceae) Leaves. Int J Phytomed. 2012; 2: 22-25.
11. Prakash V, Natarajan CP. Studies on Leaf. Food Sci Technol. 1974; 11(6): 284-286.
12. Narasimha NS, Paradkar MV, Chitguppi VP, *et al.* Alkaloids of *Murraya koenigii*: Structures of Mahanimbine, Koenimbine, (-) Mahanine, Koenine, Koenigine, Koenidine And (+)-Isomahanimbine. Ind J Chem. 1975; 13(10): 993-999.
13. Joshi BS, Kamat VN, Gawd DH. Structures of Girinimbine, Mahanimbine, Isomahanimbine, Koenimbidineand Murrayacine. Tetrahedron. 1970; 26(6): 1475-1482.
14. Kureel SP, Kapil RS, Popli SP. Two Novel Alkaloids Form Murraya Koenigii: Mahnimbicine and Bicyclomahanimbicine. Chem Ind. 1970; 29: 958.
15. Sindhu RK, Arora S. Phytochemical and Pharmacognostical Studies on *Murraya koenigii*(L.) Spreng roots. Drug Inven Today. 2012; 4(1): 325-333.
16. Dutta NL, Quasim C, Wadia MS. Constituents of *Murraya koenigii*: Structure of Angin. Ind T Chem. 1969; 7: 1061-1062.

17. Ganesan P, Phaiphan A, Murugan Y, *et al.* Comparative Study of Bioactive Compounds in and Coriander Leaves: An update. JChemPharmaceut Res. 2013; 5(11): 590-594.
18. Gahlawat DK, Jakhar S, Dahiya P. *Murraya koenigii*(L.) Spreng: An Ethnobotanical, Phytochemical and Pharmacological Review. J Pharmacog Phytochem. 2014; 3(3): 109-119.
19. Leela KS, Natarajan AV, Devi K, *et al.* Chemical Composition of Aqueous Leaf extract of *Murraya koenigii.* Int JPharmaceutBiol Arch. 2013; 4(3): 493-497.
20. Prabhu KA, Tamilanban T. Investigation of Anti-diabetic Activity of Stem of *Murraya koenigii.* Int J ResPharmacol Pharmacotherapeut. 2012; 1(2): 165-168.
21. Rana VS, Juyal JP, Rashmi, *et al.* Chemical Constituents of the Volatile Oil of *Murraya koenigii*Leaves. Int J Aromather. 2004;14(1): 23-25.
22. Ahmad, Kartini. Chemical Constituents of *Murraya koenigii*(Rutaceae) and their Biological Activities. Malaysia: Uni Putra Malaysia. 1999. p. 1-25.
23. Pagariya A, Chatur S, Nawab F. In vitro Anthelmintic Activity of Root extract of *Murraya koenigii*(linn) spreng. Int J PharmaceutInnov. 2013; 3(1): 111-114.
24. Pagariya A, Maithili V. Anti-diarrhoeal Activity of *Murraya koenigii*Linn Root Extracts. J Nat Remedies. 2009; 9(1): 8-11.
25. Susanna D, Bhavana D, Mounika D, *et al.* Study of Synergistic Anti-inflammatory Activity of *Murraya koenigii* and Aeglemarmelos. Annals of Biol Res. 2015; 6(6): 33-38.
26. Bhattacharya P, Chowdhury BK. 2-Methoxy-3-Methyl Carbazole from *Murraya koenigii.* Ind J Chem Sect. 1984; 24B(4): 452.
27. Fiebig M, Pezzuto JM, Soejarto DD. Part-40 Koenoline a further Cytotoxic Carbazole Alkaloid from *Murraya koenigii.* Phytochem. 1985; 24(12): 3041-3043.
28. Chakraborty DP, Bhattacharyya P, Roy S, *et al.* Structure and Synthesis of Mukonine, a new Carbazole Alkaloid from *Murraya koenigii.* Phytochem. 1978; 17: 834-835.
29. Adebajo AC, Avoola OF, Iwalewa EO, *et al.* Anti-trichomonal, Biochemical and Toxicological Activities of Methanolic extract and some Carbazole Alkaloids Isolated from the Leaves of *Murraya koenigii* Growing in Nigeria. Phytomed. 2006; 13(4): 246-254.
30. Patidar DK, Yadav N, Nakra V, *et al.* Wound Healing Activity of *Murraya koenigii* Leaf Extract. Int J Compr Pharm. 2010; 4(9): 1-2.
31. Vasudevan M, Parle M. Antiamnesic Potential of *Murraya koenigii* Leaves. Phytother Res. 2009; 23(3): 308-316.
32. Ningappaa MB, Dineshaa R, Srinivasa L. Antioxidant and Free Radical Scavenging activities of Polyphenol-enriched Leaf (*Murraya koenigii*L.) extracts. Food Chem. 2008; 106(2): 720-728.
33. Rageeb MD, Usman MD, Barhate SD. Phytochemical Evaluation and Effect of Antipyretic Activity on *Murraya koenigii* Spreng. Leaves extract. Int JPharmaceut Chem Sci. 2012; 1(1): 231-236.
34. Jain M, Gilhotra R, Singh RP, *et al.* Leaf (*Murraya koenigii*): A Spice with Medicinal Property. MOJ Biol Med. 2017; 2(3): 236-256. doi: 10.15406/mojbm.2017.02.00050
35. Saini SC, Reddy GBS. A Review on Leaves (*Murraya koenigii*): Versatile Multi-Potential Medicinal Plant Am J PharmamedClinTherapeut 2015; 3(04): 363-368.
36. Iyer D, Uma DP. Phyto-pharmacology of *Murraya koenigii.* Pharmacog. Reviews. 2008; 2: 180-184.
37. Gupta S, Paarakh PM, Gavani U. Isolation of Phytoconstituents from the Leaves of *Murraya koenigii*Linn. J Pharm Res. 2009, 2(8): 1313-1314.
38. Gupta GL, Nigamurraya SS. Chemical Examination of the Leaves of *Murraya koenigii.* Planta Med. 197; 19: 83-87.

39. Adebajo AC, Olayiwola G, Verspohl EJ, Iwalewa EO, Omisore NOA, Bergenthal D, *et al*. Evaluation of the Ethnomedical Claims of *Murraya koenigii*. Pharm Biol. 2004; 42(8): 610-620.
40. Chakrabarty M, Nath A, Khasnobis S, Chakrabarty M, Konda Y, Harigaya Y, Komiyama K. Carbazole Alkaloids from *Murraya koenigii*. Phytochem. 1997; 46(4): 751-755.
41. Nutan MTH, Hasnat A, Rashid MA. Antibacterial and Cytotoxic Activities of *Murraya koenigii*. Fitoterapia, 1998; 69(2): 173-175.
42. Kumar VS, Sharma A, Tiwari R, Kumar S. *Murraya koenigii* (leaf): A Review. J Med Arom Plant Sci. 1999; 21(4): 1139-1141.
43. Rana VS, Juyal JP, Rashmi, Blazquez MA. Chemical Constituents of the Volatile Oil of *Murraya koenigii* Leaves. Int J Aromather. 2004; 14(1): 23-25.
44. Rao BRR, Rajput DK, Mallavarapu GR. Chemical Diversity in Leaf (*Murraya koenigii*) Essential Oils. Food Chem. 2011; 126(3): 989-994.
45. Goutam MP, Purohit R. Murraya Antimicrobial Activity of the Essential Oil of the Leaves of *Murraya koenigii*. Ind J Pharm. 1974; 36: 11-15.
46. Narasimhan NS, Paradkar M V, Chitguppi VP, Kelkar SL. Alkaloids of *Murraya koenigii*, Structures of Mahanimbine, Koenimbine, Mahanine, Koenine, Koenigine and Koenidine. Ind.Chem. 1975; 13: 993-997.
47. Nayak A, Mandal S, Banerji A, Banerji J., Review on Chemistry and Pharmacology of *Murraya koenigii* Spreng (Rutaceae), Journal of Chem Pharmaceut Res. 2010; 2(2), 286-299.
48. Saini SC, Reddy GBS. *Murraya koenigii*, J Pharm Biol Sci. 2013; 7(6): 15-18.
49. Sivakumar CHV, Meera I, Antioxidant and Biological Activities of Three Morphotypes of *Murraya koenigii*L. from Uttarakhand, J Food Process Technol. 2013; 4(7): 1-7.
50. Kumar S.R, Loveleena D, Godwin S., Medicinal Property of *Murraya koenigii*- A Review, Int ResJ Biol Sci. 2013; 2(9): 80-83.
51. Sindhu RK, Arora S. Evaluation of Phenolic contents and Antioxidant Potential of *Murraya koenigii*(L) Spreng Roots, JAppl Pharmaceut Sci. 2012; 2(11): 120-122.
52. Parul S, Javed A, Neha B, Honey J, Anuj B.leaves- A Medicinal Herb, Asian J Pharmaceut Res. 2012; 2(2): 51-53.
53. Singh S, More PK, Mohan SM., Leaves (*Murraya koenigii*Linn. Sprengal)- a Mircale Plant, IndJ Scient Res. 2014; 4(1): 46-52.
54. Ganesan P, Phaiphan A, Murugan Y, Baharin BS. Comparative Study of Bioactive Compounds in and Coriander Leaves: An Update, J ChemPharmaceut Res. 2013; 5(11): 590-594.
55. Handral HK, Jha PK, Shruthi SD. Pharmacognostic and Phytochemical Studies on the Leaves of *Murraya koenigii*(L) Spreng, Pharmacophore. 2010; 1(3): 231-238.
56. Malwal M, Sarin R. Antimicrobial Efficacy of *Murraya koenigii*(Linn.) Spreng. Root Extracts, Ind J Nat Prod Resour. 2011; 2(1): 48-51.
57. Rageeb MD, Usman MD, Barhate SD. Phytochemical Evaluation and Effect of Antipyretic Activity on *Murraya koenigii* Spreng. Leaves Extract, Int JPharmaceut Chem Sci. 2012; 1(1): 231-236.
58. Prabhu KA, Tamilanban T. Investigation of Antidiabetic Activity of Stem of *Murraya koenigii*, Int J Res Pharmacol Pharmacotherapeut. 2012; 1(2): 165-168.
59. Prasad GBKS, Dua VK. Anti-inflammatory Activity of Leaves extract of *Murraya koenigii* L. Int J Pharma Bio Sci. 2011; 2(1): 541-544.
60. Handral HK, Pandith A, Shruthi SD. A Review on *Murraya koenigii*: Multipotential Medicinal Plant, Asian JPharmaceut ClinRes. 2012; 5(4): 5-14.

61. Tembhurne SV, Sakarkar DM. Anti-obesity and Hypoglycemic Effect of Ethanolic Extract of *Murraya koenigii*(L) Leaves in High Fatty Diet Rats, Asian Pac J Trop Dis. 2012; 2(1): 166-168.
62. Swati D, Pathak A, Burande M.D., Antigenotoxic effect of *Murraya koenigii* towards Cyclophosphamide Induced Cytogenetic Damage in Mouse Bone Marrow Cells, International Journal of Pharmacognosy and Phytochemical Research., 2012; 4(2): 59-63.
63. Sharma US, Sharma UK, Singh A, Sutar N, Singh PJ. In vitro antihelminth Activity of *Murraya koenigii*Linn. Leaves extracts, Int J PharmBio Sci. 2010; 1(3):1-4.
64. Kumar A, Tripathi A, Dora J, Tripathi R., Antihelmintic activity of Methanolic extract of *Murraya koenigii* leaves (Linn), Int J Res Pharmaceut Biomed Sci. 2011; 2(4): 1698-1700.
64. Ajay S, Rahul S, Sumit G, Paras M, Mishra A, Gaurav A., Comprehensive Review: *Murraya koenigii* Linn, Asian Journal of Pharmacy and Life Sciences., 2011;1(4): 417-425.
66. Ilangovan SS, Krishna P, Das K, Sen S (2016) A Review on Antimicrobial Properties of *Murraya koenigii*. J PharmaceutRes. 2016; 6(12): 7260-7268
67. Jain M, Jain M, Gilhotra R, Singh RP leaf (*Murraya koenigii*): A Spice with Medicinal Property. MOJ Biol Med. 2017; 2(3): 236-256. doi: 10.15406/mojbm.2017.02.00050
68. Handral H.K., Pandith A., Shruthi S.D. A Review on *Murraya koenigii*: Multipotential Medicinal Plant. Asian. Pharm. Clin. Res. 2012; 5: 5-14.
69. Bhandari P. Leaf (*Murraya koenigii*) or Cure Leaf: Review of its Curative Properties. J Med Nutr.2012; 2: 92-97. doi: 10.4103/2278-019X.101295

CHAPTER

15

An Comprehensive Appraisal on Traditional uses, Phytochemistry and Pharmacology of Fennal (*Foeniculum vulgare*)

ABSTRACT

Apart from being used for adding flavor, it is also used for various health benefits that are derived from its anti-oxidants. These anti-oxidants are essential to curb unwanted free radical reactions in the body. This phenomenon also prevents many diseases that can get serious at a later stage. Some of the antioxidants listed in these seeds are kaempferol and quercetin that are known to prevent degenerative reactions. Fennel seeds contain a good amount of dietary fiber that is essential for the body. The fiber content helps improve digestion in the body, by facilitating timely breaking down of food molecules that make energy reactions possible. The carcinogenic diseases should be treated at the right stage so that their effect can be curbed or eliminated in the future. Fiber present in fennel seeds decreases reabsorption of cholesterol, thereby preventing any heart-related diseases. A number of volatile oil compounds like myrcene, fenchone, chavicol and cineole are present in these seeds that assist in digestive, carminative, and antioxidant reactions in the body. Production of Red Blood Cells is enhanced by the consumption of Fennel Seeds. Copper, which is required by the body for the production of red blood cells, is present in these seeds. Zinc, found in the fennel seeds, promotes regular growth and development. The potassium content helps in maintaining the blood pressure and hence the heart rate is also maintained. The review aims to gather the fragmented information available in the literature regarding morphology, ethnomedicinal applications, phytochemistry, pharmacology, and toxicology of *Foeniculum vulgare*. It also compiles available scientific evidence for the ethnobotanical claims and to identify gaps required to be filled by future research. Findings based on their traditional uses and scientific evaluation indicates that *Foeniculum vulgare* remains to be the most widely used herb globally.

Keywords: Cholesterol, Myrcene, Fenchone, Chavicol, Cineole, Carminative.

Introduction

Fennel is an aromatic herb belonging to the parsley family. It is used as a spice and possesses a sweet taste that is similar to anise. It is an essential ingredient in the Mediterranean cuisine. It is native to the South European region but is consumed well in all of the European regions. It is a two-meter plant with dark green leaves and yellow flowers. Fennel seeds are not only tasty but are also very healthy owing to their nutritional content. Fennel bulb is also eaten as a vegetable in some parts of the Mediterranean region [1-4]. Saunf or Fennel seeds are an edible and healthy seeds used for many years in cooking as well as medicinal purposes. It is also called as moti saunf in India. It belongs to the Apiaceae or Umbelliferae family and Foeniculum genus, cultivated in many countries all over the world. India is the top producer of the saunf however it is cultivated in average amount in Iran, Mexico, China, Canada, Syria, Bulgaria, United States, Australia and etc. Saunf or Fennel seeds are an edible and healthy seeds used for many years in cooking as well as medicinal purposes. It is also called as moti saunf in India. It belongs to the Apiaceae or Umbelliferae family and *Foeniculum* genus, cultivated in many countries all over the world. India is the top producer of the saunf however it is cultivated in average amount in Iran, Mexico, China, Canada, Syria, Bulgaria, United States, Australia and etc. [5-8].

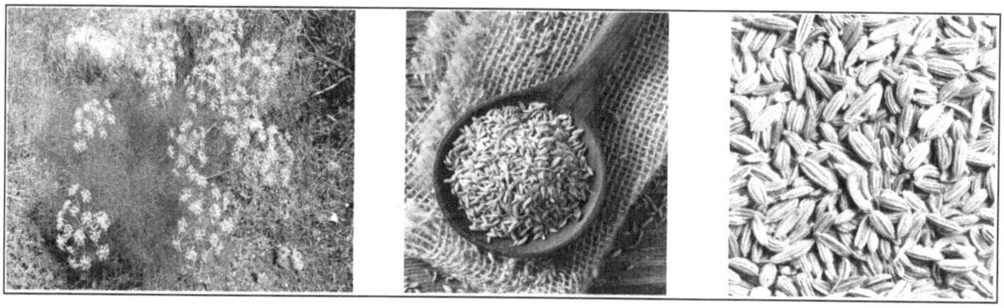

Fennel herb and seeds

In India, it is an old and most common trend of offering some fennel seeds with mishri (or sugar coated saunf) after a meal to chew. It is mostly carried out in hotels, restaurants and parties in order to prevent after eating problems like gas, indigestion, acid reflux, abdominal cramps, flatulence, and constipation. Do not be confused with the fennel seeds (moti saunf with green or yellowish color, used for cooking purpose) and aniseeds (patli or chhoti saunf with green color, used for raw eating purpose after meal) [9-10].

Phytochemical Constituents

Phytochemical research carried out on *Foeniculum vulgare* has led to the isolation of fatty acids, phenolic components, hydrocarbons, volatile components, and few other classes of secondary metabolites from its different parts. Mostly these phytochemicals [(a, b, c, d) 1-60] are found in essential oil [11-20].

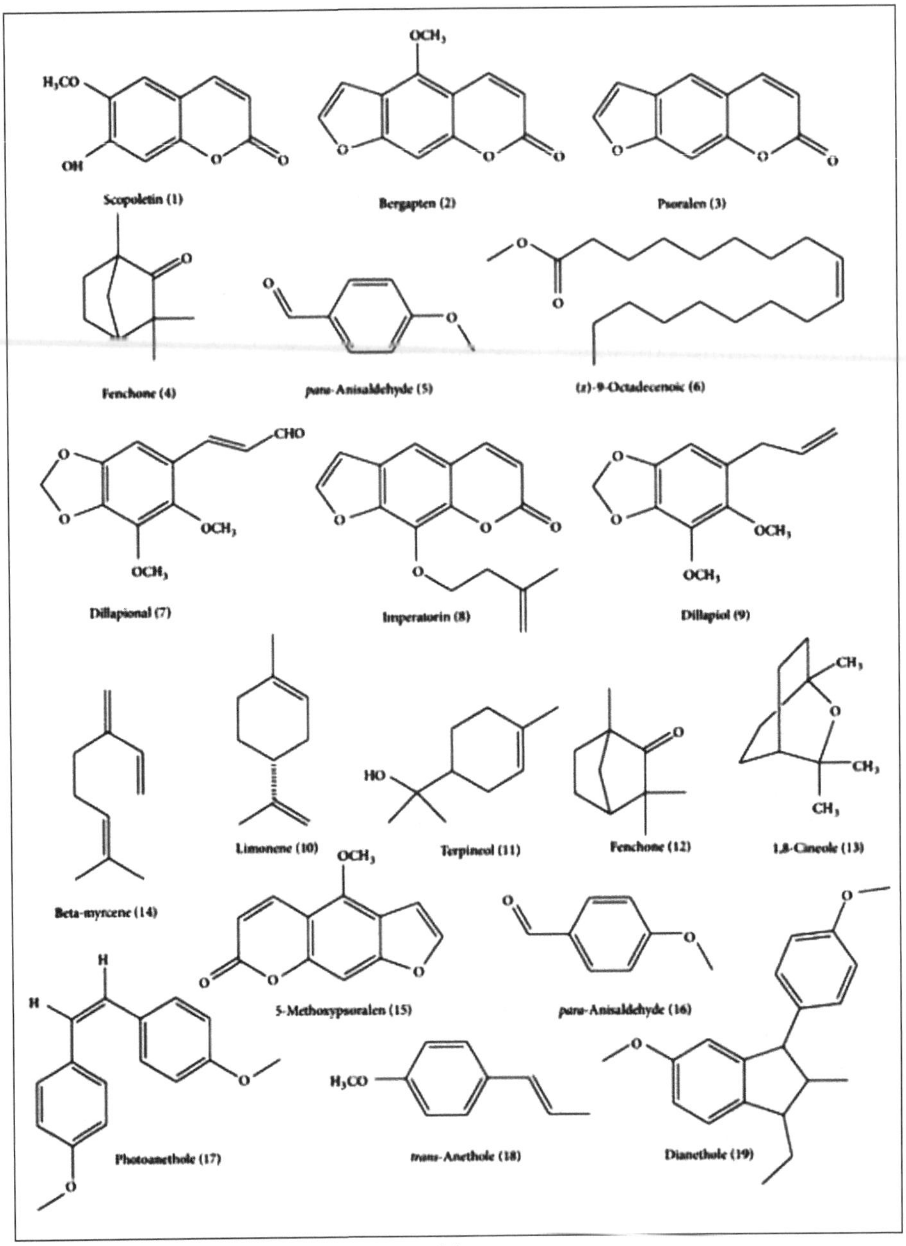
Scopoletin (1)
Bergapten (2)
Psoralen (3)
Fenchone (4)
para-Anisaldehyde (5)
(z)-9-Octadecenoic (6)
Dillapional (7)
Imperatorin (8)
Dillapiol (9)
Limonene (10)
Terpineol (11)
Fenchone (12)
1,8-Cineole (13)
Beta-myrcene (14)
5-Methoxypsoralen (15)
para-Anisaldehyde (16)
Photoanethole (17)
trans-Anethole (18)
Dianethole (19)

(a)

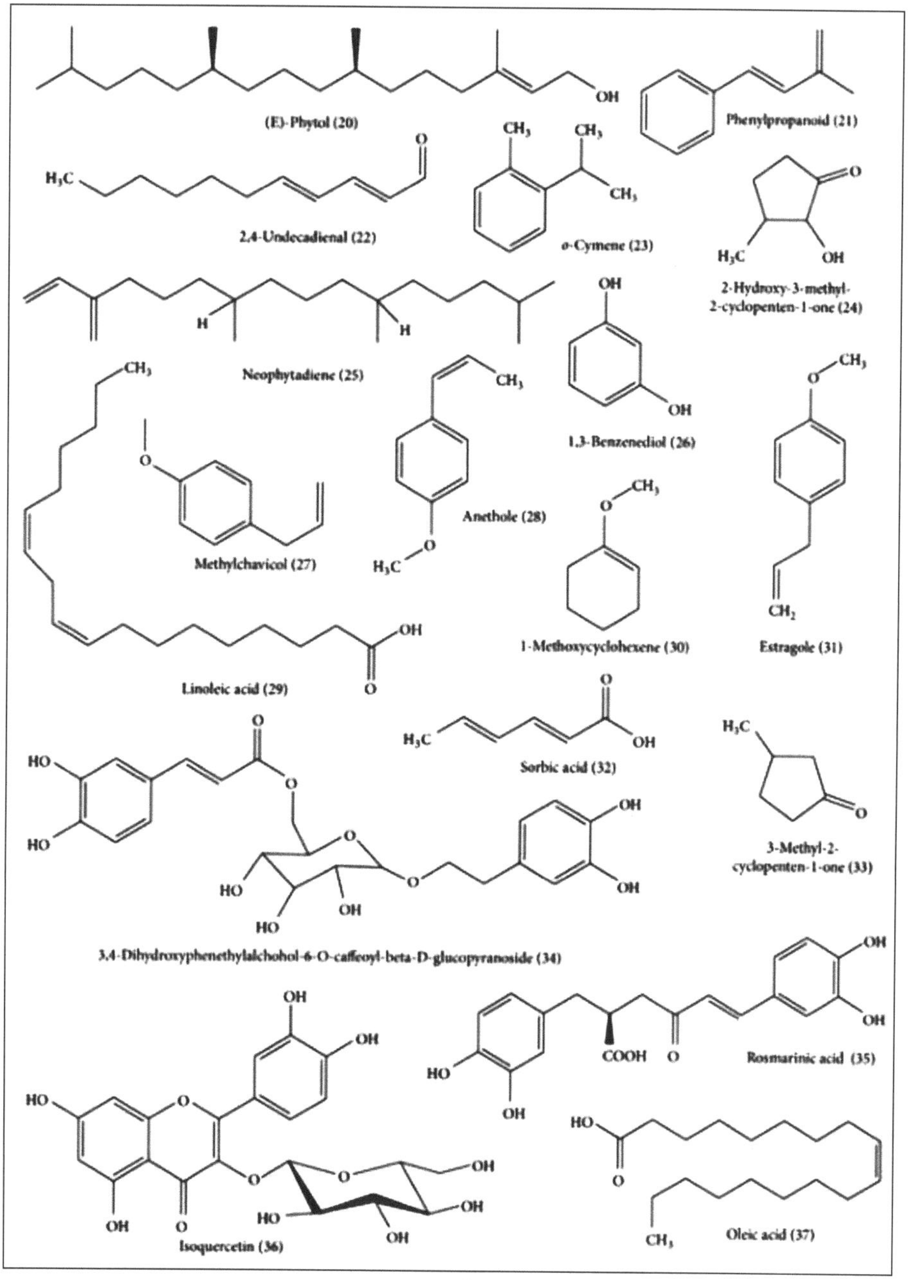
(E)-Phytol (20)
Phenylpropanoid (21)
2,4-Undecadienal (22)
o-Cymene (23)
2-Hydroxy-3-methyl-2-cyclopenten-1-one (24)
Neophytadiene (25)
1,3-Benzenediol (26)
Methylchavicol (27)
Anethole (28)
Linoleic acid (29)
1-Methoxycyclohexene (30)
Estragole (31)
Sorbic acid (32)
3-Methyl-2-cyclopenten-1-one (33)
3,4-Dihydroxyphenethylalchohol-6-O-caffeoyl-beta-D-glucopyranoside (34)
Rosmarinic acid (35)
Isoquercetin (36)
Oleic acid (37)

(b)

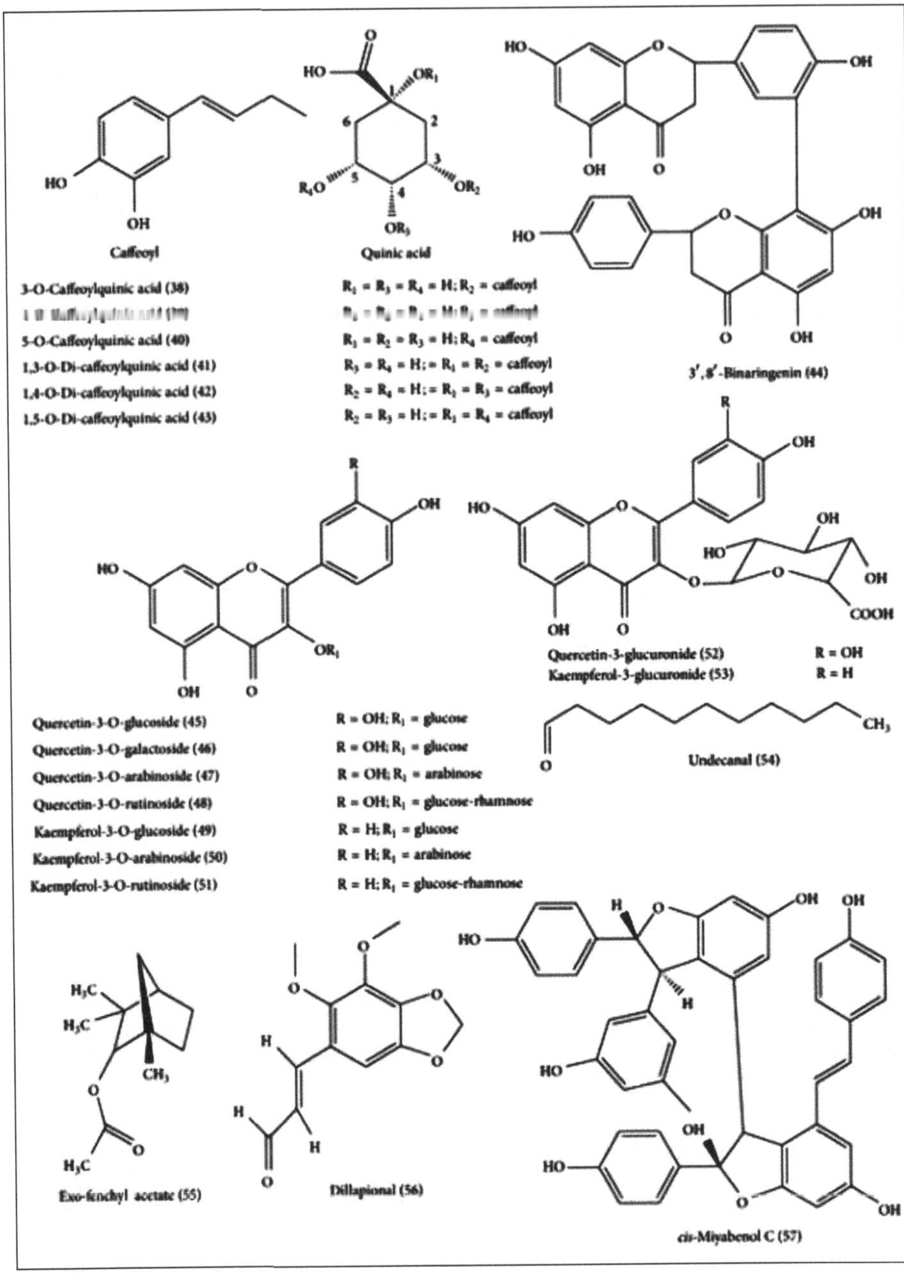
Caffeoyl
Quinic acid
3-O-Caffeoylquinic acid (38)
5-O-Caffeoylquinic acid (40)
1,3-O-Di-caffeoylquinic acid (41)
1,4-O-Di-caffeoylquinic acid (42)
1,5-O-Di-caffeoylquinic acid (43)
$R_1 = R_3 = R_4 = H; R_2$ = caffeoyl
$R_1 = R_2 = R_3 = H; R_4$ = caffeoyl
$R_3 = R_4 = H; = R_1 = R_2$ = caffeoyl
$R_2 = R_4 = H; = R_1 = R_3$ = caffeoyl
$R_2 = R_3 = H; = R_1 = R_4$ = caffeoyl
3′,8′-Binaringenin (44)
Quercetin-3-glucuronide (52) R = OH
Kaempferol-3-glucuronide (53) R = H
Quercetin-3-O-glucoside (45) R = OH; R_1 = glucose
Quercetin-3-O-galactoside (46) R = OH; R_1 = glucose
Quercetin-3-O-arabinoside (47) R = OH; R_1 = arabinose
Quercetin-3-O-rutinoside (48) R = OH; R_1 = glucose-rhamnose
Kaempferol-3-O-glucoside (49) R = H; R_1 = glucose
Kaempferol-3-O-arabinoside (50) R = H; R_1 = arabinose
Kaempferol-3-O-rutinoside (51) R = H; R_1 = glucose-rhamnose
Undecanal (54)
Exo-fenchyl acetate (55)
Dillapional (56)
cis-Miyabenol C (57)

(c)

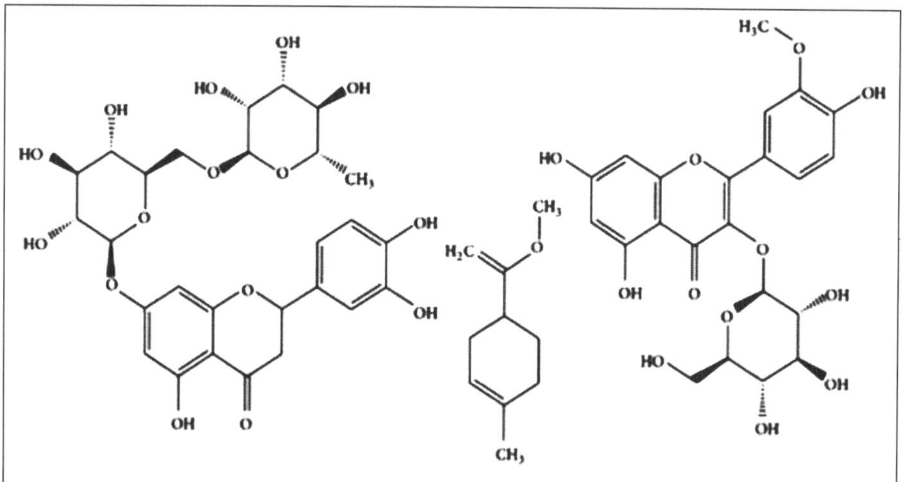

Eriodictyol-7-rutinoside (58) Limonene-10-ol (59) Isorhamnetin-3-O-glucoside (60)

(d)

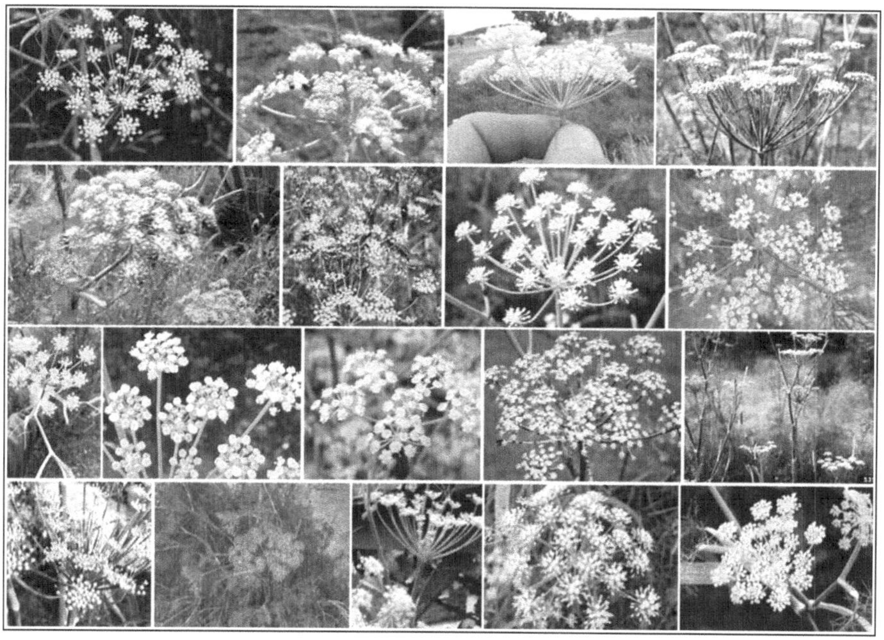

Medicinal Properties

Apart from being used for adding flavor, it is also used for various health benefits that are derived from its anti-oxidants. These anti-oxidants are essential to curb unwanted free radical reactions in the body. This phenomenon also prevents many diseases that can get serious at a later stage. Some of the antioxidants listed in these seeds are kaempferol and quercetin that are known to prevent degenerative reactions. Fennel seeds contain a good amount of dietary fiber that is essential for the body. The fiber content helps improve digestion in the body, by facilitating timely breaking down of food molecules that make energy reactions possible. The carcinogenic diseases should be treated at the right stage so that their effect can be curbed or eliminated in the future. This is made possible by the anti-oxidant capabilities of the fennel seeds [21-23]. Another effect of prevention of free radical reactions by fennel seeds – Neurological diseases are helpfully kept at bay. Cholesterol absorption in the arteries is prevented by the action of the fiber binding to the bile salts. Fiber present in fennel seeds decreases reabsorption of cholesterol, thereby preventing any heart-related diseases. A number of volatile oil compounds like myrcene, fenchone, chavicol and cineole are present in these seeds that assist in digestive, carminative and antioxidant reactions in the body. Production of Red Blood Cells is enhanced by the consumption of Fennel Seeds. Copper, which is required by the body for the production of red blood cells, is present in these seeds. The growth and development of the body are geared up. Zinc, found in the fennel seeds, promotes regular growth and development. These days, when people face tensions in their day to day lives, it is very important to maintain the blood pressure and keep the heart rate balanced. Fennel Seeds help a lot in this process. The potassium content helps in maintaining the blood pressure and hence the heart rate is also maintained [24-26].

Fennel juice is an extremely nutritional beverage. It contains vitamin A, B, C, E, and beta-carotene. It is a rich source of minerals like magnesium, iron, cobalt, potassium, phosphorus, sodium, silicon, and zinc. It also provides high levels antioxidants, carotenoids, and flavonoids. It contains anethole, a phytonutrient that provides fennel juice its strong aroma. The high levels of antioxidants neutralize free radicals in the body, preventing cell damage. Fennel juice has a calming effect on the intestine. The anti-spasmodic properties of fennel juice can reduce intestinal cramps, bloating, and flatulence. The essential oils present in fennel juice stimulate the secretion of digestive juice, reducing stomach inflammation. It also improves the absorption of nutrients from the foods we eat. Fennel juice is widely used as an antacid. The roughage in fennel juice balances the digestive tract, promoting regular bowel movements. Fennel also reduces bad bacteria and increases good bacteria in the gut [27-29].

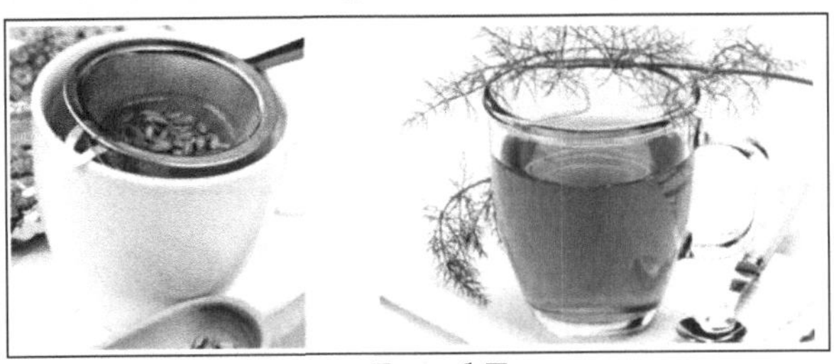

Fennel Tea

The high concentration of iron and histamine in fennel juice makes it a good natural remedy for anemia. Regular consumption of fennel juice increases the production of hemoglobin in the body, reversing anemia. It also prevents the formation of blood clots in the body. Fennel contains several essential nutrients, which helps to improve vision. The antioxidants and amino acids in fennel juice rejuvenate the eyes, preventing macular degeneration. Fennel juice, when applied to the eye, can reduce eye irritations and fatigue. The flavonoids present in fennel juice are very useful in preventing oxidative stress, which helps to prevent macular degeneration. The diuretic properties of fennel juice help to remove the toxic substance from the body through frequent urination. This helps to reduce inflammation that causes rheumatism and swelling. It also prevents the formation of kidney stones. Fennel juice contains phyto-estrogen, a chemical that is similar to the hormone estrogen in structure. Thus, fennel juice is very useful for women suffering from menopause and pre-menstrual problems. It also contains folate, which prevents birth defects in unborn babies. Fennel juice eases menstruation problems by regulating hormonal actions in the body. Lactating mothers can regularly drink fennel juice to increase milk production. Fennel juice is believed to release endorphins into the bloodstreams, which relieve depression associated with certain diseases and creates a mood of euphoria. Potassium in fennel juice increases brain function and the cognitive abilities of the brain. In addition to this, fennel juice is also a vasodilator, which increases oxygen supply to the brain and delays the onset of dementia. Fennel essential oil is an aperitif. It helps boost appetite. So if you think you aren't feeling hungry when it is required, fennel essential oil is what you should turn to! Spasms are violent and involuntary contractions of the organs, respiratory tract, intestines, muscles, and nerves. It can lead to chronic cough and acute pain and inflammation. Severe cases of spasms can lead to fainting and even death. Fennel essential oil is an active antispasmodic agent, which relaxes the intestines, muscles and nerves. It provides instant relief from spasms [30-34].

Fennel essential oil contains many chemicals, which exhibit antiseptic and bactericidal characteristics. Fennel oil helps prevent wounds from turning septic. Fennel essential oil prevents tetanus and other post-surgical infections as well.

Fennel essential oil is an active carminative agent. It helps release gas from intestines and provides relief from stomach problems like pain, restlessness, heartburn and indigestion. It also inhibits the formation of gas and helps treat excessive flatulence. Fennel bulb exhibits strong anti-inflammatory properties. Whether you talk of inflammation that is internal or external, fennel bulb cures both. This magic food contains anethole. Anethole serves as a very strong anti-inflammatory flavonoid. It easily cures inflammation caused in humans without causing any side-effects. Fennel bulb offers natural cooling and neutralizing benefits. Thus, it is used to treat the problem of acidity in the duodenum. It makes intestines active and eases the process of absorption. Hence, the toxins get separated from useful minerals. The separated toxins are easily flushed out of the body. Hence, the normal pH level is restored which results in relief from acidity. Vitamin C is a natural immunity boosting vitamin for humans. Fennel bulb is highly rich in vitamin C. Hence; its regular intake strengthens the immune system. It keeps the body safe from minor infections naturally. It also increases the body's capacity to fight back major infections. This is because – stronger immune system means active WBCs. As soon as some infection enters the body, the WBCs engulf all the disease-causing bacteria and viruses and destroy them. Fennel bulb is a rich source of cineole [35-37]. Cineole is an active agent that potentially clears nasal blockages. Thus, it is a boon for people suffering from congestion, asthma, and bronchitis. Cineol efficiently clears and controls the formation and accumulation of phlegm in the chest and nasal passage. Hence, it eases respiration. Fennel bulb is a rich source of potassium. Potassium is an active component of cranial nerves. It is also an active compound that maintains the electrolytic balance of the brain. Moreover, potassium is also a memory charger. In short, fennel bulb ensures proper functioning of the human brain by regulating the levels of potassium. It sharpens the memory and improves focus and concentration. Fennel bulb can regulate hormonal changes in the human body. Its mild analgesic benefits work like a boon to control and cure menstrual pain in women. We all want to have healthy skin and hair but the mere thought of money and time involved in a beauty regime is enough to put us off. But what if I told you that you can stay beautiful with the help of a tiny thing called the fennel seed? Fennel seeds not only impart a special flavor to those gastronomic delights brewing in your kitchen, but can also be utilized for achieving a flawless skin and healthy hair. Yes, you got that right! Fennel seeds can be beneficial for your skin and hair. Fennel seeds are inexpensive and readily available. Loaded with minerals like iron, copper, selenium, potassium, magnesium, zinc and even vitamins like Vitamin C, Vitamin A, and Vitamin E, fennel seeds are also known to be a rich storehouse of dietary fibers, active compounds, and antioxidants. Fennel seeds offer amazing effects for the skin. Not only fennel seeds are antiseptic by nature, but also are loaded with antioxidants. As a result, they help prevent acne, cell damage, while keeping the skin toned. Using fennel seeds as a part of your skin care will help you delay the onset of lines, dark spots and wrinkles. When you consume fennel seeds in one form or the other, you get glowing and flawless skin in return. When consumed, fennel imparts a cooling effect to the skin. It soothes inflammation and skin irritation. Fennel tea, when consumed on a daily basis, helps in improving the overall texture of the skin. It treats acne and makes your skin look youthful. Fennel seeds, when consumed daily, provide the body with minerals like iron, zinc, selenium and calcium. These minerals are effective in maintaining the oxygen balance, thus imparting healthy skin [38-40].

Fennel Home Remedies

Saunf is an aromatic and sweet flavored seed acts as a mouth freshener and helps in removing bad breath, relief from toothache and gum problems. Eating saunf seeds provides relief from the common cold and cough problems. It is rich source of essential nutrients, fibers, anti-oxidants, vitamins and minerals which promotes courage and strength if consumed regularly. It is a powerful anti-oxidant as it contains some natural antioxidant compound called kaemferol and quercetin which helps in combating with harmful free radicals thus prevents from various degenerative diseases like cancer, aging, neurological diseases and etc. Regular intake of saunf helps in getting relief from the constipation and other digestive problems as it contains high level of dietary fibers which absorbs more water and makes stool soft and ease passage. Dietary fibers found in it helps in lowering the serum cholesterol level as it gets binded with bile salts and reduces its absorption in the colon. Its antioxidant nature protects colon and its mucus membrane from the cancer by inhibiting the growth and development of the cancerous cells. Fennel seed is rich source of essential oil compounds like limonene, anisic aldehyde, myrcene, pinene, fenchone, chavicol, anethole, cineole and etc. which make it able to prevent from various health disorders. It is rich source of copper which is highly required by the body to produce red blood cells thus it protects from anemia and other problems caused due to decreased amount of hemoglobin.

It is rich source of zinc mineral which acts as a co-factor for many enzymes regulating the growth and development of body, sperm production, nucleic acid synthesis and etc. Fennel seed is rich source of potassium electrolyte which is very necessary for the balance of cells and body fluid as well as controlling heart rate and blood pressure. It is also a rich source of manganese mineral which is the important co-factor for various powerful antioxidant enzymes. Its antibacterial nature protects from the infection of various harmful bacteria including *Bacillus subtilis, Cladosporium cladosporiodes, Aspergilus niger* and etc. It provides relief from the problems of stomach, intestine, colon, irritable bowel syndrome, spleen, kidney and etc. It helps in curing fever by increasing perspiration. Washing mouth with the warm saunf water is very helpful in removing bad breath.

Massaging the muscles on lower abdominal area with the mixture of saunf oil, whole fatty milk, geranium oil and clary sage oil helps in reducing menstrual pain, cramps and PMS disorders. It contains good level of phytoestrogens improving food digestion by soothing the irritable gastric glands. Fennel seed is a good blood purifier helps in purifying blood if a handful of raw saunf is eaten two times a day, morning and evening. It helps in curing heat stroke if saunf water (soaked into water for whole night) is taken by adding a pinch of salt. It helps in promoting proper bowel movements if one teaspoon of the roasted saunf is taken after meals. It is diuretic in nature helps in removing toxic materials from the body as well as provides relief from the body swelling and joints pain during rheumatism and arthritis. It stimulates the secretion of digestive enzymes and juices as well as reduces inflammation of digestive tract thus promote more absorption of the essential nutrients from the food while passing through the alimentary canal. Regular intake of it helps in recovering digestive system functioning after getting long radiation or chemotherapy treatments. Saunf water acts as a vasodilator thus keeps mind and body stress free and calm by enhancing oxygenated blood flow to the brain and all through the body thus keeps away from depression, dementia and other memory loss problem.

Fennel seed is a most common mouth freshener used in the paan (betel leaf) to make it delicious and flavored to chew. Fennel seed is a natural home remedy to suppress appetite and go for weight maintenance. It has been used for years by the women during their fasting periods to reduce hunger. It is a fat digester and hunger suppressor thus helps in decreasing weight among obese and overweight people if saunf tea or saunf water is taken in the early morning with empty stomach. It helps in preventing from the eye disorders (optic nerves weakness, glaucoma and night blindness) and improving eye sight if carrot juice is taken with half tsf powdered saunf regularly. Regular consumption of saunf helps in maintaining clear vision. Fennel seed promotes blood vessels dilation in the eye by reducing the eye pressure thus prevents from glaucoma (caused due to increased eye pressure), retinopathy (vision loss in diabetics), vision impairment diseases and etc.

It is good source of all the minerals required for bone growth such as calcium, phosphorus, magnesium and etc. thus helps in improving bone strength and development. Fennel seed naturally slows down process of bone destroying cells production in the body as well as reduces occurrence of age related bone problems like osteoporosis. Applying the mixture of saunf water (boil two tsf of saunf into a glass of water for at least one hour at low heat) and whey (or dahi water) to the face for 15 to 20 minutes then wash, helps in getting fair look with smooth skin. Whether it is applied directly to the skin or eaten, helps in getting acne and spots free skin as it has antiseptic and antioxidant properties.

It slows down the aging process by preventing cell damage and reducing the effects of free radicals thus keeps skin flawless without wrinkles and fine lines. Applying fennel seed water to the skin helps in getting toned, flexible and soft skin as it hydrates the skin by enhancing blood circulation to the face. Regular use of fennel seeds tea (drinking or applying to hair) helps in getting strong and lengthy hair as it prevents unusual hair loss and premature hair graying.

It prevents from hair fall by providing relief from itchy scalp and dandruff. Saunf has emmenagogue property which helps in regulating the regular menstrual flow among women. Its availability with essential phytoestrogens helps in curing menstrual disorders such as premenstrual syndrome, early menopause, unusual breast enlargement and etc. It prevents from the cardiovascular diseases, hormone or estrogen dependent cancer, menopausal disorders, hot flashes, dysmenorrheal (painful menstruation) and etc. Fennel seed keeps mind very calm and stress free by reducing the level of anxiety, depression, stimulating proper menstruation, lowering blood pressure, and etc. It helps in relieving morning sickness, weakness, fatigue and other symptoms during pregnancy. Regular use of fennel seeds helps in improving milk production among women on breast feeding or nursing mothers because of its galactagogue property. Drinking saunf water with little honey (boil saunf into water and add honey) helps in increasing the breast milk production.

It is aphrodisiac in nature helps in enhancing libido as well as maintaining sexual power in both men and women. It is a better home remedy to enhance breast at home than other surgical breast enlargement procedures. It is loaded with the natural hormones which involve in the developing and growing breast tissues to make breasts large and firm without any side effects. Saunf is used in manufacturing many creams and pills having estrogenic effects which are used by most of the women for years to get their enhanced breast. Its natural phytoestrogens availability prevents abnormal growth of the breast tissues thus protects from breast cancer. Fennel seeds availability with high amount of flavonoids helps in promoting the production of estrogen hormone which in turn promotes breast enlargement. Massaging breast with saunf oil for 10-15 minutes each (100-300 circular rubs for each) once a day in the morning or before going to bed helps in enhancing breast size. This procedure needs time and dedication but result oriented. It is very beneficial for the newborn babies as it helps in relieving from the colic pain as well as improving digestion. Massaging joints with the fennel seed oil or saunf oil helps in relieving joints pain (caused due to arthritis) and cellulite. It also provides relieve from the respiratory problems like cough, bronchitis and etc.

It contains essential oil required for the health of liver thus protects from the liver disorders. Drinking jeera and saunf water on daily basis (boil jeera and saunf seeds powder into a glass of water till it remains half) helps in getting wrinkles and acne free skin as well as helps in good digestion by keeping acidity away. Eating one tsf of powdered mixture of saunf, almonds and mishri at every night before going to bed with a glass of warm milk for one and half months helps in improving eyesight by curing all the eye disorders. Avoid drinking water after having this mixture. Taking this mixture with milk also helps in enhancing the memory and concentration level by curing headache and eye pain. A fennel seed tea is a natural detoxifier (when used regularly) helps in releasing body toxins by detoxifying the body as well as prevents from water retention in the body. It can be prepared at home by boiling one or two tsf saunf seeds or leaves into a cup of water till it remains half and add some sweetener (sugar, honey or jaggery) and milk according to the need and taste. Taking saunf tea on daily basis helps in relieving gastrointestinal disorders including gas, acid reflux, bloating, loss of appetite, indigestion, acidity and etc. Generally it is used by the people during summer season as a home remedy to get relief from the summer heat. It improves digestion by curing intestinal worms problem among kids. It helps in regulating menses by easing menstrual spasms. Regular intake of saunf tea aids in proper digestion and assists in weight loss. It helps in keeping body fit and youth look. It helps in curing bloating, gas, indigestion and digestive tract inflammation which helps in decreasing belly fat and thus weight loss. Fennel leaves are used to reduce the effect of snake bite and neutralize the vegetable poison like mushroom etc. Inhaling the steam of boiled fennel leaves helps in treating respiratory infections of bronchitis and asthma [35-44].

On account of its carminative properties, fennel is chiefly used medicinally with purgatives to allay their side effects and for this purpose forms one of the ingredients of the well-known compound liquorice powder. Fennel water has properties similar to those of anise and dill water: mixed with sodium bicarbonate and syrup, these waters constitute the domestic 'gripe water', used to correct flatulence of infants. Fennel tea, also employed as a carminative, is made by pouring boiling water on a teaspoonful of bruised fennel seeds. In the Indian Subcontinent, fennel seeds are eaten raw, sometimes with some sweetener to improve eyesight. Extracts of fennel seeds have been shown in animal studies to have a potential use in the treatment of glaucoma, as a diuretic and a potential drug for the treatment of hypertension. It has been used as a galactagogue improving the milk supply of a breast feeding mother. This is suggested to be due to the presence of phytoestrogens present in fennel which promote growth of breast tissue.

Nutritional benefits of Saunf/Fennel Seeds per 100 G

(*Source:* USDA Nutrient Database)

Energy: 345 Kcal Carbohydrate: 52.29 g Protein: 15.80 g

Fat: 14.87 g

Dietary Fibers: 39.8 g

Vitamins

Thiamin (B1): 0.408 mg

Riboflavin (B2): 0.353 mg

Niacin (B3): 6.050 mg

Pyridoxine (B6): 0.470 mg
Vitamin A: 135 IU
Vitamin C: 21 mg

Electrolytes

Sodium: 88 mg
Potassium: 1694 mg

Minerals

Calcium: 1196 mg
Copper: 1.067 mg
Iron: 18.54 mg
Magnesium: 385 mg
Manganese: 6.533 mg
Phosphorus: 487 mg
Zinc: 3.70 mg

Conclusion

Foeniculum vulgare has shown that it is an important medicinal plant used in a wide range of ethnomedical treatments, especially for abdominal pains, antiemetic, aperitif, arthritis, cancer, colic in children, conjunctivitis, constipation, depurative, diarrhea, dieresis, emmenagogue, fever, flatulence, gastralgia, gastritis, insomnia, irritable colon, kidney ailments, as a laxative, leucorrhoea, liver pain, mouth ulcer, and stomachache. This plant has been in use for a long period of time without any documented serious adverse effects. Studies carried out in the past and present indicate that fennel possesses diverse health benefits and are an important constituent of food. Studies have shown that various extracts of fennel possess a range of pharmacological actions, such as antiaging, antiallergic, anticolitic, antihirsutism, anti-inflammatory, antimicrobial and antiviral, antimutagenic, antinociceptive, antipyretic, antispasmodic, antistress, antithrombotic, anxiolytic, apoptotic, cardiovascular, chemomodulatory action, cytoprotection and antitumor, cytotoxicity, diuretic, estrogenic properties, expectorant, galactogenic, gastrointestinal effect, hepatoprotective, human liver cytochrome P450 3A4 inhibitory, hypoglycemic, hypolipidemic, memory-enhancing property, nootropic, and oculohypotensive activity supporting its traditional use. The observed health benefits may be credited to the presence of the various phytochemicals like volatile compounds, flavonoids, phenolic compounds, fatty acids, and amino acids. Fennel also contains mineral and trace elements like aluminum, barium, calcium, cadmium, cobalt, chromium, copper, iron, magnesium, manganese, nickel, lead, strontium, and zinc; fat soluble vitamins such as vitamins A, E, and K; water soluble vitamins like ascorbic acid, thiamine, riboflavin, niacin, and pyridoxine; essential amino acids like leucine, isoleucine, phenylalanine, and tryptophane may contribute to the myriad health beneficial effects at least in part. Among several classes of chemical constituents identified in fennel, volatile components of fennel essential oil and phenolic compounds are assumed to be the main bioactive compounds responsible for the majority of its pharmacological effects. However, the vast traditional use and proven pharmacological activities of fennel indicate that an immense scope still exists for its chemical exploration.

REFERENCES

1. Ono M, Ito Y, Kinjo J, Yahara S, Nohara T, Niiho Y. Four New Glycosides of Stilbene Trimer from Foeniculi fructus (fruit of Foeniculum vulgare Miller)., Chem Pharmaceut Bull. 1995; 43(5): 868-871.
2. Muckensturm B, Foechterlen D, Reduron J P, Danton P, Hildenbrand M. Phytochemical and Chemotaxonomic Studies of *Foeniculum vulgare*. *Biochemical Systematics and Ecology*. 1997; 25(4): 353-358.
3. Kaur GJ, Arora DS. Antibacterial and Phytochemical Screening of Anethum Graveolens, Foeniculum Vulgare and Trachyspermum ammi. *BMC Complementary and Alternative Medicine*. 2009; 9: 123-126.
4. Manonmani R, Abdul Khadir VM. Antibacterial Screening on *Foeniculum vulgare* Mill. *International Journal of Pharma and Bio Sciences*. 2011; 2(4): 390-394.
5. Orhan IE, Özçelik B, Kartal M, Kan Y. Antimicrobial and Antiviral Effects of Essential Oils from Selected Umbelliferae and Labiatae Plants and Individual Essential Oil Components. *Turkish Journal of Biology*. 2012; 36(3): 239-246.
6. Dua A, Garg G, Mahajan R. Polyphenols, Flavonoids and Antimicrobial Properties of Methanolic extract of Fennel (*Foeniculum vulgare Miller*) *European Journal of Experimental Biology*. 2013; 3(4): 203-208.
7. Ozbek H, Ugras S, Dülger H, *et al*. Hepatoprotective effect of *Foeniculum vulgare* Essential Oil. *Fitoterapia*. 2003; 74(3): 317-319.
8. Oktay M, Gülçin I, Küfrevioglu ÖI. Determination of in vitro Antioxidant Activity of Fennel (*Foeniculum vulgare*) Seed extracts. *LWT-Food Science and Technology*. 2003; 36(2): 263-271.
9. Barros L, Carvalho AM, Ferreira ICFR. The Nutritional Composition of Fennel (*Foeniculum vulgare*): Shoots, Leaves, Stems and Inflorescences. *LWT: Food Science and Technology*. 2010; 43(5): 814-818.
10. Garg C, Khan SA, Ansari SH, Suman A, Garg M. Chemical Composition, Therapeutic Potential and Perspectives of *Foeniculum ulgare*. *Pharmacognosy Reviews*. 2009; 3(6): 346-352.
11. He W, Huang B. A Review of Chemistry and Bioactivities of a Medicinal Spice: *Foeniculum vulgare*. *Journal of Medicinal Plants Research*. 2011; 5(16): 3595-3600.
12. Jamwal NS, Kumar S, Rana AC. Phytochemical and Pharmacological review on Foeniculum Vulgare; 2013; 327-341.
13. Grover S, Malik CP, Hora A, Kushwaha HB. Botany, Cultivation, Chemical Constituents and Genetic Diversity in Fennel (*Foeniculum vulgare* Mill): A Review. *International Journal of Life Sciences*. 2(2): 128-139.
14. Rahimi R, Ardekani MRS. Medicinal Properties of *Foeniculum vulgare* Mill. In Traditional Iranian Medicine and Modern Phytotherapy. *Chinese Journal of Integrative Medicine*. 2013; 19(1): 73-79.
15. Krishnamurthy KH. Medicinal Plants: Madhurika, Saunf or Fennel (*Foeniculum vulgare*, Gaertn) *Journal of New Approaches to Medicine and Health*. 2011; 19(1): 1-4.

16. Akgül A, Bayrak A. Comparative Volatile Oil Composition of Various Parts from Turkish bitter fennel (*Foeniculum vulgare* var. *vulgare*) *Food Chemistry.* 1988; 30(4): 319-323.
17. Damjanovic B, LepojevicŽ, Živkovic V, Tolic A. Extraction of Fennel (*Foeniculum vulgare* Mill.) Seeds with Supercritical CO_2: Comparison with Hydrodistillation. *Food Chemistry.* 2005; 92(1): 143-149.
18. Fang L, Qi M, Li T, Shao Q, Fu R. Headspace Solvent Microextraction-gas Chromatography-mass Spectrometry for the Analysis of Volatile Compounds from *Foeniculum vulgare* Mill. *Journal of Pharmaceutical and Biomedical Analysis.* 2006; 41(3): 791-797.
19. Singh G, Maurya S, de Lampasona MP, Catalan C. Chemical Constituents, Antifungal and Antioxidative Potential of *Foeniculum vulgare* Volatile Oil and its Acetone Extract. *Food Control.* 2006; 17(9): 745-752.
20. Tognolini M, Ballabeni V, Bertoni S, Bruni R, Impicciatore M, Barocelli E. Protective Effect of Foeniculum Vulgare Essential Oil and Anethole in an Experimental Model of Thrombosis. *Pharmacological Research.* 2007; 56(3): 254-260.
21. Telci I, Demirtas I, Sahin A. Variation in Plant Properties and Essential Oil Composition of Sweet Fennel (*Foeniculum vulgare* Mill.) Fruits during Stages of Maturity. *Industrial Crops and Products.* 2009; 30(1): 126-130.
22. Díaz-Maroto MC, Pérez-Coello MS, Esteban J, Sanz J. Comparison of the Volatile Composition of Wild Fennel Samples (*Foeniculum vulgare* Mill.) from Central Spain. *Journal of Agricultural and Food Chemistry.* 2006; 54(18): 6814-6818.
23. Gross M, Lewinsohn E, Tadmor Y, *et al.* The Inheritance of Volatile Phenylpropenes in Bitter Fennel (*Foeniculum vulgare* Mill. var. *vulgare,* Apiaceae) Chemotypes and their Distribution within the Plant. *Biochemical Systematics and Ecology.* 2009; 37(4): 308-316.
24. Guillén MD, Manzanos MJ. A Study of Several Parts of the Plant *Foeniculum vulgare* as a Source of Compounds with Industrial Interest. *Food Research International.* 1996; 29(1): 85-88.
25. Senatore F, Oliviero F, Scandolera E, *et al.* Chemical Composition, Antimicrobial and Antioxidant Activities of Anethole-rich Oil from Leaves of Selected Varieties of Fennel [Foeniculum Vulgare Mill. ssp. vulgare var. *azoricum* (Mill.) Thell] *Fitoterapia.* 2013; 90: 214-219.
26. Esquivel-Ferriño PC, Favela-Hernández JMJ, Garza-González E, Waksman N, Ríos MY, del Rayo Camacho-Corona M. Antimycobacterial activity of Constituents from *Foeniculum Vulgare* Var. Dulce grown in Mexico. *Molecules.* 2012; 17(7): 8471-8482.
27. Diao W, Hu Q, Zhang H, Xu J. Chemical Composition, Antibacterial Activity and Mechanism of action of Essential Oil from Seeds of Fennel (*Foeniculum vulgare* Mill.) *Food Control.* 2014; 35(1): 109-116.
28. Faudale M, Viladomat F, Bastida J, Poli F, Codina C. Antioxidant Activity and Phenolic Composition of Wild, Edible, and Medicinal Fennel from different Mediterranean Countries. *Journal of Agricultural and Food Chemistry.* 2008; 56(6): 1912-1920.
29. Nassar MI, Aboutabl EA, Makled YA, ElKhrisy EA, Osman AF. Secondary Metabolites and Pharmacology of *Foeniculum vulgare* Mill. Subsp. *Piperitum* . *Revista Latinoamericana de Química.* 2010; 38(2): 103-112.
30. Cherng J, Chiang W, Chiang L. Immunomodulatory Activities of Common Vegetables and Spices of Umbelliferae and its related Coumarins and Flavonoids. *Food Chemistry.* 2008; 106(3): 944-950.
31. Ghanem MTM, Radwan HMA, Mahdy EM, Elkholy YM, Hassanein HD, Shahat AA. Phenolic Compounds from *Foeniculum vulgare* (Subsp. *Piperitum*) (Apiaceae) herb and Evaluation of Hepatoprotective Antioxidant Activity. *Pharmacognosy Research.* 2012; 4(2): 104-108.

32. Albert-Puleo M. Fennel and Anise as Estrogenic Agents. *Journal of Ethnopharmacology.* 1980; 2(4): 337-344.
33. Abdul-Ghani AS, Amin R. The Vascular action of Aqueous extracts of *Foeniculum vulgare* Leaves. *Journal of Ethnopharmacology.* 1988; 24(2-3): 213-218.
34. Choi E, Hwang J. Antiinflammatory, Analgesic and Antioxidant Activities of the Fruit of *Foeniculum vulgare. Fitoterapia.* 2004; 75(6): 557-565.
35. Joshi H, Parle M. Cholinergic basis of Memory-strengthening Effect of *Foeniculum vulgare* Linn. *Journal of Medicinal Food.* 2006; 9(3): 413-417.
36. Gulfraz M, Mehmood S, Minhas N, *et al*. Composition and Antimicrobial Properties of Essential Oil of *Foeniculum vulgare. African Journal of Biotechnology.* 2008; 7(24): 4364-4368.
37. Özcan MM, Chalchat J, Arslan D, Ates A, Ünver A. Comparative Essential Oil Composition and Antifungal effect of Bitter Fennel (*Foeniculum vulgare* ssp. *piperitum*) Fruit Oils Obtained during different Vegetation. *Journal of Medicinal Food.* 2006; 9(4): 552-561.
38. Anwar F, Ali M, Hussain AI, Shahid M. Antioxidant and Antimicrobial Activities of Essential Oil and Extracts of Fennel (*Foeniculum vulgare* Mill.) Seeds from Pakistan. *Flavour and Fragrance Journal.* 2009; 24(4): 170-176.
39. Park SH, Seong I. Antifungal effects of the Extracts and Essential Oils from *Foeniculum vulgare* and *Illicium verum* against *Candida albicans. Korean Journal of Medical Mycology.* 2010; 15(4): 157-164.
40. Thakur N, Sareen N, Shama B, Jagota K. Studies on *in vitro* Antifungal Activity of *Foeniculum vulgare* Mill. against Spoilage Fungi. *Global Journal of Bio-Science and BioTechnology.* 2013; 2(3): 427-430.
41. Taie HAA, Helal MMI, Helmy WA, Amer H. Chemical Composition and Biological Potentials of Aqueous extracts of Fennel (*Foeniculum vulgare* L) *Journal of Applied Sciences Research.* 2013; 9(3): 1759-1767.
42. Kwon YS, Choi WG, Kim WJ, *et al.* Antimicrobial Constituents of *Foeniculum vulgare. Archives of Pharmacal Research.* 2002; 25(2): 154-157.
43. Zellagui A, Gherraf N, Elkhateeb A, *et al*. Chemical Constituents from Algerian Foeniculum Vulgare Aerial Parts and Evaluation of Antimicrobial Activity. *Journal of the Chilean Chemical Society.* 2011; 56(3): 759-763.
44. Yoshioka M, Tamada T. Aromatic Factors of Anti-platelet Aggregation in Fennel Oil. *Biogenic Amines.* 2005; 19(2): 89-96.

CHAPTER 16

Amazing Health benefit of Fenugreek (*Trigonella foenum-graecum* Linn.)

ABSTRACT

Fenugreek is known for its medicinal qualities such as antidiabetic, anticarcinogenic, hypocholesteremic, antioxidant, and immunological activities. Beside its medicinal value, it is also used as a part of various food product developments as food stabilizer, adhesive, and emulsifying agent. More importantly it is used for the development of healthy and nutritious extruded and bakery product. The main chemical components of fenugreek are fibers, lavonoids, polysaccharides, saponins, fixed oils and some identified alkaloids. Mature seeds mainly contain amino acid, fatty acid, vitamins, saponins and a large quantity of folic acid. It also contains disogenin, gitogenin, neogitogenin, homorientin saponaretin, neogigogenin, and trigogenin. The endosperm of the seed is rich with galactomannan. The young seeds mainly contain carbohydrates. In this review paper, the potential of fenugreek for disease prevention and health improvement has been emphasized.

Keywords: Diabetes; Fenugreek Lactone, Dietary fibres, Nutraceutical, Hypoglycemic, Gum extrudate.

Introduction

Fenugreek (*Trigonella foenum-graecum*) is a leguminous, herbaceous, rainfed crop included among the seed spices is about 30-60 cm tall, leaflets are about 2-2.5 cm long, flowers are 1-2 cm long, axillary, sessile and cultivated throughout the country and have been used as a spice throughout the world to enhance the sensory quality of foods. Fenugreek, a short-living, self-pollinating crop, is a native to Indian subcontinent and the Eastern Mediterranean region. It belongs to Fabaceae family and is used extensively in various parts of the world as herb, food, spice, and traditional medicine. It is an annual herb with white flowers and hard, yellowish brown and angular seeds, known from ancient times, for nutritional value beside of it medicinal attributes. Fenugreek seeds are rich source of gum, fiber, alkaloid, flavonoids, saponin and volatile content. Due to its high content of fiber, fenugreek could be used as food stabilizer, adhesive and emulsifying agent to change food texture for some special purposes. The present article is aimed to review the potential applications of fenugreek as a functional food and nutraceutical. This novel legume source provides soluble fiber along with other glucose-, cholesterol-, and triglyceride-lowering compounds [1-3]. This seed spice is employed for medicinal purpose in many traditional systems as antibacterial, gastric stimulant, against anorexia, antidiabetic agent and as a galactogogue. In recent decades, several health beneficial physiological attributes of fenugreek seeds have been seen in animal studies as well as human trials. Not only therapeutic, Fenugreek also used as spices worldwide. The leaves are used as green leafy vegetables in the diet. Fenugreek seeds are bitter in taste and have been in use for over 2500 years. In different languages it has different names, as *Fenugrec* (French), *Methi* (Hindi), *Bockshorklee* (German), *Fienogreco* (Italian), *Pazhitnik* (Russian), *Alholva* (Spanish), *Koroha* (Japanese), *Hulba* (Arabian), *Halba* (Malaya), and *K'u –Tou* (China). India is the major producer of Fenugreek and its main consumers are culinary and medicinal users. In the indigenous system, it is effective against anorexia and as gastric stimulant. Fenugreek having antidiabetic, antifertility, anticancer, antimicrobial, antiparasitic, lactation stimulant, hypocholesteremic influence, antioxidant potency, digestive stimulant action and hepatoprotective effect [4-6]. Among these beneficial physiological effects, the antidiabetic and hypocholesteremic property of fenugreek, both of which are mainly attributable to the intrinsic dietary fiber constituent, possess promising nutraceutical value, have been discussed in this comprehensive review paper.

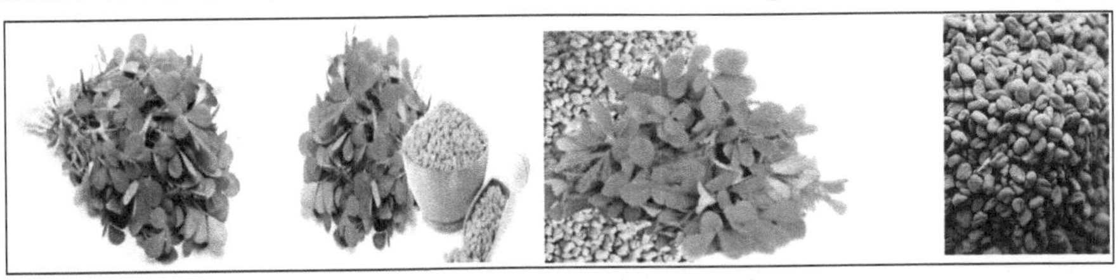

Phytochemistry and Pharmacology

Plant-derived natural products have long-standing utility toward treating degenerative diseases. Fenugreek is considered as one of the oldest medicinal plants and its health-promoting effects have been cited in Ayurveda and traditional Chinese medicine. In recent decades, several health beneficial physiological attributes of fenugreek seeds have been seen in animal studies as well as human trials. These include antidiabetic effect, hypocholesteremic influence, antioxidant potency, digestive stimulant action, and hepatoprotective effect. The investigations into the chemical composition and pharmacological actions have seen a renaissance in recent years. Extensive preclinical and clinical research have outlined the pharmaceutical uses of fenugreek as antidiabetic, antihyperlipidemic, antiobesit y, anticancer, anti-inflammatory, antioxidant, antifungal, antibacterial, galactogogue and for miscellaneous pharmacological effects, including improving women's health. The pharmacological actions of fenugreek are attributed to diverse array of phytoconstituents [5-8]. The phytochemical analysis reveals the presence of steroids, alkaloids, saponins, polyphenols, flavonoids, lipids, carbohydrates, amino acids, and hydrocarbons. It is also used for conditions that affect heart health such as "hardening of the arteries" (atherosclerosis) and for high blood levels of certain fats including cholesterol and triglycerides. Fenugreek is used for kidney ailments, a vitamin deficiency disease called beriberi, mouth ulcers, boils, bronchitis, infection of the tissues beneath the surface of the skin (cellulitis), tuberculosis, chronic coughs, chapped lips, baldness, cancer, Parkinson's disease and exercise performance. Fenugreek has been associated with increased testosterone levels and enhanced sexual function in middle age men with androgen deficiency symptoms, as well as with a reduced severity of both menopausal symptoms and dysmenorrhea, including menstrual pain, fatigue, headache, nausea, and lack of energy. These hormone-regulating actions, equally beneficial for both men and women, are attributed to a high content of phytoestrogens (stearic acid, palmitic acid, and beta-sitosterol) and steroidal saponins (diosgenin, tigogenin, neotigogenin, and yamogenin). The presence of phytomenadione (a vitamin K derivative that aids coagulation), as well as alkaloids, aminoacids (such as lysine), also contributes to the galactagogue, hypoglycemic, and hormone balancing properties of fenugreek. Additionally, fenugreek's omega-3 fatty acids and dietary fiber, as well as a water-soluble polysaccharide called galactomannan, are thought to contribute with the beneficial effects of fenugreek on metabolic functions. Galactomannan has been shown to help regulate digestive enzymes, also inhibiting the absorption of glucose in the gastrointestinal tract. Fenugreek seeds contain no essential oil and their characteristic scent and flavor are due to the presence of fenugreek lactone (sotolone), an extremely powerful odorant agent [6-9].

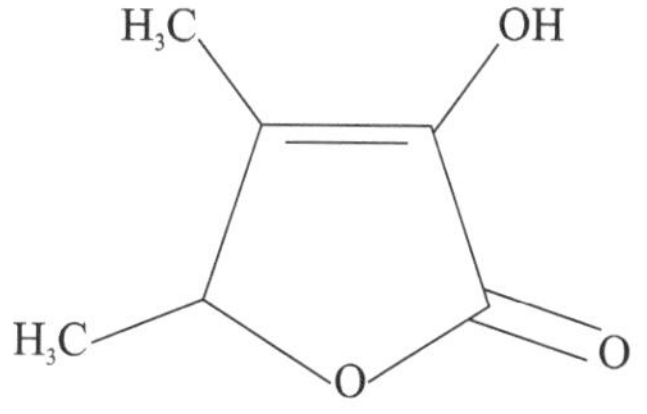

Galactomannan structure

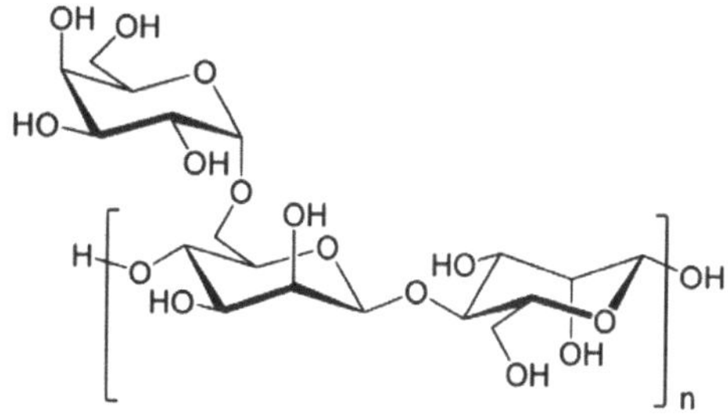

Structure of Fenugreek Lactone

Fenugreek contains a number of chemical constituents including steroidal sapogenins. Diosgenin component has been found in the oily embryo of fenugreek. There are two furastanol glycosides, F-ring opened precursors of diosgenin that have been reported in fenugreek also as hederagin glycosides. Alkaloids such as trigocoumarin, nicotinic acid, trimethyl coumarin and trigonelline are present in stem. The mucilage is a standing out constituent of the seeds. There is about 28% mucilage; a volatile oil; 2 alkaloids such as trigonelline and Choline, 5% of a stronger-smelling, bitter fixed oil, 22% proteins and a yellow coloring substance are present in stem. Fenugreek contains 23-26% protein, 6-7% fat and 58% carbohydrates of which about 25% is dietary fiber. Fenugreek is also a rich source of iron, containing 33 mg/100 g dry weight [10-14].

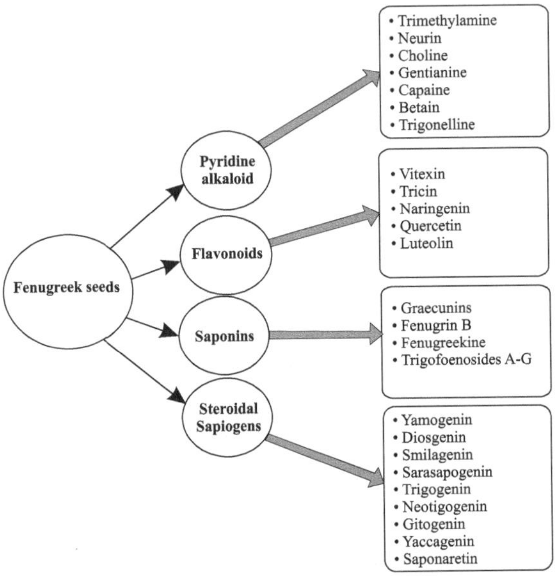

The leaves contain seven saponins, known as graecunins. These compounds are glycosides of diosgenin. Leaves contain about 86.1% moisture, 4.4% protein, 0.9% fat, 1.5% minerals, 1.1% fiber, and 6% carbohydrates. The mineral and vitamins present in leaves include calcium, zinc iron, phosphorous, riboflavin, carotene, thiamine, niacin and vitamin C. It has been found that fresh leaves of fenugreek contain ascorbic acid of about 220.97 mg per 100 g of leaves and β-carotene is present about 19 mg/100 g. On the other side, it was reported that 84.94% and 83.79% ascorbic acid were reduced in sun and oven-dried fenugreek leaves respectively. Fresh leaves are used as vegetables in the diets. It was found that there was a better retention of nutrients in the leaves of fenugreek. Fenugreek is known for its pleasantly bitter, slightly sweet seeds. The seeds are available in any form whether whole or ground form is used to flavor many foods mostly curry powders, teas and spice blend. Fenugreek seed has a central hard and yellow embryo which is surrounded by a corneous and comparatively large layer of white and semi-transparent endosperm. The chemical composition of fenugreek (such as seeds, husk and cotyledons) showed that endosperm had the highest (4.63 g/100 g) saponin and (43.8 g/100 g) protein content. As against this, husk contains higher total polyphenols. The seeds of fenugreek contain about 0.1-0.9% of diosgenin and are extracted commercially. The plant tissue cultures from seeds of fenugreek when grown under optimal conditions have been found to produce as much as 2% diosgenin with smaller amounts of trigogenin and gitongenin [12-16]. Seeds also contain the saponin (fenugrin B). Fenugreek seeds have been found to contain several coumarin compounds as well as a number of alkaloids (e.g., trigonelline, gentianine, carpaine). The large amount of trigonelline is degraded to nicotinic acid and related pyridines during roasting. The major bioactive compounds in fenugreek seeds are believed to be polyphenol compounds, such as rhaponticin and isovitexin. Small amount of volatile oils and fixed oil has been found in fenugreek seeds have found the odor active compounds based on the fenugreek aroma detection with the help of Gas Chromatograph and these includes the olfactometry diacetyl, 1-Octene-3-one, sotolon, acetic acid; 3-Isobutyl-2-methoxypyrazine, butanoic acid, isovaleric acid, 3-isopropyl-2-methoxypyrazine, caproic acid, eugenol, 3-Amino-4,5-dimethyl-3, linalool, (Z)-1,5-Octadiene-3-one, 4-dihydro-2(5H)-Furanone with characteristic aroma of buttery like, roasty/earthy, metallic, pungent, paprika like, sweaty/rancid, flowery, musty, spicy respectively. Out of all these volatile compounds, sotolon was reported to be found most predominantly in (5s)-enantiomeric form (95%) in fenugreek. A study was conducted on sweat of human after fenugreek ingestion and it has been concluded that compounds responsible for the strong maple-syrup odor present in sweat after fenugreek ingestion are due to the following components including the following: pinene; 3-octen-2-one, 2,5-dimethylpyrazine, β-; camphor; terpinen-4-ol; 4- isopropyl-benzaldehyde; neryl acetate and β-caryophyllene but it was observed that 2,5-dimethylpyrazine to be a major component responsible for sweat odor contributing compound [15-18].

Odorous compound	Aroma quality
l-Octen-3-one	Mushroom-like
(Z)-l,5-Octadiene -3-one	Metallic
3-Isopropyl-2-methoxy pyrazine	Roasty, earthy
Acetic acid	Acidic, pungent
3-Isobuty-2-methoxy pyrazine	Roasty, paprika-like
Linalool	Flowery
Butanoic acid	Sweaty, rancid
Isovaleric acid	Sweaty, rancid
Caproic acid	Musty
Eugenol	Spicy
3-Amino-4,5-dimethyl 3, 4-dihydro-2-(5*H*) furanone	Seasoning-like
Stolon	Seasoning-like

Odorous chemical constituents occurring in aroma extract of fenugreek seeds

Chemical structures of (1) Diosgenin (2) rhaponticin and (3) isovitexin (Volatile contents)

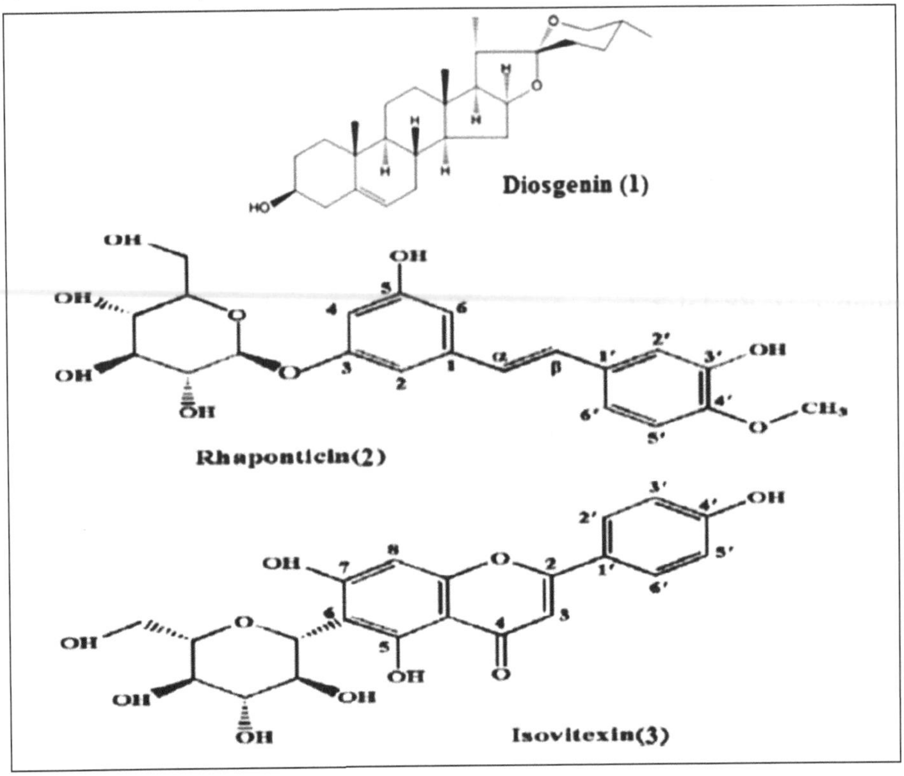

Use of Fenugreek in Day to day life

Methi seeds are a great remedy for diabetics. Methi helps in controlling the blood sugar level. The amino acid compounds in fenugreek seeds increase insulin secretion in the pancreas which helps in lowering the blood sugar level in the body. Consumption of fenugreek helps in treating kidney stones. Methi seeds help in improving kidney health. Drinking methi water will keep you full for long. Methi is packed with fiber which gives you a feeling of fullness. This helps you manage your weight. When you feel full, you don't eat many calories and also prevents you from bingeing on unhealthy snacks. It also prevents bloating. Fenugreek seeds have nutrients that help in hair growth. Consuming fenugreek water will promote hair growth, improve hair volume and keep hair problems such as dandruff, roughness at bay. Fenugreek or methi water helps in flushing out the harmful toxins from your body and it helps in improving your bowel movement. It helps you fight against digestive problems. It prevents constipation, indigestion among other digestion problems [17-20]. Methi is immensely useful for your skin and hair too.

Fenugreek is taken for digestive problems such as loss of appetite, upset stomach, constipation, inflammation of the stomach (gastritis). Fenugreek is also used for painful menstruation, polycystic ovary syndrome and obesity. Some men use fenugreek for hernia, erectile dysfunction, male infertility, and other male problems. Both men and women use fenugreek to improve sexual interest. Fenugreek is used for a variety of purposes. Fenugreek seed extract is the principal flavoring ingredient of simulated maple syrup. It is also used as a tobacco-flavoring ingredient, hydrolyzed vegetable protein flavor, perfume base, and a source of steroid sapogenin in drug manufacturing industries. The leaves are commonly consumed as a vegetable [18-22]. Currently, there is not enough conclusive evidence to fully support the use of fenugreek for any medical purpose. However, people have been using fenugreek in varying forms for hundreds or potentially thousands of years to treat a very wide range of conditions, such as: digestive problems, including constipation, loss of appetite, and gastritis; breast milk production and flow; diabetes; low testosterone or libido; painful menstruation; menopause; arthritis; high blood pressure; obesity; breathing problems; boils; low exercise; performance; ulcers; open wounds; muscle pain; migraines and headaches; childbirth pains. Of all the reported health benefits of fenugreek, only a few have been substantially backed by scientific evidence. Among other benefits, some research suggests that fenugreek may: Quite a few studies in animals have shown that at least four compounds in fenugreek have antidiabetic properties. They primarily: reduce intestinal glucose absorption; delay gastric emptying; improve insulin sensitivity and action; reduce concentrations of lipid-binding protein. Fenugreek may help stimulate breast milk production and ease the flow. Practitioners of traditional Asian medicine have long recommended fenugreek for this purpose. Fenugreek may suppress the appetite and increase feelings of fullness, which could help reduce overeating and lead to weight loss. Fenugreek may help increase low testosterone and sperm levels. Fenugreek may help regulate cholesterol levels and improve blood pressure, which can reduce the risk of developing heart conditions and improve heart health. Fenugreek has long been used for pain relief in traditional systems of medicine. Researchers think that compounds called alkaloids in the herb help block sensory receptors that allow the brain to perceive pain [19-23].

Traditional uses

The medicinal value of fenugreek seeds is mentioned in Ayurvedic texts as well as in Greek and Latin pharmacopoeia. The Ayurvedic texts praise this herb for its power as an aphrodisiac, but modern vaidyas seem to be using it more for digestive and respiratory problems stemming from an excess of kaph (phlegm) and vat (wind). In ancient Egypt, methi was used to ease childbirth and to increase milk flow and modern Egyptian women are still using it today to relieve menstrual cramps, as well as making hilba tea out of it to ease other kinds of abdominal pain. The Chinese call it hu lu ba, and also use it for treating abdominal pain. Though this cool season crop is grown in most corners of the world, its uses and people's awareness of its value vary considerably.

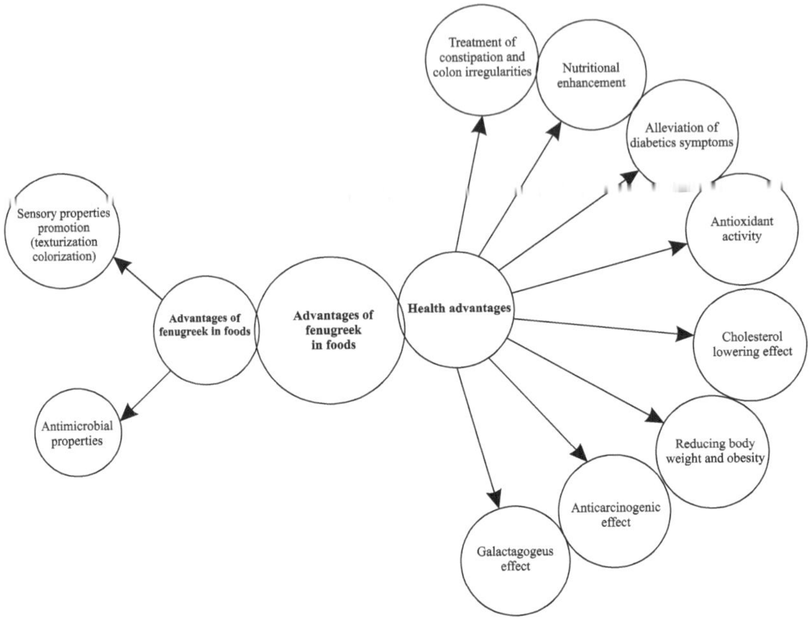

In India, fresh methi ka saag (the stems and leaves of the plant) is very commonly cooked as a winter vegetable, and the seeds are used year-round as a flavoring agent for various dishes. The seeds are also eaten raw as sprouts and used medicinally. In Egypt and Ethiopia, methi is used in baking bread, and the Swiss use it for flavoring cheese. In the USA, it is mainly used to make spice blends for soups and stews [22-24]. The herb of fenugreek has been used for centuries as a cooking spice in European countries and it remains a popular ingredient in curry powders, pickles and spice mixtures in India Pakistan, Bangladesh and other Asian countries. Fenugreek has been used in the folk medicines for the treatment of cellulitis, boils, and tuberculosis. Fenugreek remained a key ingredient in a 19th century patent medicine for dysmenorrheal and postmenopausal symptoms. It also has been recommended for the promotion of lactation. The seeds of fenugreek have been used as an orally as insulin substitute for reduction in blood glucose and the extracts from seed have been reported to lower blood glucose levels. The maple aroma and flavor of fenugreek have led to its use in imitation maple syrup [23-25].

Fenugreek usage in Bakery and extruded Products

The interaction of fenugreek protein with the food constituents determines its ability to stabilize and emulsify the food constituents. The effect of fenugreek gum on solubility and emulsifying properties of soy protein isolate has been evaluated and reported that the emulsifying activity of soy protein isolate with fenugreek gum was four times higher than that of soy protein isolate with fenugreek gum or fenugreek gum alone and the results were to those of bovine serum albumin. The emulsifying stability of soy protein isolate with fenugreek gum dispersions was respectively three times higher than that of soy protein isolate with fenugreek gum and bovine serum albumin. Emulsifying properties and solubility of soy protein isolate with fenugreek gum dispersions were also stable over wide ranges of high temperature, pH and ionic strength. Fenugreek contains higher dietary fiber content which acts as probiotic in functional food. The soluble fiber of fenugreek acts as an excellent substrate for fermentation done by the microorganisms in the large intestine. The dietary fiber of fenugreek has potential for widespread use in the food industry because its galactomannan composition has emulsifying and stabilizing properties. Flour supplemented with a percentage of 8% and 10% of fenugreek dietary fiber has been used in the production of baked goods such as bread, pizza, muffins and cakes. This application of fenugreek to flour allows for the production of functional foods that may be widely acceptable to consumers observing western diets [24-26]. Fenugreek paste, locally termed as "Cemen" is a popular food in Turkey which is prepared from ground fenugreek seeds. Crushed fenugreek seed or coarse fenugreek powder is used to make ball for making clarified butter. Adding fenugreek fiber to refined flours helps to fortify with a balance of soluble and insoluble fiber. Flour fortified with 8-10% fenugreek fiber has been used to prepare bakery foods such as pizza, bread, muffins, and cakes with acceptable sensory properties. Fenugreek seed husk is a rich source of dietary fiber and several important minerals. This fiber-rich functional ingredient can be incorporated in the manufacture of high-fiber muffins. The fiber-rich muffins possessed good volume, soft texture and medium-fine grain with twice the amount of DF incorporated fenugreek in bread and demonstrated that fenugreek in food helps in reduction of blood sugar but due to its bitterness and strong odor its use is restricted. They did not find significant variation in color, texture, proximate composition, firmness, and flavor intensity between the wheat and fenugreek bread, but level of glucose and insulin was found to be lower in the fenugreek bread. Fenugreek's functional property of reducing insulin resistance was maintained in the bread. Therefore, it is evident from this study that fenugreek can be incorporated in baked products in acceptable limit which will reduce insulin resistance and treat diabetic patients as well. Fenugreek flour has been incorporated up to a 10% level in the formulation of biscuits without affecting their overall quality. The physical, sensory and nutritional characteristics generally revealed that biscuits containing 10% germinated fenugreek flour were the best among all the composite fenugreek flour biscuits. Hence, development and utilization of such functional foods will not only improve the nutritional status of the general population but also helps those suffering from degenerative diseases. In a study incorporation of fenugreek flour up to 10% level has been used in the formulation of biscuits [25-27]. Baking quality, color attributes and organoleptic evaluation revealed that wheat flour can be replaced using 10% Soaked Fenugreek and 20% Germinated Fenugreek flours to produce acceptable and high nutritional value biscuits. The study confirmed that fenugreek seed (raw, soaked and germinated) significantly reduced total lipids, serum total cholesterol, and LDL-cholesterol but non-significant changes in triglycerides and serum HDL-cholesterol were observed. It can be recommended that fenugreek may be used for lipid lowering purposes. Supplementation of basal diets with fenugreek leaves, seeds (dry and germinated) and wheat flour supplemented with germinated fenugreek powder at 5-10% levels increased the total proteins, fibers, iron, zinc, calcium, vitamin B_2, carotene, vitamin E and vitamin C contents. These dietary supplements also improve the blood picture of anemic rats so they have nutritive and restorative properties. The daily use of fenugreek products as a dietary supplement is proved to be safe and healthy. Therefore, this study recommends that intake of fenugreek products may be beneficial for patients who suffer from iron deficiency anemia owing to their nutritive and restorative values. In the same way 10% germinated fenugreek seed flour has been incorporated into the wheat based biscuits formula resulted in improving their chemical and nutritional quality and additionally also complimented the deficiency of lysine, isoleucine, leucine, threonine and valine, and hence neutralizes the amino acid imbalance. Fenugreek seed flour and fenugreek leave powder have been used for the development of extruded snacks. In a study a mixture of about 1.78% fenugreek seed flour and 0.66% fenugreek leaves powder with the base material was found to have high preference levels for parameters of physical, functional and color and could be extruded with acceptable quality characteristics. The effects of fenugreek flour and debittered fenugreek polysaccharide inclusion on the physical and sensory quality characteristics and glycemic index (GI) of chickpea–rice based extruded products were studied. Due to the distinct bitter taste, inclusion of fenugreek flour was not acceptable at levels more than 2% in extruded chickpea based products. Addition of fenugreek polysaccharide resulted in slight reduction in radial expansion, while longitudinal expansion increased. Water absorption index increased while water solubility index decreased compared to the control. The mean scores of sensory evaluation indicated that all products containing fenugreek polysaccharide up to 15% were within the acceptable range. There were no significant differences between products containing 5-15% fenugreek polysaccharide in their color, flavor, texture and overall quality. Fenugreek, in the form of debittered polysaccharide could be incorporated up to a level of 15% in a chickpea–rice blend to develop snack products of acceptable physical and sensory properties with low GI. In another study, fenugreek gum was extruded in a twin-screw extruder without an exit die to minimize a decrease in molecular weight of fenugreek gum during extrusion process. Both the steady and dynamic shear rheological tests revealed that extrusion process did not substantially influence the steady and dynamic shear properties of the gum. The power law model was applied to describe the flow behavior of the extruded gum solutions. The extrusion modified fenugreek gum solutions exhibited a shear thinning flow behavior at 25 °C, and the values of consistency index and apparent viscosity increased with an increase in the gum concentration. The magnitudes of storage modulus and loss modulus for the extrusion modified fenugreek gum solutions increased with increasing frequency and with increasing gum concentration. Fenugreek gum (extruded and non-extruded) was substituted for wheat flour at 0%, 5% and 10% (w/w) and the rheological effects and bread making characteristics were determined [22-26]. Bread containing fenugreek gum (FG) at 5% and 10% showed volumes and texture comparable with control bread. Extruding FG also improved its solubility in bread. Fenugreek gum resulted in an increase in dough farinograph water absorption compared with the control, but extruding the gum caused an even greater increase in water absorption when compared with the non-extruded gum. The addition of FG to bread dough caused an increase in storage modulus (*G*2) and loss modulus (*G*3). Starch pasting using RVA showed an increase in peak viscosity, final viscosity, breakdown and setback in a dose-related response when compared with a control. Another study showed the addition of fenugreek gum (FG) to the extruded pea–rice snack products. In addition to fenugreek gum, two more gums (guar gum and locust bean gum) were added to it. When these three gums were added to the formulations at levels of up to 20%, good expansion of the products occurred. The WAI of the extrudates containing FG increased with increasing inclusion levels. In addition to the high contents of starch that serve to provide energy, these snacks are good sources of protein and dietary fiber, and are low in fat, qualifying them as low GI snack products. In particular, the reduction in GI was the greatest with fenugreek gum extrudates [23-29].

Discussion and Conclusion

Fenugreek is the famous spices in human food. The seeds and green leaves of fenugreek are used in food as well as in medicinal application that is the old practice of human history. Fenugreek seeds are rich with vitamin E. Fresh Fenugreek leaves are beneficial for indigestion, flatulence and in sluggish liver treatment. Regular use of fresh Fenugreek leaves paste helps hair grow, preserves natural color, keeps hair silky and also cures dandruff. Fenugreek Seeds made in gruel are given to nursing mothers to increase the flow of milk and also reduce the amount of calcium oxalate in the kidney which causes kidney stones. In animal studies, Fenugreek appeared to lowering the chance of developing colon cancer by blocking the action of certain enzymes. Fenugreek is currently used as a source of the steroid diosgenin, one of its active constituent from which other steroids can be synthesized. Not only that Fenugreek has a broad range of pharmacological profile but also it has antidiabetic activity, antiplasmodic activity, hypolipidemic activity, immunological activity, antibacterial activity, anthelmintic activity, anti-inflammatory, analgesic activity and antioxidant activity. These beneficial physiological effects including the antidiabetic and hypocholesteremic effects of fenugreek are mainly attributable to the intrinsic dietary fibers constituent which have promising nutraceutical value. It has been used to increase the flavoring and color, and also modifies the texture of food materials. It is well known for its fiber, gum, other chemical constituents and volatile contents. Dietary fiber of fenugreek seed is about 25% which changes the texture of food. These days, it is used as food stabilizer, adhesive and emulsifying agent due to its high fiber, protein and gum content. The protein of fenugreek is found to be more soluble at alkaline pH. Fenugreek is having beneficial influence on digestion and also has the ability to modify the food. Fenugreek has been found to have important bioactive compounds. From this review, it was observed that fenugreek has been used as food stabilizer, food adhesive, food emulsifier and gum. Fenugreek has been used to produce various types of bakery products and extruded product. Based on these several health usefulness as discussed in review, based on various past reported scientific findings, fenugreek can be recommended and must be taken as a part of our daily diet as its liberal use is safe and various health benefits can be drawn from this natural herb. The above-mentioned studies on fenugreek suggest that the functional, nutritional and therapeutic characteristics of fenugreek can be exploited further in the development of healthy products. Wonderful functional and medicinal values of fenugreek are attributed to its chemical composition proteins, dietary fiber, mucilaginous soluble fiber, fixed fatty acids and essential oils, and steroidal saponins. Moreover, some minor components such as alkaloids (trigonolline, cholin, gentianine, carpaine, etc.), free unnatural amino acids (4-hydroxyisoleucine), and individual spirostanols and furastanols like diosgenin, gitogenin and yamogenin have also been identified and determined as the main component for its various biological effects. Regarding the composition of fenugreek seeds, husk and cotyledons it has been reported that endosperm had the highest saponin and protein content, whereas husk had higher total polyphenols and total dietary fiber, comprising insoluble dietary fiber and soluble dietary fiber. It has been shown that fenugreek has antidiabetic, anticancer, hypocholesteremic, anti-inflammatory, antioxidant and chemopreventive activity due to its useful chemical constituents. Fenugreek has strong flavor and aroma. The plants leaves and seeds are widely consumed in Indo-Pak subcontinent as well as in other oriental countries as a spice in food preparations and as an ingredient in traditional medicine. A wide range of uses were found for fenugreek in ancient times. Medicinally, it was used for the treatment of wounds, abscesses, arthritis, bronchitis, ulcer and digestive problems. Traditional Chinese herbalists used it for kidney problems and conditions affecting the male reproductive tract. Fenugreek was, and remains, a food and a spice commonly eaten in many parts of the world. Among the spices, the Fenugreek is used as esoteric food adjacent to enhance the flavor and colour of the food and make it tasty and also used to modify the texture of food. The seeds and plants are basically hot and dry and also they are suppurative, aperient, and diuretic. They have some useful aspect in dropsy, chronic cough, enlargement of the liver and the spleen. The leaves of Fenugreek are useful for both internal and external swellings and burns and also used to prevent the hair falling off. The seeds are considered as carminative, tonic and aphrodisiac. Fenugreek is used to ease child birth as well as it helps to increase the milk flow of mother. Egyptian women are still taking Fenugreek for menstrual pain and tourist use it as hilba tea to remove stomach problem. Not only that the plant is also recommended for use in dyspepsia with loss of appetite, in diarrhea of puerperal women and in rheumatism. An infusion of seeds is given to small-pox patients as a cooling drink. Fenugreek seed contains various bioactive compounds like flavonoids (quercetin, rutin, vetexin), saponins (graecunins, fenugrin B, Fenugreekine), amino acids (isoleucine, 4- hydroxyisoleucine, histidine, leucine, lysine). As medicinal plant, it shows its activity against allergies, appetite/loss of catarrh, bronchial, cholesterol, diabetic retinopathy, gas, gastric disorders, lung infections, mucus excessive, throat/sore, abscesses, anemia, asthma, boils, body odour, bronchitis, cancer, swollen eyes, fevers, gallbladder problems, heartburn, inflammation, sinus problems, ulcers, uterine problems etc. A study in India showed that Fenugreek seed is used to reduce the blood sugar and other harmful fats. The evidence to date suggests that fenugreek can be a potential natural health product for the prevention and treatment of type II diabetes. This novel legume source provides soluble fiber along with other glucose-, cholesterol- and triglyceride-lowering compounds. It would be a significant contribution to the daily management and stabilization of blood glucose and lipid levels for non-insulin-dependent diabetics. Fenugreek has antioxidants and anti-inflammatory properties. Among the spices that are esoteric food adjuncts being used to enhance flavoring and color, fenugreek also modifies the texture of food. This seed spice is also employed for medicinal purpose in many traditional systems as antibacterial, gastric stimulant, against anorexia, antidiabetic agent and as a galactogogue. It is important to increase awareness of the public, dieticians, and other health professionals as to the unique properties of fenugreek and to recommend it for the prevention of hyperglycemia and hyperlipidemia.

REFERENCES

1. Srinivasan K. Fenugreek (Trigonella foenum-graecum): A Review of Health Beneficial Physiological Effects.Food Rev Int. 2006; 22(2): 203-224doi; 10.1080/875591 20600586315222K
2. Mooventhan A, Nivethitha L. A Narrative Review on Evidence-based Antidiabetic Effect of Fenugreek (Trigonella Foenum-Graecum). Int J Nutr Pharmacol Neurol Dis. 2017; 7: 84-87.
3. Sharma RD, Sarkara A., Hazra DK, Mishra B, Singh JB, Sharma, SK, Maheshwari BB, Maheshwari PK. Use of Fenugreek Seed Powder in the Management of Non-insulin Dependent Diabetes Mellitus. Nutr Res. 1996; 16: 1331-1339.
4. Sharma RD. Effect of Fenugreek Seeds and Leaves on Blood Glucose and Serum Insulinresponses in Human Subjects. Nutr. Res. 1986; 6: 1353-1364.
5. Srinivasan K. Role of Spices beyond Food Flavouring: Nutraceuticals with Multiple Healheffects. Food Rev Int. 2005; 21: 167-188.
6. Srinivasan K, Sambaiah K, Chandrasekhara N. Spices as Benefical Hypolipidemic Foodadjuncts: A Review. Food Rev Int. 2004; 20: 187-220.
7. Singhal RD, Glatzel H. Physiological aspects of Flavour Compounds. Ind spices. 1968; 5: 13-21.
8. Venkata KCN, Swaroop A , Debasis Bagchi D, Bishayee A. A Small Plant with Big Benefits: Fenugreek (Trigonella foenum-graecum Linn.) for Disease Prevention and Health Promotion. Mol Nutr Food Res doi: 10.1002/mnfr.201600950
9. Wani SA Kumar P. Fenugreek: A Review on its Nutraceutical Properties and Utilization in Various Food Products.J Saudi Soc Agri Sci. 2018; 17, Issue (2): 97-106. https://doi.org/10.1016/j.jssas.2016.01.007
10. Basch EC. Ulbricht C, Kuo G, Szapary P, Smith M. Therapeutic Applications of Fenugreek. Altern Med Rev. 2003; 8 (1): 20-27.
11. Blank J, Lin S, Devaud, R. Fay FLB. The Principal Flavour Components of Fenugreek (*Trigonella foenum graecum*) S.J. Risch, T.H. Chi (Eds.), 1997; Spices: Flav Chem Antioxi Proper, ACS, Washington, DC.
12. Bukhari SB, Muhammad IB, Shahabuddin M. Antioxidant Activity from the Extract of Fenugreek Seeds. Pak J Anal Environ. Chem. 2008; 9 (2): 78-83.
13. Chang YH, Cui SW, Roberts KT, Ng PKW, Wang Q. Evaluation of Extrusion-modified Fenugreek GumFood Hydro Colloid. 2011; 25: 1296-1301.
14. Chatterjee, S.Variyar P, Sharma A. Bioactive Lipid Constituents of Fenugreek. Food Chem. 119 (2010), pp. 349-353
15. Chauhan G, Sharma M, Varma A, Khanrkwal H. Phytochemical Analysis and Anti-inflammatory Potential of Fenugreek, Medicinal Plants Int J Phytomed Rel Ind. 2010; 2 (1): 39-44.
16. Im KK, Maliakel B. Fenugreek Dietary Fibre a Novel Class of Functional Food Ingredient. Agro Food Ind Hi-Tech. 2008; 19: 18-21.

17. Meghwal M, Goswami TK. A Review on the Functional Properties, Nutritional Content, Medicinal Utilization and Potential Application of Fenugreek. J Food Process Technol. 2012; 3: 9-12.
19. Passano P. The many uses of Methi. Manushi. 1995; 2: 31-34.
20. Snehlata HS, Payal DR. Fenugreek (*Trigonella foenum-graecum* L.): An Overview. Int. J Curr Pharm Rev Res. 2012; 2 (4): 169-187.
21. Ghosh B, Chandra I, Chatterjee S. Fenugreek (Trigonella foenum-graecum L.) and its necessity [Review paper]. Fire J Eng Technol. 2025; 1(1): 60-67.
22. Akbari M, Rasouli H, Bahdor T. Physiological and Pharmaceutical Effect of Fenugreek: A Review. IOSR J Pharm 2012; 2(4): 49-53.
23. Khorshidian N, Asli MY, Arab M, Mirzaie AA, Mortazavian AM. Review Article Fenugreek: Potential Applications as a Functional Food and Nutraceutical. Nutr Food Sci Res. 2016; 3(1): 5-16.
24. Naidu M, Shyamala B, Naik JP, Sulochanamma G, Srinivas P. Chemical Composition and Antioxidant Activity of the Husk and Endosperm of Fenugreek Seeds. Food Sci Technol-Leb. 2011; 44(2): 451-456.
25. Youssef M, Wang Q, Cui S, Barbut S. Purification and Partial Physicochemical Characteristics of Protein free Fenugreek Gums. Food Hydrocolloid. 2009; 23(8): 2049-2053.
26. El Nasri NA, El Tinay A. Functional Properties of Fenugreek (Trigonella foenum graecum) Protein Concentrate. Food Chem. 2007; 103(2): 582-589.
27. Srinivasan K. Fenugreek (Trigonella foenum-graecum): A Review of Health Beneficial Physiological Effects. Food Rev Int. 2006; 22(2): 203-224.
28. Shang M, Cai S, Han J, Li J, Zhao Y, Zheng J, *et al*. Studies on Flavonoids from Fenugreek (Trigonella foenumgraecum L.). China journal of Chinese Materia Medica. 1998; 23(10): 614-616.
29. Yadav UC, Baquer NZ. Pharmacological Effects of Trigonella foenum-graecum L. in Health and Disease. Pharm Biol. 2014; 52(2): 243-54.

CHAPTER

17

Engrossing Dietetic régime of Prophylactic Flaxseeds (*Linumusita tissimum* L.)

ABSTRACT

Preventing the occurrence of CVD with nutritional interventions is a therapeutic strategy that may warrant greater research attention. The increased use of omega ω-3 fatty acids is a powerful example of one such nutritional strategy that may produce significant cardiovascular benefits. Marine food products have provided the traditional dietary sources of ω-3 fatty acids. Flaxseed is an alternative to marine products. It is one of the richest sources of the plant-based ω-3 fatty acid, ALA. Based on the results of clinical trials, epidemiological investigations and experimental studies, ingestion of ALA has been suggested to have a positive impact on CVD. Because of its high ALA content, the use of flaxseed has been advocated to combat CVD. Amongst its other incredible nutrition facts, flax seeds are also packed with antioxidants. Lignans are unique fiber-related polyphenols that provide us with antioxidant benefits for anti-aging, hormone balance and cellular health. The purpose of the present review was to identify chemical constituents of flaxseeds and their exemplary therapeutic usage with special reference to ALA and, just as importantly, what is presently unknown.

Keywords: ALA, ω-3 fatty acid, Lignans, CVD, Phytoesterogens

Introduction

Flaxseed, or linseed (*Linumusita tissimum* L.), comes from the flax plant, which is an annual herb. The ancient Egyptians used flaxseed as both food and medicine. The Latin name of flaxseed means "very useful", and it has two basic varieties: brown and yellow or golden (also known as golden linseeds). The flax plant is a small, single-stemmed annual that grows to about 2 ft. (0.6 m) tall and has grayish green leaves and sky-blue flowers. Historically, flax has been cultivated for thousands of years. Linen made from flax has been found in the tombs of Egyptian pharaohs and is referred to in the Bible and in Homer's Odyssey. The Roman naturalist Pliny wrote about the laxative and therapeutic powers of flax in the first century AD, and many authorities believe it has been used as a folk remedy since ancient times. Flax is believed to be native to Egypt, but its origins are questionable since it has been used widely around the world. It is cultivated in many places, including Europe, South America, Asia, and parts of the United States1-3 Flaxseed is one of the most important oilseed crops for industrial as well as food, feed, and fiber purposes [1-3]. Almost every part of the flaxseed plant is utilized commercially, either directly or after processing. The stem yields good quality fiber having high strength and durability. The seed provides oil rich in omega-3, digestible proteins, and lignans. In addition to being one of the richest sources of α-linoleic acid oil and lignans, flaxseed is an essential source of high quality protein and soluble fiber and has considerable potential as a source of phenolic compounds. Flaxseed is emerging as an important functional food ingredient because of its rich contents of lignans, and fiber. Lignans appear to be anti-carcinogenic compounds [4-5]. The omega-3s and lignan phytoestrogens of flaxseed are in focus for their benefits for a wide range of health conditions and may possess chemo-protective properties in animals and humans.

Flax seeds come from flax which is a fiber crop that dates back to ancient Egypt. Flax seeds are thus, high in fiber. In addition to their fiber content, they are a rich source of antioxidants as well as healthy fats. There are two kinds of flax seeds, golden and brown, that have very similar nutritional make ups. Flax seeds contain high concentrations of two essential polyunsaturated fatty acids— linoleic acid (*x*-6) and *a*-linolenic acid (*x*-3), which cannot be produced by the human body. Their oxidation occurs rapidly in the air. [3-6]

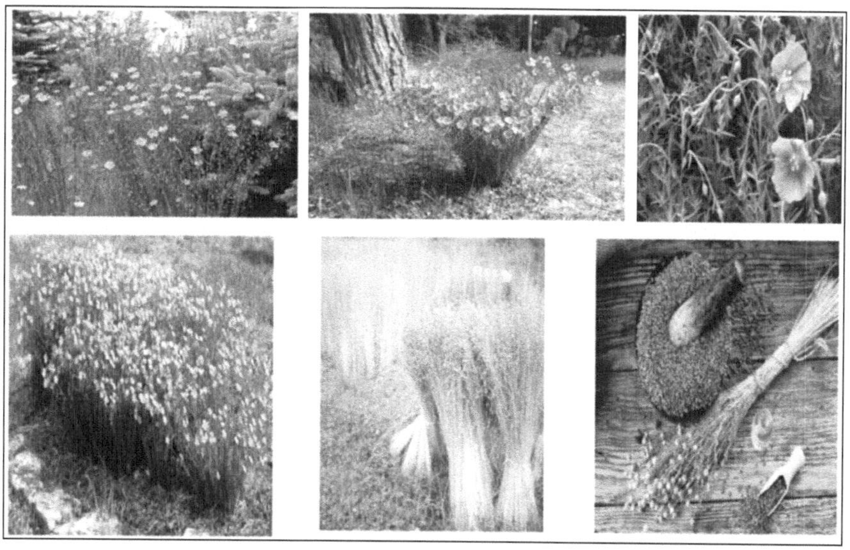

Types of Seeds

There are two main types of flaxseed: golden flaxseed and brown flaxseed. Their nutritional profiles are very similar and both contain the same number of short-chain omega-3 fatty acids. The ANA (American Nutrition Association) highlighted the importance of this "neglected food," stating that flaxseed is not only "an excellent source of two fatty acids that are essential for human health - linoleic acid and alpha-linolenic acid," but also, "an excellent source of fiber and a good source of minerals and vitamins.

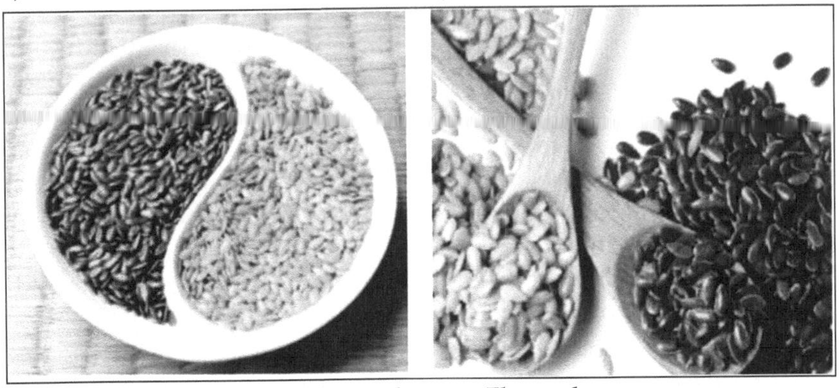

Golden and Brown Flaxseeds

Flaxseed Nutrition Facts

One of the most extraordinary benefits of flax seeds is that they contain high levels of mucilage gum content. Mucilage is a gel-forming fiber that is water soluble and has incredible benefits on the intestinal tract. The mucilage can keep food in the stomach from emptying too quickly into the small intestine which can increase the absorption. Also, flax is extremely high in both soluble and insoluble fiber which can support colon detoxification, fat loss and reduce sugar cravings. The ALA fats in flax seeds benefits the skin and hair by providing essential fats as well as b-vitamins which can help reduce dryness and flakiness. It can also improve symptoms of acne, rosacea, and eczema. This also applies to eye health as flax can reduce dry eye syndrome. The soluble fiber content of flax seeds trap fat and cholesterol in the digestive system so that it unable to be absorbed [7-9].

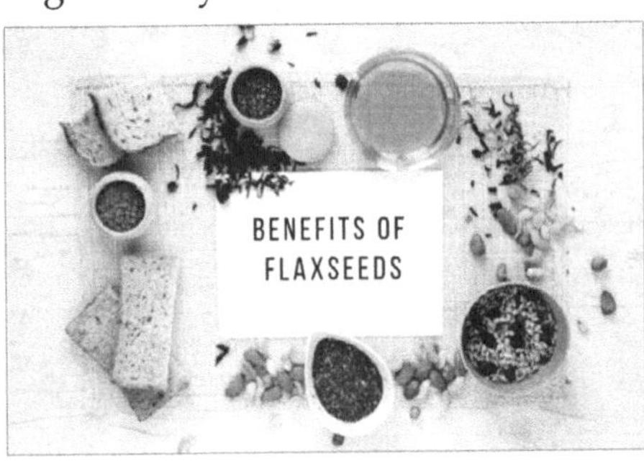

Soluble fiber also traps bile, which is made from cholesterol in the gallbladder. The bile is then excreted through the digestive system, forcing the body to make more, using up excess cholesterol in the blood and lowering cholesterol overall. Using flax is a great way to naturally replace gluten-containing grains which are inflammatory where flax is anti-inflammatory [9-11]. So, flax seeds are great for those who have Celiac disease or have a gluten-sensitivity. They may also be a good alternative to omega-3 fats in fish for people with a seafood allergy. Amongst its other incredible Nutrition facts, flax seeds are also packed with antioxidants. Lignans among all commonly eaten foods, researchers now rank flaxseeds as the no.1 source of lignans in human diets, containing about 7x as many lignans as the closest runner-up food (sesame seeds). They contain about 338x as many lignans as sunflower seeds, 475x as many as cashew nuts and 3,200x as many lignans as peanuts) are unique fiber-related polyphenols that provide us with antioxidant benefits for anti-aging, hormone balance and cellular health. Polyphenols support the growth of probiotics in the gut and may also help eliminate yeast and candida in the body. Lignans are also known for their anti-viral and antibacterial properties, therefore consuming flax regularly may help reduce the number or severity of colds and flus. Maybe the biggest flax seed benefits come from its ability to promote digestive health. The ALA in flax can help protect the lining of the digestive tract and maintain GI health. It has been shown to be beneficial for people suffering from Crohn's disease or other digestive ailments, as it can help reduce gut inflammation. Flax is also very high in soluble and insoluble fiber which can also improve digestive health and is one of the highest magnesium foods in the world. Flax seed benefits have been proven time and time again and even including fighting breast, prostate, ovarian and colon cancer [12-15]. The three lignans found in flaxseeds can be converted by intestinal bacteria into enterolactone and enterodiol which naturally balance hormones which may be the reason flax seeds reduce the risk of breast cancer. The lignans in the flax have been shown to have benefits for menopausal women. It can be used as an alternative to hormone replacement therapy because lignans do have estrogenic properties. These properties may also help reduce the risk of osteoporosis. It can even help menstruating women by helping maintain cycle regularity. A study published in *Nutrition Reviews* has shown that approximately 20% of ALA can be converted into EPA, but only 5% of ALA is converted into DHA. Also, surprisingly gender may play a big role in conversion where young women had a 2.5-fold greater rate than men. Regardless of conversion, ALA is still considered a healthy fat and should be included in a balanced diet [16-18]. Flaxseeds or *Alsi* are not commonly included in our daily diet, but those tiny, brown seeds pack a lot of health benefits that you might not know about. Containing Omega-3 fatty acids (also known as 'good fat'), lignans (rich in antioxidants and estrogen content) and fiber, flaxseeds are great for your health, here's why.

Lignans present in flaxseed, are known to improve the blood sugar levels in type 2 diabetics having flaxseed on a daily basis can help maintain your blood sugar levels over an extended period of time. Flaxseeds are great for your heart health. Not only do they help prevent the formation of plaque within your arteries, but they also prevent atherosclerosis (when the arteries become stiff and less elastic), reduce blood pressure, heart rate and beat oxidative stress (due to its antioxidant properties). Apart from that flaxseeds can help lower the levels of bad cholesterol (or LDL cholesterol) in check, protecting your heart. The high content of antioxidants and Omega 3 fatty acids protect against breast cancer, prostate cancer and colon cancer. The lignin content in flaxseed especially protects against tumors that are hormone sensitive e.g. estrogen-sensitive breast tumors [19-21]. The omega 3 fatty acids, lignans and ALA (alpha-linolenic acid) present in flaxseeds are known to block the release of inflammatory agents and are especially beneficial for patients who suffer from diseases such as arthritis, and Parkinson's disease. Hot flashes are a problem that is commonly associated with menopausal women. If you suffer from this condition then flaxseeds can help. The antioxidant properties of flaxseeds help regularize the hormonal imbalance responsible for hot flashes and a study found that women who had a spoon of flaxseeds regularly experienced a 57% drop in the intensity of hot flashes they experienced [22-25]. Flaxseed may also help to lower cholesterol, control high blood pressure, protect against heart disease, control constipation, heal hemorrhoids, prevent painful gallstones and dissolving existing ones, it promotes healthy hair and nails, treats acne, eczema, reduces cancer risk, treats menopausal symptoms, infertility and male impotence! Make sure to include any form of flax in your daily diet, it is a must for the gout sufferer. Flaxseed's oil is very high in Omega-3 fatty acids and levels vary from the types and colors of the flax seed, usually in a yellow or brownish color. Just one teaspoon contains about 2.5 grams, the equivalent of more than twice the amount most people get through their diets! Flaxseeds also provide you with calcium, magnesium and potassium, all of which are needed in any gout diet. Flaxseeds also have omega-6 fatty acids in the form of linoleic acid. Flaxseed oil only contains alpha-linolenic acid (Omega 3 oils), and not the fiber or lignan components. Flaxseed is also good for gout sufferers that can't eat any fish which is on the higher end in the purines scale since it may trigger gout attacks for them [26-27]. Fish oil or flax seed oil supplements are into existence for obtaining health benefits from omega 3 fatty acids. Omega 3 fatty acids are essential fatty acids as these cannot be synthesized in our body and must be obtained from food or supplements. Three types of omega-3 fatty acids are ALA (alpha-linolenic acid), EPA (eicosapentaenoic acid) and DHA (docosahexaenoic acid). Omega-3 supplements in the form of EPA and DHA are what offers many of the evidence based benefits when used in the body and can be supplemented with fish oil. Flax seed oil contains omega-3 in the form of ALA from which the body can make EPA and EPA is finally converted to DHA but the ratio of conversion is not efficient [28-30].

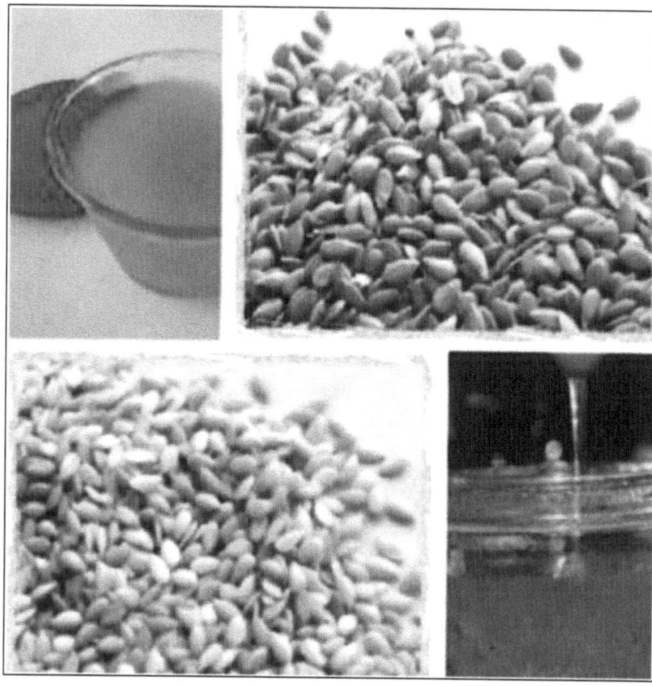

Estimates of the rate of conversion range from 5% to 25%. Several factors further reduce the ability to convert ALA to EPA. For example, with growing age this rate of conversion is diminished. ALA also competes metabolically with the other essential fatty acid omega-6. Too much of omega-6 in the diet leading to unbalanced fatty acid ratios also negatively affects the conversion. Looking at typical Indian diet excess of omega-6 through grains, cereals and cooking oil like sunflower oil is undeniable. Other factors like gender (conversion of ALA to EPA is limited in men and further transformation to DHA is very low.), medications, alcohol consumption, deficiency of certain micronutrients etc. also affect the conversion rate. Thus, omega-3 fatty acid from flax seed cannot be considered substitute for omega-3 fatty acids from fish oil [31-32]. The best option for those who cannot have fish oil can be DHA rich algae oil. Fish consume algae and therefore are rich in DHA and EPA. Algae are the primary producers of DHA and EPA in the ecosystem, and several refined algal oils are rich sources of DHA. DHA is retroconverted to EPA following supplementation. Due to nontrivial retroconversion efficiency between omnivores and vegetarians, DHA supplementation represents an alternative to fish oil to increase blood and tissue levels of EPA, and DHA.

Nutritional value of flaxseed per 20 g (2 tbsp)

Energy - 54.7 kcal (DV = 3%)	Carbohydrates - 3.0 g (DV = 1%)
Sugars - 0.2 g	Dietary fiber - 2.8 g (DV = 11%)
Fat - 4.3 g (DV = 7%)	Saturated fat - 0.4 g (DV = 2%)
Monounsaturated fat - 0.8 g	Polyunsaturated fat - 2.9 g
Protein - 1.9 g (DV = 4%)	Thiamine (vit B1) - 0.2mg (DV = 11%)
Riboflavin 0.0mg	Niacin (vit. B3) - 0.3mg (DV = 2%)
Pantothenic acid (B5) - 0.1mg (DV = 1%)	Vitamin B6 - 0.0 mg
Folate - 8.9 mcg (DV = 2%)	Vitamin C - 0.1 mg (DV = 0%)
Calcium - 26.1mg (DV = 3%)	Iron - 0.6mg (DV = 3%)
Magnesium - 40.2 mg (DV = 10%)	Phosphorus - 65.8mg (DV = 7%)
Potassium - 83.3 mg (DV = 2%)	Zinc - 0.4mg (DV = 3%)

Source: USDA Database

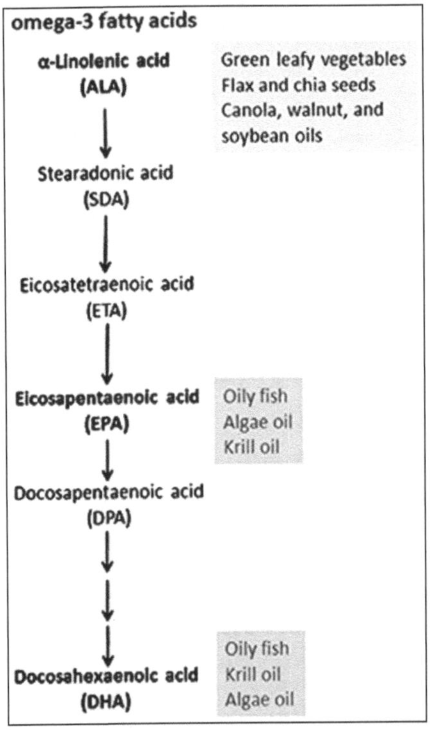

Therapeutic Importance of Flaxseed Oil

Flaxseed oil is used medicinally. Linseed oil is the term usually used for the oil found in polishes, varnishes, and paints. Flaxseed oil is derived from the flax plant's crushed seeds, which resemble common sesame seeds but are darker. The amber oil is very rich in a type of fat called alpha-linolenic acid (ALA), an omega-3 fatty acid that is good for the heart and found in certain plants. High amounts of omega-3 fatty acids are found in fish and smaller amounts are found in green leafy vegetables, soy-derived foods, and nuts. Studies suggest that they can lower triglyceride levels and reduce blood pressure. Omega-3 fatty acids may also decrease the risk of heart attacks and strokes by preventing the formation of dangerous blood clots within arteries. In high dosages, the fatty acids may help to alleviate arthritis, though flaxseed products have not yet been shown to be effective for this purpose. In addition to omega-3 fatty acids, flaxseed products also contain potentially therapeutic chemicals called lignans. Lignans are believed to have antioxidant properties and may also act as phytoestrogens, very weak forms of estrogen found in fruits, vegetables, whole grains, and beans. Unlike human estrogen, phytoestrogens have dual properties: they can mimic the effects of the hormone in some parts of the body while blocking its effects in others. Many herbalists believe that phytoestrogens can be useful in the prevention or treatment of a variety of diseases, including cancer , CVD and osteoporosis . The estrogen-blocking effects of phytoestrogens may be particularly effective at combating certain cancers that depend on hormones, such as cancers of the breast or uterus. Women who consume large amounts of lignans appear to have lower rates of breast cancer. The fact that heart disease and certain cancers occur less frequently in Asian countries is sometimes attributed to a diet rich in plant foods containing phytoestrogens [32-34]. Flaxseed is sometimes referred to as a nutraceutical, a recently coined term that includes any food or food ingredient thought to confer health benefits, including preventing and treating disease. Several studies, some conducted in people, suggest that flaxseed products (or agents contained in them) may help to keep the heart and cardiovascular system healthy. Flaxseed products may lower cholesterol levels, help control blood pressure and may reduce the buildup of plaque in arteries. Test tube and rat studies suggest that chemicals in flaxseed may help to prevent or shrink cancerous tumors. Due to its estrogen-like effects, some women use flaxseed oil to ease breast tenderness, alleviate symptoms of PMS (premenstrual syndrome), and help control menopausal symptoms. Flaxseed oil has also been recommended to treat skin conditions, inflammation, and arthritis. It is usually taken internally for all the purposes mentioned above. The oil may be used externally to help the healing of scalds and burns. More recently, flaxseed has been shown to be beneficial for people suffering from digestive disorders. It is now recommended as an "effective herbal agent" for treating IBS [30-34].

Culinary Asset

Finding creative ways to add flaxseeds to your meals can be a challenge. One popular technique is to incorporate ground flaxseeds into your muffin, cookie, or bread recipes. Recent research studies have shown that ground flax can be added to baked foods without sacrificing large amounts of alpha-linolenic acid (ALA), their showcase omega-3 fatty acid that accounts for over half of their total fat content. Oven temperatures of 300° F (150°C) -

even over several hours of baking time - do not appear to substantially reduce the amount of ALA in baked products. This outcome has been demonstrated for breads, muffins and cookies. Even when flaxseeds are ground prior to incorporatation into breads and pastas, these preparation methods - involving grinding prior to heating - only appear to lower ALA levels by about 4-8%. Interestingly, bread enriched with ground flaxseed has also been shown to have a greater antioxidant capacity and a much lower GI (glycemic index) value (of ~ 51) than the same bread without the ground flaxseed addition. These research findings are great news for anyone who wants to include flaxseeds in baked dishes, in either whole or ground form.You could start off by having one tablespoon of ground flaxseed powder every morning on an empty stomach with a glass of warm water. Alternatively, you can even add it to your energy drink or fresh juice or include it in your meals by sprinkle one tablespoon of flaxseed powder on the dish you cook.Remember to not put the powder directly into hot oil, as the excess heat tends to deactivate the beneficial properties of flaxseed and may add a bitter taste to your food. Also do not have more than 2 tablespoons per day, as it can be detrimental to your health.

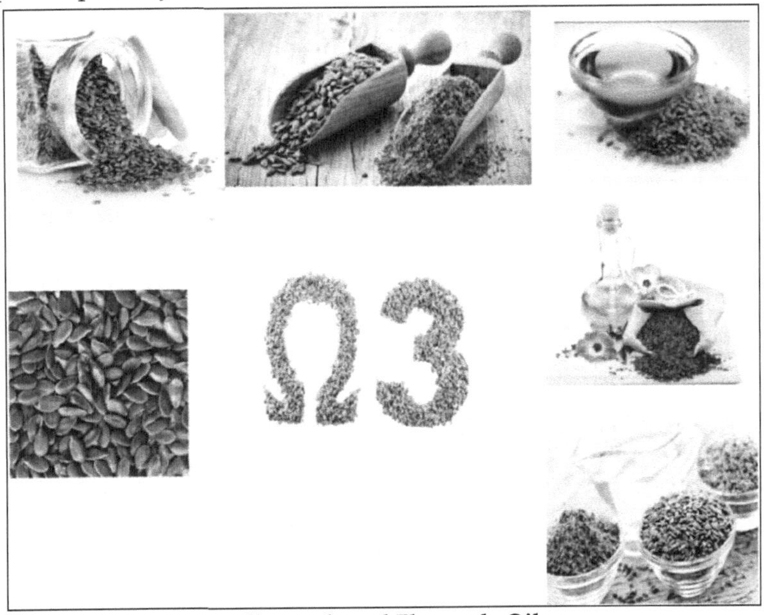

Flaxseeds and Flaxseeds Oil

Conclusion

Flaxseeds are extremely good for one's health. They are a prime source of ω-3 fatty acids which makes them a must-have in one's diet especially if you are a vegetarian. Flax seeds also rich in Fe, Zn, Ca, Ca, K, Mg, protein, folate, soluble fiber and even B. They are high in antioxidants which prevent free-radical damage by protecting healthy cells from getting damaged. Flax may be beneficial in suppressing the growth of breast and prostate cancers because when consumed, tumor cell proliferation goes down, cancer cell death increases, and c-erbB2 score is reduced. Combining flaxseed with dietary fat restriction may have an even greater effect on prostate cancer. Eating only 1 tbs of ground flaxseed a day may help prevent and reverse diabetes. Eating flaxseeds may also diminish skin sensitivity and improve skin barrier function and condition. Because lignans are activated by our gut bacteria, taking antibiotics may impair the production of the lignans. They also contain dietary fibre which is essential for regulating proper bowel movements. Fibre prevents constipation and also keeps you fuller for a longer time. So people who are on a weight loss diet should eat flaxseeds regularly. When flaxseeds are compared with other commonly eaten foods in terms of their total polyphenol content (polyphenols are one very important group of antioxidants), flaxseeds rank 9th among 100 commonly eaten foods. Flaxseeds turn out to be significantly higher in polyphenol antioxidants than fruits like blueberries or vegetables like olives. The antioxidant benefits of flaxseeds have long been associated with prevention of cardiovascular diseases and have recently also been tied to decreased insulin resistance. Flaxseeds also help keep lifestyle diseases like diabetes, high BP, heart disease at bay.

REFERENCES

1. Gebauer SK, Psota TL, Harris WS, Kris-Etherton PM. n-3 Fatty Acid Dietary Recommendations and Food Sources to Achieve Essentiality and Cardiovascular Benefits. Am J Clin. 2006; 83: 1526S-35S.
2. Francois CA, Connor SL, Bolewicz LC, Connor WE. Supplementing Lactating Women with Flaxseed Oil does not Increase Docosahexaenoic Acid in their Milk. Am J Clin. 2003; 77: 226-33.
3. Burdge GC, Calder PC. Dietary α-linolenic Acid and Health-related Outcomes: A Metabolic Perspective. Res Rev. 2006; 19: 26-52.
4. Zhao G, Etherton TD, Martin KR, West SG, Gillies PJ, Kris-Etherton PM. Dietary Alpha-linolenic Acid Reduces Inflammatory and Lipid Cardiovascular Risk Factors in Hypercholesterolemic Men and Women. J. 2004; 134: 2991-7.
5. Seidelin KN, Jensen B, Haugaard SB, Reith J, Olsen TS. Ischemic Stroke and n-3 Fatty Acids. J Stroke Cereb Dis. 1997; 6: 405-9.
6. Stuglin C, Prasad K. Effect of Flaxseed Consumption on Blood Pressure, Serum Lipids, Hemopoietic System and Liver and Kidney Enzymes in Healthy Humans. J CardiovascPharmacolTher. 2005; 10: 23-7.
7. Lemay A, Dodin S, Kadri N, Jacques H, Forest JC. Flaxseed Dietary Supplement versus Hormone Replacement Therapy in Hypercholesterolemic Menopausal Women. Obstet Gynecol. 2002; 100: 495-504.
8. Harper CR, Edwards MC, Jacobson TA. Flaxseed Oil Supplementation does not Affect Plasmlipoprotein Concentration or Particle Size in Human Subjects. J. 2006; 136: 2844-8.
9. Bloedon LT, Szapary PO. Flaxseed and Cardiovascular Risk. Rev. 2004; 62: 18-27.
10. Rise P, Marangoni F, Galli C. Regulation of PUFA Metabolism: Pharmacological and Toxicological Aspects. Prostaglandins LeukotEssent Fatty Acids. 2002; 67: 85-9.

11. Hallund J, Tetens I, Bügel S, Tholstrup T, Bruun JM. The Effect of a Lignan Complex isolated from Flaxseed on Inflammation Markers in Healthy Postmenopausal Women. MetabCardiovasc Dis. 2008; 18: 497-502.
12. Tohgi N. Effect of Alpha-linolenic Acid-containing Linseed Oil on Coagulation in Type 2 Diabetes. Diabetes Care. 2004; 27: 2563-4.
13. Allman MA, Pena NM, Pang D. Supplementation with Flaxseed Oil versus Sunflower Oil in Healthy Young Men Consuming a Low Fat Diet: Effects on Platelet Composition and Function. Eur J Clin. 1995; 49: 169-78.
14. Akabas SR, Deckelbaum RJ. Summary of a Workshop on n-3 Fatty Acids: Current Status of Recommendations and Future Directions. Am J Clin. 2006; 83 (Suppl): 1536S-8S.
15. Spence JD, Thornton T, Muir AD, Westcott ND. The Effect of Flax Seed Cultivars with Differing Content of α-linolenic Acid and Lignans on Responses to Mental Stress. J Am Coll. 2000; 22: 494-501.
16. Chaudhary K, Agarwal M, Rani B, Jat BL, Abid M, Khan MMAA, Naqvi MS, Maheshwari RK. (2015). Experimental Optimization of Extraction Conditions of Phenolic Compounds from Flax Seed, *Pisum*peel, *Aloe* peel. J BiolChem Res2015; 33(1): 1-23.
17. Rani B, Bhati I, Dhawan NG, Rajnee, Sharma S,Tyagi SN, Maheshwari RK. Dietary Antioxidants to Prop up Vigour & Vitality: An Overview. J Drug DiscovTherapeut. 2013; 1 (7): 106-122.
18. Rani B, Singh U, Maheshwari R. Natural Antioxidants and their Intrinsic Worth for wellbeing. Glob J Med Res.2013; XIII (B-VII): 54-69.
19. Daun JK, Barthet VJ, Chornick TL, Duguid. Structure, Composition, and Variety Development of Flaxseed. Flaxseed in Human Nutrition Thompson LU, Cunnane SC. 2003; 1-40.
20. Singh KK, Mridula D, Rehal J, Barnwal P. Flaxseed: A Potential Source of Food, Feed and Fiber. Crit Rev Food Sci Nut. 2011; 51(3): 210-222.
21. Leyva DR, Dupasquier C, McCullough R, Pierce G. The Cardiovascular Effects Offlaxseed and its Omega-3 Fatty Acid, Alpha-linolenicacid. The Canadian J Cardiol. 2010; 26(9), 489-496.
22. Harper CR, Edwards MJ, Filippis APD. Jacobson TA. Flaxseed Oil Increases the Plasmaconcentrations of Cardioprotective (n-3) Fatty Acids in Humans. J Nut.2006; 136: 83-87.
23. Rabetafika HN, Remoortel V, Danthine S, Paquot M, Blecker C. Flaxseed Proteins: Fooduses and Health Benefits. Int J Food Sci. Technol. 2011; 46: 221-228.
24. Chung MWY, Lei B, Chan ECYL.Isolation and Structural Characterization of the Major Protein Fraction from NorMar Flaxseed (Linumusitatissi-mum L.). Food Chem. 2005; 90: 271-279.
25. HoC, Cacace J, Mazza G. Extraction of Lignans, Proteins and Carbohydrates from Flaxseedmeal with Pressurized Low Polarity Water. LWT FoodSci Technol. 2007; 40: 1637-1647.
26. Rubilar M, Gutierrez C, Verdugo M, Shene C, Sineiro J. Flaxseed as a Source of Functional Ingredients. J Soil Sci Plant Nut. 2010; 10: 373-377.
27. Thompson LU, Rickard SE, Orcheson L.J, Seidl MM. Flaxseed and its Lignan and Oil Components reduce Mammary Tumor Growth at a Late Stage of Carcinogenesis. Carcinogenesis. 1996; 17: 1373-1376.
28. Thompson LU, Seidl MM, Rickard SE, Orcheson LJ, Fong HH. Antitumorigenic Effect of a Mammalian Lignan Precursor from Flaxseed. Nut Cancer, 1996; 26: 159-165.

29. Bloedon L, Szapary P. Flaxseed and Cardiovascular Risk. Nut Rev. 2004; 62(1): 18-27.
30. Oomah BD, Mazza G. Flaxseed Proteins: A Review. Food Chem. 1993 48: 109-114.
31. Bourre JM. Dietary Omega-3 Fatty Acids and Psychiatry: Mood, Behaviour, Stress, Depression, Dementia and Aging." J Nut Health Aging. 2005; 9(1): 31-8.
32. Lowcock EC1, Cotterchio M, Boucher BA. Consumption of Flaxseed, a Rich Source of Lignans, is Associated with Reduced Breast Cancer Risk. Cancer Causes Contr. 2013; 24(4): 813-6. doi: 10.1007/s10552-013-0155-7.
33. Kislev ME, Simchoni O, Melamed Y, Maroz L. Flax Seed Production: Evidence from the Early Iron Age site of Tel Beth-Shean, Israel and from Written Sources VegetHist Archaeobot. 2011; 20: 579-584doi: 10.1007/s00334-011-0303-5.
34. Shisty S, Monika. Health Benefits and Nutritional Value of Flaxseed- a Review.Ind J Appl Res. 2016; 6(1): 243-245.

CHAPTER

18

Hing (*Ferula asafoetida* Linn.) for overall Health benefits

ABSTRACT

Ferula asafoetida Linn. is a main source of asafoetida, a strong, tenacious and sulfurous odor, and oleogum resin of medicinal and nutritional importance. Asafoetida has been consumed as a spice and a folk medicine for centuries. Recent studies have shown several promising activities particularly relaxant, neuroprotective, memory enhancing, digestive enzyme, antioxidant, antispasmodic, hypotensive, hepatoprotective, antimicrobial, anticarcinogenic, anticancer, anticytotoxicity, antiobesity, anthelmintic and antagonistic effect. Plant *F. asafetida* is herbaceous, monoecious, perennial herb that belongs to the family Apiaceae (Umbelliferaceae). The plant has a fetid smell due to the presence of sulfur constituents. Asafoetida or Hing is the dried latex or oleogum resin extracted from the rhizomes or roots of this perennial herb. It is a native species of Iran, Afghanistan and Pakistan. It carries a strong, tenacious and sulfurous odor. It is also used as a spice or as a condiment in various cookeries as a flavor like in curries, fresh vegetables, meat, pickles and pulses. Traditionally, the plant is used to treat diseases like whooping cough, asthma, bronchitis, epilepsy, ulcer, stomachache, flatulence, bronchitis, antispasmodic, intestinal parasites, influenza and weak digestion. The main active constituents present in the *Ferula asafetida* plant are resins, gums and essential oils. This review effectively deals with phytochemistry and various pharmacological and clinical studies of asafoetida.

Keywords: Oleo-gum-resin, Sulfur compounds, antispasmodic, stomacache.

Introduction

Asafoetida is used as a flavoring agent in food and as a traditional medicine for many diseases in many parts of the world. Asafoetida (*Ferula asafoetida*) is an oleogum-resin obtained from the stems of *Ferula* plants belonging to the family *Umbelliferae.* Out of more than 170 species, sixty spices of *Ferula* are widely distributed in Central Asia, particularly West Afghanistan, Iraq, Turkey and Eastern Iran, Europe and North Africa. *F. asafoetida* is one of the important species of *Ferula* and is more native to

Afghanistan and Iran than grows about 2 m in height and is in two types bitter and sweet. It is commonly called Hing/Hingua or Devil's dung [1-3]. Asafoetida is extracted from the *Ferula* plants which have massive taproots or carrot-shaped roots, around 15 cm in diameter at the crown when they are 4-5 years old. Before the plants flower, the upper part of the living rhizome root is laid bare and the stem cut off close to the crown. A dome- shaped structure made of twigs and earth covers the exposed surface. A milky juice exudes from the cut surface. The exudates are scraped off and a fresh slice of the root cut when more latex exudes, sometimes the resin is removed along with the slice. The collection of resin and slicing of the root are repeated until exudation ceases. Asafoetida has a strong, tenacious and sulfurous odor. Nowadays it is a popular ingredient in the Indian cuisine, most probably because its odor is reminiscent of the flavor of garlic and onion, two sprouting vegetables, as well as meat. Asafoetida is traditionally used for the treatment of different diseases, such as whooping cough, asthma, ulcer, epilepsy, stomachache, flatulence, bronchitis, intestinal parasites, antispasmodic, weak digestion and influenza. Asafoetida is an effective remedy for several diseases of the stomach [4-7]. The digestive stimulant actions of asafoetida are the most commonly experimented beneficial physiological effect via enhanced secretion of saliva and activity of salivary amylase. It plays an important role in the digestion of dietary lipids by stimulating bile flow and enhances the bile acid secretion and also enhances the activities of digestive enzymes of the pancreas and small intestine. Moreover, it is used for low acid levels in the stomach, stomach pressure, flatulence and loose stools. It is specially considered an ailment for women. It is used as a treatment of several problems such as unwanted abortion, unusual pain, sterility, difficult and excessive menstruation and leucorrhoea. Recent pharmacological and biological studies have also shown several activities, such as antioxidant, antimicrobial, antiviral, antifungal, cancer chemopreventive, anti-diabetic, anticarcinogenic, antispasmodic and hypotensive, relaxant effect, neuroprotective and molluscicidal from this asafoetida. The present review deals with phytochemistry, various pharmacological and clinical studies of asafoetida [8-10].

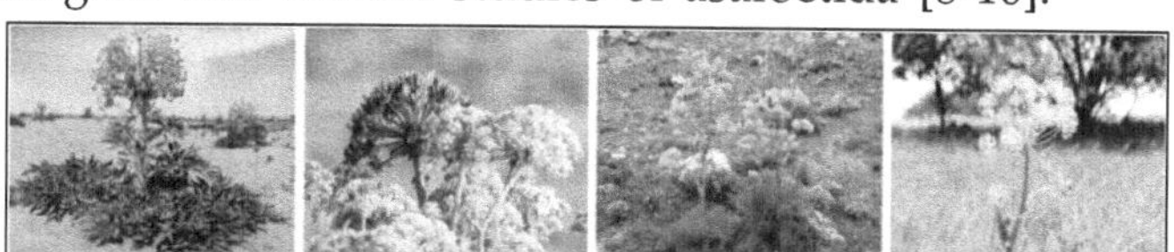

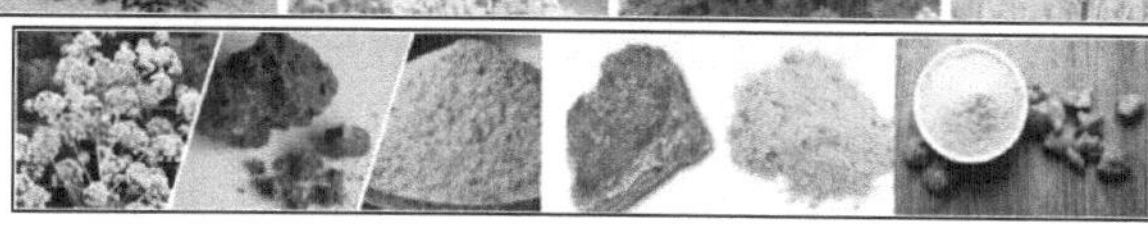

Chemical Constituents

There are various chemical constituents present in the Ferula asafoetida plant includes carbohydrates (68%), moisture (16%), protein (4%), fats (1%), minerals (7%) and fibers (4%). The major chemical constituent consist of three main fractions which include resins (40-64%), gums (25%) and essential oil (10-17%). The phenolic compound and diterpenes are also present in the F. asafetida plant which includes vanillin, dimethoxycinnamyl-3-(3, 4-diacetoxyphenyl) acrylate, picealactone C, 7-oxocallitristic acid. Resins include coumarins, sesquiterpene coumarins, ferulic acids and their esters, and other terpenoids. The coumarin and sesquiterpene constituents include umbelliprenin, 5-hydroxyumbelliprenin, 8-hydroxyumbelliprenin, ludohiferin, galbanic acid, 8-acetoxy-5-s-hydroxyumbelliprenin, conferol, gummosin, epi-samarcandin, epi-samarcandin acetate, franesiferol, Asacoumarin. Assfoetidin, ferocaulicin, assafoetidinol A and B, polyanthinin, komolonol, foetidine, saradaferin. 10-R-acetoxy-11-hydroxyumbelliprenin, 10-R-karatavicinol, methyl galbanate, lehmferin, feselol, ligupersin A, epi-conferdione, microglobulin, umbelliferone, taraxacin,fetidone A and B. Gum includes glucose, rhamnose, galactose, 1-arabinose,glucuronic acid, polysaccharides and glycoproteins. The volatile fraction contains a sulfur-containing compound which includes 2-butyl 1-propenyl disulfide, 1-(methyl thio)-2-propenyl disulfide, 2-methyl-2-propanethiol, 2-butyl 3-(methylthio)-2-propenyl disulfide, 2, 3-dimethylthiirane, s-methylpropanethioate, dimethyltrisulfide, dipropyldisulfiefoetisulfide A and C, monoterpenes and other volatile terpenoids that are responsible for biological activities. The other compounds found in the *Asafetida* plant includes oleic acid, beta-sitosterol, falcarinolone, arabinose, rhamnose, ferulic acid, luteolin 7-beta-d-glucopyranoside and glucuronic acid [11-20].

Traditional and Contemporary Uses

Ferula asafetida is considered as the most important remedial plant in Ayurveda. *F. asafoetida* plant has a characteristic sulfurous odor and has a bitter taste. In Ayurveda, it is used to treat gastrointestinal disorders and is useful as an effective remedy against flatulency. It is used in roasted form because the unprocessed as a *fetida* causes irritation and inflammation. It is used to treat nervous disorders and is considered an effective remedy for hysteria. It is also useful as an aphrodisiac agent and is used to treat impotence. It balances the Kapha and Vatadosha and increases Pitta dosha. It is used to treat diseases like impotence, whooping cough, asthma, skin disorders, gastrointestinal disorders like stomachache, acidity, nervine disorders, reproductive disorders and is used as a carminative, diuretic and laxative agent [21-22]. The *F. asafetida* plant is used to treat various types of diseases. It helps in treating gastrointestinal disorders and is used mainly in the roasted form. In the eastern region of Shimoga of India, it is used to cure stomachache. It is used as a condiment in various dishes as well in meat.

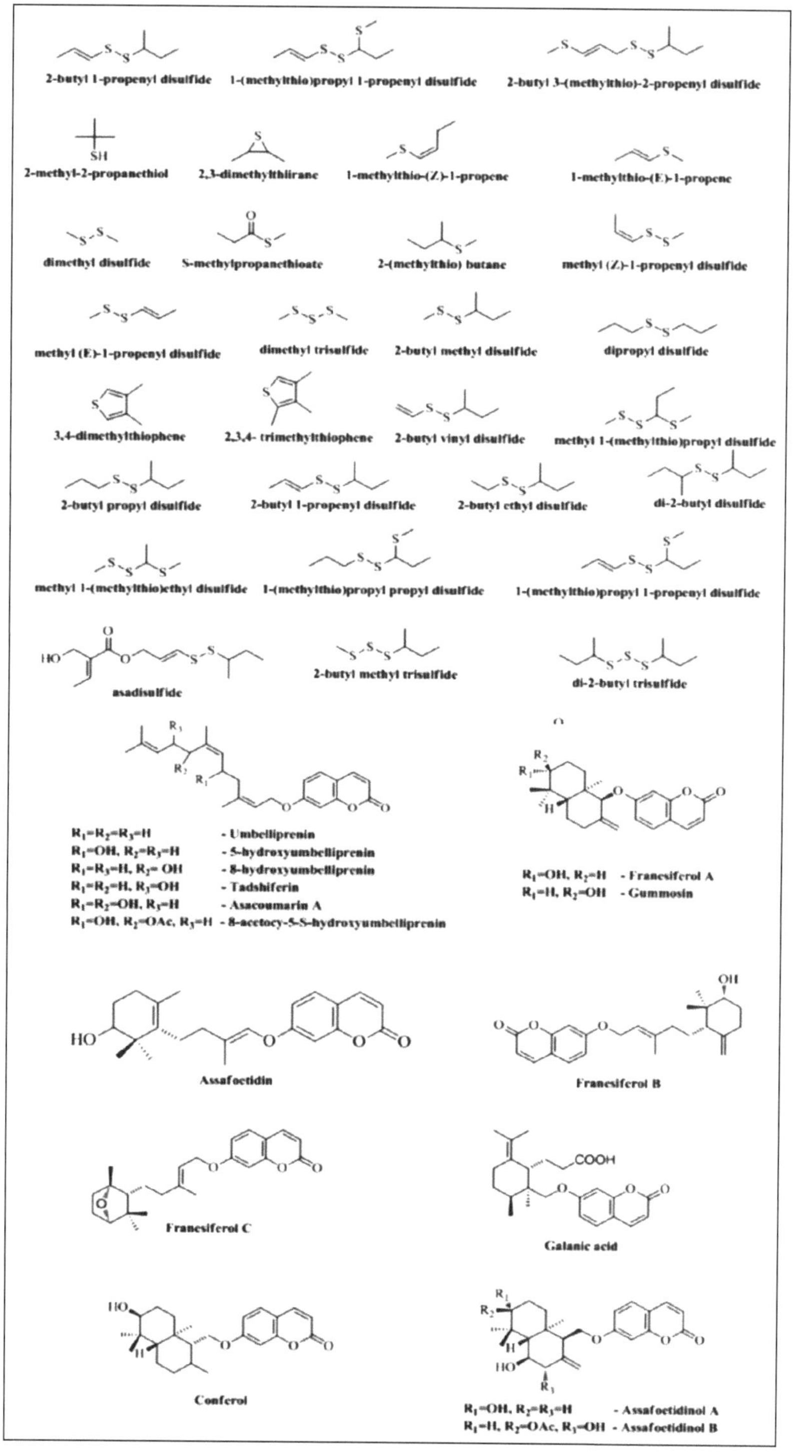
2-butyl 1-propenyl disulfide
1-(methylthio)propyl 1-propenyl disulfide
2-butyl 3-(methylthio)-2-propenyl disulfide
2-methyl-2-propanethiol
2,3-dimethylthiirane
1-methylthio-(Z)-1-propene
1-methylthio-(E)-1-propene
dimethyl disulfide
S-methylpropanethioate
2-(methylthio) butane
methyl (Z)-1-propenyl disulfide
methyl (E)-1-propenyl disulfide
dimethyl trisulfide
2-butyl methyl disulfide
dipropyl disulfide
3,4-dimethylthiophene
2,3,4- trimethylthiophene
2-butyl vinyl disulfide
methyl 1-(methylthio)propyl disulfide
2-butyl propyl disulfide
2-butyl 1-propenyl disulfide
2-butyl ethyl disulfide
di-2-butyl disulfide
methyl 1-(methylthio)ethyl disulfide
1-(methylthio)propyl propyl disulfide
1-(methylthio)propyl 1-propenyl disulfide
asadisulfide
2-butyl methyl trisulfide
di-2-butyl trisulfide
R1=R2=R3=H - Umbelliprenin
R1=OH, R2=R3=H - 5-hydroxyumbelliprenin
R1=R3=H, R2= OH - 8-hydroxyumbelliprenin
R1=R2=H, R3=OH - Tadshiferin
R1=R2=OH, R3=H - Asacoumarin A
R1=OH, R2=OAc, R3=H - 8-acetocy-5-S-hydroxyumbelliprenin
R1=OH, R2=H - Francsiferol A
R1=H, R2=OH - Gummosin
Assafoetidin
Francsiferol B
Francsiferol C
Galanic acid
Conferol
R1=OH, R2=R3=H - Assafoetidinol A
R1=H, R2=OAc, R3=OH - Assafoetidinol B

Major chemical constituents of *Ferula asafoetida*

Traditionally, it is used as an antibacterial, antispasmodic, diuretic and as a laxative agent in India. The water extract of the dried gum of the *F. asafetida* plant carries anthelmintic property. In Afghanistan, the hot water extract of the dried gum is used to treat hysteria, whooping cough and ulcers. In China, the infusion of the plant is used to treat vermifuge when taken orally. In Brazil, the oleoresin powder is used as a condiment in a crushed form. The oral administration of the hot water extract of the dried leaf and stem of the plant is used as an aphrodisiac agent in males and its extracts are also used as a general and nerve tonic. 52% of the Egyptian people used the dried gum of the plant as a contraceptive agent. They applied the dried gum vaginally before or after the coitus. The oral administration of the decoction prepared from dried root is used as an antispasmodic, diuretic, a vermifuge and as an analgesic agent [23-25]. Fiji people use the dried resin of the plant in paste form to treat whooping cough (application of the paste over the chest). *Asafetida* plant is also used to cleanse a new mother with *Allium sativum*. The decoction of the dried resin is used to treat stomach problems. In India, the dried extracts of the *F. asafetida* along with *Brassica alba* and rock salt when diluted with vinegar are used as an abortifacient agent when taken orally. The decoction of the dried gum is used as a carminative, antispasmodic and as expectorant in chronic bronchitis diseases. It is also used to treat cholera when mixed with cayenne pepper and sweet flag. The dried gum resin in the paste form is taken orally to anticipate guinea worm disease. Gum resins are used to cure stomachache when applied externally with salt and the bark juice of *Moringa pterygosperma*. It is also used to cure diseases like gallstones, kidney stones and the hot water extract of the dried resin is administered orally as an emmenagogue. In Malaysia and Morocco, the gum is chewed by the females for amenorrhea and is used as an antiepileptic. Nepal people used the water extract of the resin as an anti-helminthic agent. Saudi Arabia people used the dried gum of the *F. asafetida* plant against whooping cough, asthma and bronchitis [26-27]. The fluid extract of the plant is used by the US people as a stimulating expectorant, an anthelminthic, aphrodisiac, as a stimulant to the brain and nerves and as an antispasmodic agent. In Ayurveda, it is used as an appetizer and is used to restore consciousness. The plant is also utilized as an antidote for opium. Traditionally, the plant is used to treat a variety of diseases like whooping cough, stimulates the intestinal, nervous and respiratory system, asthma, epilepsy, ulcer, stomachache, flatulence, bronchitis, antispasmodic, intestinal parasites, influenza and weak digestion 9, 10, 11. In Europe and the United States, Hing is used in perfumes and flavoring. Also, it is used as an effective treatment against women to cure problems like unwanted abortion, abnormal pain, sterility, painful menstruation and leucorrhoea. The active constituents of the *Asafetida* plant are mainly resins, gum and essential oil. Due to the presence of phytochemical constituents, it carries various therapeutic and pharmacological properties like antioxidant, antimicrobial antifungal, antiviral, antitumor, antimicrobial, anti-diabetic, antispasmodic, hypertensive, hepatoprotective, neuroprotective and antiviral properties. Ancient Romans used to store Asafetida in jars with pine nuts, which is used as a flavor in delicate dishes which enhances the taste in mushroom and vegetable dishes and adds a unique flavor to barbecued or fried meat. It is utilized in dissolved, solid and in powder form [28-29]. Adulteration is the major problem faced by the herbal drug industry in the present scenario. It is not only affecting the herbal drug industry but also the life of a well-being. Adulteration can be done by substitution or addition of the toxic materials which results in the degradation of the quality of the original herbal medicines. Due to the increased demand for herbal products, the risk with the herbal medicines also rises as the quality of the end product compromises because of the contaminated raw material with toxic metals, microbes, and other residues, adulteration (addition of fake or inferior plant material, orthodox drugs, foreign material) which results in the poor quality of raw material and end product. Lack of standardization techniques is also responsible for the poor quality of drugs as it fails to detect the original drug which exploits its usage in the conventional system of medicines. So, it is necessary to develop an Herbal Authentication System (HAS) which can serve as a regulator and also helps in improving the quality of herbal trade [24-30].

Conclusion

Asafetida is used as a condiment in various regions of the world which provides a great flavor in cookery items like curries, meat, vegetables and other food items. From the reported studies, it is clear that the *Asafetida* plant contains various phytochemical constituents like sesquiterpenes and coumarins that play a vital role in the pharmaceutical and industrial applications to produce modern herbal formulations. Besides this, the plant is used traditionally to treat several ailments like cough, asthma, gastrointestinal disorders, impotency, fever, epilepsy, paralysis and many more. In Ayurveda, the asafetida plant plays a significant role as it contains various medicinal properties and is used by several Ayurvedic practitioners to treat diseases like asthma, bronchitis, infertility, reproductive problems, flatulence, stomachache, analgesic, digestive disorders, etc. In recent studies of pharmacological and biological activities have also shown that asafoetida acquire numerous activities such as a relaxant, neuroprotective, memory enhancing, digestive enzyme, antioxidant, antispasmodic, hypotensive, hepatoprotective, antimicrobial, anticarcinogenic, anticancer, anticytotoxicity, antiobesity, anthelmintic and antagonistic effect. Even though Asafoetida has very good medicinal significance, detailed studies are also very much needed.

REFERENCES

1. Amalraj A. Gopi S. Biological Activities and Medicinal Properties of Asafoetida: A ReviewJTradit Complement Med. 2017; 7(3): 347-359. doi: 10.1016/j.jtcme.2016.11.004
2. Sahebkar A, Iranshahi M. Biological Activities of Essential Oils from the Genus *Ferula* (*Apiaceae*) *Asian Biomed.* 2010; 4: 835-847.
3. Duan H.Takaishi Y, Tori M. Polysulfide Derivatives from Ferula Foetida. *J Nat Prod.* 2002; 65: 1667-1669.
4. Lee CL, Chiang CL, Cheng LH, Liaw CC. Influenza A (H1N1) Antiviral and Cytotoxic Agents from *Ferula asafoetida*. *J Nat Prod.* 2009; 72: 1568-1572.
5. Mahendra P, Bisht S. *Ferula asafoetida*: Traditional uses and Pharmacological Activity. *Pharmacogn Rev.* 2012; 6: 141-146.
6. Dehpour AA, Ebrahimzadeh MA, Fazel NS. Mohammad N.S. Antioxidant Activity of the Methanol Extract of *Ferula asafoetida* and its Essential Oil Composition. *GrasasAceites.* 2009; 60: 405-412.
7. Kavoosi G, Rowshan V. Chemical Composition, Antioxidant and Antimicrobial Activities of Essential Oil Obtained from *Ferula asafoetida* oleo-gum-resin: Effect of Collection Time. *Food Chem.* 2013; 138: 2180-2187.
8. Shrivastava V, Bhardwaj U, Sharma V, Mahajan N, Sharma V, Shrivastava G. Antimicrobial Activities of Asafoetida Resin Extracts (A Potential Indian Spice) *J Pharm Res.* 2012; 5: 5022-5024.
9. Divya K, Ramalakshmi K, Murthy PS, Rao LJ.M. Volatile Oils from *Ferula asafoetida* Varieties and their Antimicrobial Activity. *LWT Food Sci Technol.* 2014; 59: 774-779.
10. Patil SD, Shinde S, Kandpile P, Jain AS. Evaluation of Antimicrobial Activity of Asafoetida. *Int J Pharm Sci Res.* 2015; 6: 722-727.
11. Bhatnager R, Rani R, Dang AS. Antibacterial Activity of *Ferula asafoetida*: A Comparison of Red and White Type. *J Appl Biol Biotechnol.* 2015; 3: 18-21.
12. Mostafa Z, Soheil P, Mahdi J, Mahmoodi S. Antifangal Effects of Asafoetida Seed Essential Oil on *in vitro* Growth of Five Species of Plant Pathogenic Fungi. *Int Res J Appl Basic Sci.* 2013; 4: 1159-1162.
13. Saleem M., Alam A., Sultana S. Asafoetida Inhibits Early Events of Carcinogenesis: A Chemopreventive Study. *Life Sci.* 2001; 68: 1913-1921.
14. Fatehi M., Farifteh F., Fatehi-Hassanabad Z. Antispasmodic and Hypotensive Effects of *Ferula asafoetida* Gum extract. *J Ethnopharmacol.* 2004; 91: 321-324.
15. Iranshahy M, Iranshahi M. Traditional uses, Phytochemistry and Pharmacology of Asafoetida (*Ferula asafoetida* oleogum-resin) – a Review. *J Ethnopharmacol.* 2011; 134: 1-10.
16. Iranshahi M., Amin G., Salehi Sourmaghi M., Shafiee A., Hadjiakhoondi A. Sulphur-containing Compounds in the Essential Oil of the Root of *Ferula persica* Willd. var. *persica*. *Flavour Frag J.* 2006; 21: 260-261.
17. Appendino G, Tagliapietra S, Mario Nano G., Jakupovic J. Sesquiterpene coumarin ethers from Asafetida. *Phytochemistry.* 1993; 35: 183-186.
18. Kajimoto T., Yahiro K., Nohara T. Sesquiterpenoid and Disulphide Derivatives from *Ferula asafoetida*. *Phytochemistry.* 1989; 28: 1761-1763.
19. Nassar MI, Mustafa EAA, Ahmed AA. *Sesquiterpene coumarins* from *Ferula asafoetida* L. *Pharmazie.* 1995; 10: 766-767.
20. Banerji A, Mallick B, Chatterjee A, Budzikiewicz H, Breuer M. Assafoetidin and Ferocolicin, Two Sesquiterpenplatoid Coumarins from *Ferula asafoetida* Regel. *Tetrahedron Lett.* 1988; 29: 1557-1560.
21. Razek MHAE, Ohta S, Ahmed AA, Hirata T. Sesquiterpenecoumarins from the Roots of *Ferula asafoetida*. *Phytochem.* 2001; 58: 1289-1295.

22. Buddrus J., Bauer H., Abu-Mustafa E. Foetidin, a Sesquiterpenoidcoumarin from *Ferula asafoetida. Phytochem.* 1985; 24: 869-870.
23. Rajanikanth B, Ravindranath B, Shankaranarayana ML. Volatile Polysulphides of asafoetida. *Phytochem.* 1984; 23: 899-900.
24. Razek MHAE. A new ester isolated from *Ferula asafoetida* L. *Biosci Biotechnol Biochem.* 2007; 71: 2300-2303.
25. Christensen LP, Brandt K. Bioactive Polyacetylenes in Food Plants of the Apiaceae Family: Occurrence, Bioactivity and Analysis. *J Pharm Biomed Anal.* 2006; 41: 683-693.
26. Pangarova TT. Zapesochnaya GG. Flavonoids of *Ferula asafoetida. Chem Nat Compd.* 1975; 9: 768.
27. Gundamaraju R. Evaluation of Anti-helmintic Activity of *Ferula foetida* "Hing-A Natural Indian Spice" Aqueous Extract. *Asian Pac J Trop Dis.* 2013; 3: 189-191.
28. Choudhary S, Kaurav H, Chaudhary G.Hing (Ferula asafoetida). A Review Based Upon its Ayurvedic and Pharmacological Properties. *Int JPharmaceutSci Rev Res.* 2021; 68(2): 31-39. 10.47583/ijpsrr.2021.v68i02.006
29. Kareparamban JA, Nikam PH, Jadhav AP, Kadam VJ. Ferulafoetida "Hing": A Review. Res JPharmaceutBiolChem Sci. 2012; 3(2): 775-86.28.
30. Mahendra P, Bisht S. Ferula asafoetida: Traditional uses and Pharmacological Activity. *Pharmacogn rev.* 2012; 6(12): 141-145.

CHAPTER 19

Health benefits of Mango Fruit Powder (Amchur)

A Short Communication

Amchur powder is a staple of Indian concocting which adds up the delicate fruitiness flavor in the recipes. Amchur is produced using the unripe and sun-dried mangoes. Amchur has a citrus-like flavoring. Amchur originated from India and Pakistan. Amchur powder preparation is historical. Once the mangoes are harvested, they are peeled, thinly sliced, and sun-dried. The dried strips, which gradually get light brown and take after pieces of woody bark, are also available to purchase, however significantly, the strips are processed in a manner to make the fine powder. Amchur is known as mango powder and is made from dried green mangoes. It is widely used in cooking for seasoning dishes. This fruity spice is very popular in many of the Indian dishes. It adds flavor to the dishes and is the best spice to use when mangoes are not in season. Amchur Powder, which is also referred as mango powder, is one of the Indian fruity spices powder that is made from dried unripe green mangoes. Mango extract is derived from the tropical mango fruit and the liquid extract is used in cooking a variety of dishes, including desserts, salads, and poultry. It can be a safer alternative to use the often allergenic mango fruit with skin. Mangoes are known to include a variety of vitamins, and, as a result, the extract is also used in some diet supplements for weight loss. It contributes copper, calcium and iron to the diet as well as antioxidants such as zeaxanthin and beta-carotene.

Lowing intakes of vitamin K have been associated with a higher risk for bone fracture. It helps to prevent constipation and promote regularity and a healthy digestive tract.

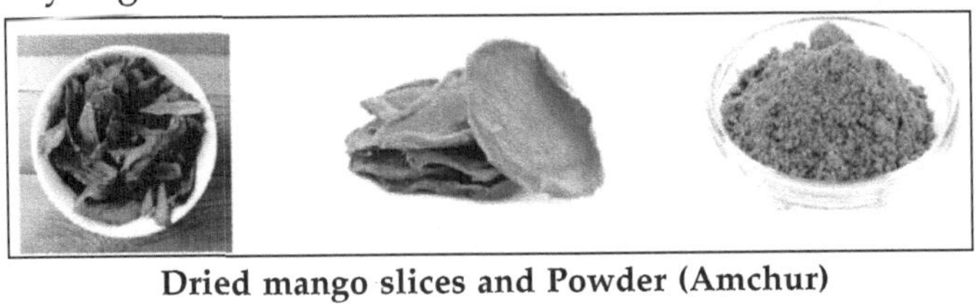

Dried mango slices and Powder (Amchur)

Mango fruit powder is used in desserts, such as pies, cakes, and ice cream; Aside from cooking, mango extracts are also used in the creation of dietary supplements.

Amchur or Amchur Powder, which is also referred as mango powder, is one of the Indian fruity spices powder that is made from dried unripe green mangoes. Amchur powder is usually used when the mangoes are out of season, to add flavor and nutritional benefits of mangoes to the foods and drinks. It is sour yet sweet to taste. Tart pale beige to brownish in color, it is used to add tanginess to the dishes and can be used as a substitute of lemon. Apart from adding flavor, color and taste to the food, amchur powder comprises various health benefits. It contains many nutrients including vitamin A, E and C, and antioxidants and is used in preparing many Ayurvedic medicines. Amchur is also rich in iron and known to be quite beneficial for pregnant women. It improves immunity system of the body and also quite beneficial for your skin and hair. It can be a great substitute for your costly beauty products and medicines also. It is believed that amchur also helps in controlling your blood pressure as well as diabetes. Amchur powder improves your digestion and helps to fight acidity. Mango contains powerful antioxidants, which ensures good bowel movement and helps combat constipation and flatulence. Mango helps your body in eliminating harmful toxins and detoxifies it, all thanks to the presence of vitamin A, C, D and B6. Hence, amchur is used in ayurvedic medicines to treat diarrhea, dysentery and urinary tract infections. Amchur supports proper functioning of your hormone and by consuming amchur regularly you can improve your eyesight. It also prevents eye related disease like cataract too. 10 grams of Amchur powder has 36 calories of which, there is zero percent fat. 13% of the quantity is made up of sodium. This accounts for 300mg. It has 2 grams of fiber, 2% of calcium and 3% of vitamin C. Amchur Powder also contains vitamin A and C in abundance. Amchur is even used in the treatment of scurvy. There are many more benefits to this raw mango powder. You can use it in a variety of recipes and reap its benefits for overall health.

It eliminates toxins, detoxifies the body and is used in treating anemia. Nervous systems disorders can also be cured by using mango powder. In Ayurveda medicine, Amchur powder used to treat conditions like diarrhoea, dysentery and urinary tract infection. Amchur powder has many benefits for the digestive system health. It will help fight acidity and improve digestion. It combats constipation, flatulence and ensures good bowel movement. Amchur have phenols and other phenolic compounds that are powerful antioxidants. It is important to have good digestion for a strong metabolic system. Amchur powder works wonders to ensure that cardiovascular health is in good condition. Amchur powder is an extremely rich source of iron. Women who suffer from iron deficiencies like anemia are advised to include food rich in iron, as part of their diet. This fruit can be a part of the diet in one form or the other. Since ripe mangoes contain high amounts of sugar, it is advisable to add amchur in your diet, as it is a healthier option. Amchur powder has high levels of Vitamin C. This proves to be very helpful in healing conditions like scurvy. It is a medical condition that is caused due to the deficiency of vitamin C. Scurvy can be treated and prevented, if amchur powder is consumed on a daily basis. One recipe that is used is the combination of amchur with jaggery. It is said to be very effective in treating scurvy. Amchur contains a high amount of Vitamin A and E. They are essential for healthy eyes and skin. This powder ensures that the hormones are functioning well. Amchur powder has an anti-aging effect on the skin. You can improve your eyesight and prevent eye-related conditions like cataract, by consuming amchur regularly.The antioxidant properties that are present in amchur can boost metabolism. This in turn, helps to increase weight loss. Mango powder or Amchur powder has low carbohydrates and are recommended in weight loss programs. You can include this powder in your diet and gain all of its multiple benefits.

One of the most amazing use of mango powder is that, it is used in treating cancer effectively. It protects the body from this life-threatening condition, as it contains high amounts of vitamin C. It eliminates free radicals that are responsible for most of the diseases. Mangoes have many health benefits and one factor is that, it helps to maintain low glycemic index. This helps to keep the fat levels in control. The potassium that is present in amchur powder will also make sure that the blood levels are regulated. Diabetes is also kept under control, if you consume amchur powder regularly. Amchur is suggested as a cure for many allergies. Anemic people are suggested to have this powder, as it contain high amount of iron. Pregnant women are advised to include them in their diet, so that they have a safe delivery. All you have to do is sprinkle some of it over your food. It will add flavor and give you can reap the many health benefits. Amchur is a great source of all the important vitamins. This includes vitamin A, C and E. These are essential for the hormones to work well. These vitamins are also good for having healthy eyes and skin. Mango seeds when crushed and made into powder can be applied on the skin, after mixing it with tomato juice. Apply it on the face and leave it on for a few minutes. Rub it off gently and wash your face. It has an exfoliating effect on the skin. Amchur powder cures breakouts, blemishes, and blackheads. It even removes the redness of the skin. Amchur acts as a mild scrub on the skin.

Amchur has many uses, when it comes to prepare dishes. It adds flavor to soups, chutneys, curries, dal, pickles, stir fried vegetables and fruit salad. The dried powder is directly added to these dishes like tomato chicken, fish tikka and stew. It is a spice that is even used in continental dishes like grilled citrus fish. But, that's not it. You may also use amchur in your smoothies and shakes to make them tasty and healthy. Amchur powder can be used to add the sweet and sour taste tinge in any dishes, pudding or dessert. There are many recipes in which you can use this powder. It is a favorite spice among children and adults alike. Let check out the health benefits of consuming amchur powder, good for digestion, prevent acidity, improves skin toning. It is great to add flavors to soups, chutneys, and curries. The dried powder is directly added to these dishes. Dishes that include chicken and fish are also enhanced with the flavor of amchur. The unique flavor that you get in amchur is irreplaceable. The many medical benefits it renders are effectively made use in ayurvedic medicines as well. It is used in medicines that improve digestion. This sweet and sour powder is consumed in keeping the heart-healthy. Amchur is recommended for women of all ages, as it has a high iron content that women require on a daily basis. It helps to maintain healthy skin and eyes, by consuming amchur regularly. Due to its high nutritional value and less side effects, amchur can be used in our daily diet.

REFERENCES

1. Kumar V. Amchur, The Secret Benefits of Spices and Condiments, New Delhi, New Dawn Press, Inc., 2006; 10-11.
2. Lauricella M, Emanuele S, Calvaruso G, Giuliano M, D'Anneo A. Multifaceted Health benefits of Mangiferaindica L.(Mango): The Inestimable Value of Orchards recently Planted in Sicilian Rural Areas. Nutrients. 2017; 9(5): 525.
3. Shah KA, Patel MB, Patel RJ, Parmar PK. Mangiferaindica (mango). Pharmacognosy Reviews. 2010 Jan; 4(7): 42.
4. Gupta C, Garg AP, Gupta S. Antimicrobial and Phytochemical Studies of Fresh Ripe Pulp and Dried Unripe Pulp of Mangiferaindica (AMCHUR) Middle-East JScient Res2010; 5 (2): 75-80.

CHAPTER 20

Nutrional Gains of Nutmeg (*Myristica fragrans* Houtt.) for Perfect Health

ABSTRACT

Nutmeg and mace are the two spices derived from several tree species in genus Myristica. They contain essential oil and is used therapeutically, cosmetic and culinary preparations. Several value addition products widen the commercial value of this tree. *Myristica fragrans* is well known as a commercial source of mace (aril) and nutmeg (seed), which have long been widely used as spices in the culinary field. From very ancient time *M. fragrans* fruit has been used as a folk medicine. It has been known to provide many medicinal properties due to its complex molecular structure. The chemical constituents of *M. fragrans* have been studied for hypocholesterolemic, hypolipidemic, antidepressant, aphrodisiac, antimicrobial, memory enhancer, antioxidant and hepatoprotective properties. Numerous studies have indicated that *M. fragrans* contains diverse phytochemicals such as lignans, neolignans, diphenylalkanes, phenylpropanoids, and terpenoids, which exhibit many of pharmacological activities. Among them, macelignan, meso-dihydroguaiaretic acid, myristicin, and malabaricone C are the most active compounds. The aim of the present review was to introduce *M. fragrans* as a potent medicinal plant by highlighting its traditional applications as well as the recent findings for novel pharmacological and clinical applications.

Keywords: Myristicin, Lignans, Hypolipidemic, Antidepressant, Twin spice, Pharmacological activities.

Introduction

Myristica fragrans Houtt. (Myristicaceae), an aromatic evergreen tree is indigenous to India, Indonesia and Srilanka. It produces two spices, nutmeg and mace. Nutmeg is the seed kernel inside the fruit and mace is the fleshy red, net like skin covering (aril) on the kernel. It is a spreading aromatic ever green tree usually growing up to 20 meters. The pointed dark green leaves are arranged alternately along the branches and are borne on leaf stems about 1 cm long. Upper leaf surfaces are shiny. Flowers are usually single sexed; occasionally male and female flowers are found on the same tree. Female flowers arise in groups of 1 to 3; males in groups of 1 to 10. Flowers are pale yellow, waxy, fleshy and bell-shaped. The fruits are fleshy, drooping, yellow, smooth, 6 to 9 cm long with a longitudinal ridge. When ripe, the succulent yellow fruit coat splits into 2 valves revealing a purplish-brown, shiny seed (nutmeg) surrounded by a red aril (mace). Seeds (nutmegs) are broadly ovoid (2 to 3 cm long), firm, fleshy, whitish and transversed by red-brown veins. When fresh, the aril (mace) is bright scarlet becoming more horny, brittle and a yellowish-brown color when dried. The trees do not give flowers until around 9 years old, but once start flowering they continue to do so for further 75 years. The trees bear 2 to 3 crops a year. The seeds (nutmegs) need 3to 6 weeks to dry before they are ready for use [1-4].

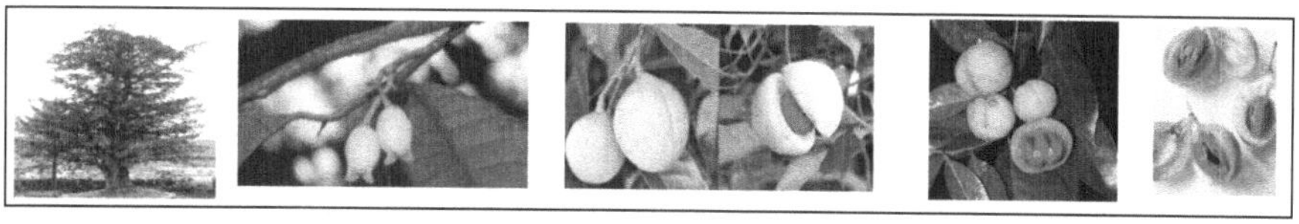

M. fragrans tree flower, fruit, kernel covered with red aril (mace)

The nutmeg is unique among tree spices as it is the donor of the two distinct spices, nutmeg and mace. Nutmeg is the seed kernel inside the fruit and mace is the covering (aril) on the kernel. Both mace and nutmeg are used as condiment and medicine. It is native of Indonesia (Moluccas Islands). In India it is cultivated in Kerala, Tamil Nadu, Karnataka, Goa, Maharashtra, North East India and Andamans. Accordingly, *M. fragrans* extract have many useful properties due to its valuable bioactive compounds and they may have potentials for drugs against pathogenic microorganisms as well as cure for different non-communicable diseases. Since *M. fragrans* is natural source, adverse effects after consumption are less and can be developed to use in many areas like drug industry, bakery industry, cosmetics industry. The objective of this review was to show the recent advances in the exploration of *M. fragrans* as phytotherapy and to illustrate its potential as a therapeutic agent. With the current information, it is evident that *M. fragrans* has pharmacological functions including anti-inflammatory, analgesic, anti-convulsant, antibacterial, antifungal and antioxidant activities, among others. [5-9]

Phytopharmacological aspects of *M. fragrans*

Jatiphala, Jaiphal or Nutmeg is a small brown-colored oval-shaped aromatic fruit. The tree of Jaiphal is an evergreen one, with small yellow-colored flowers. It is rich in oils, proteins, minerals and resins. On ripening completely, the mace outgrows the Jaiphal and it is called Javitri. Jaiphal has a sweet aroma and is a favorite in the Indian and Persian Kitchens. Adding a little nutmeg powder to the food makes it very nutritious.

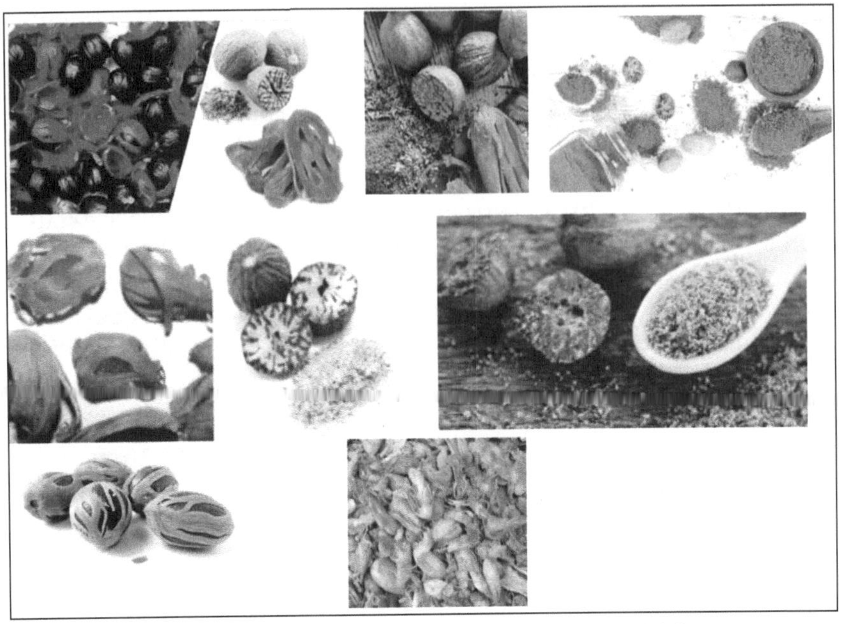

Nutmeg (Jaiphal) & its powder, and mace (javitiri)

Not only the rich taste and unique flavor of this spice that makes it a must- have ingredient in all varieties of dishes but also has therapeutic potential. Its healing properties include – it is a good appetizer, boosts immunity, improves digestion! It has astringent properties [10-13]. Jaiphal has many beneficial properties. Jaiphal has a tikhta and katurasa. Jaiphal is bitter and pungent in taste. Jaiphal is a light and strong fruit. So, it has a laghu and teekshnaguna. Jaiphal has ushnavirya or a hot potency. It has a Katu or pungent vipaka, post digestion. It acts like trutahara – to relieve thirst, and vaktrakledahara – aiding excess secretions in the mouth. It helps to fight bad breath. It is said to have properties to treat sore throat as artijit. Being prameha, regulates diabetes. It is vrushya – potent aphrodisiac, hridaya-optimizes cardiac health, shwasahara – promotes respiratory health and treats COPD and asthma, and vishahara – cleanses the system). Jaiphal helps to balance the Vata and Kapha Doshas. It helps to treat anorexia with healthy weight management. It promotes the digestive fire and facilitates good digestion. It pacifies the vatadosha by keeping the throat, nose, and respiratory system healthy. It helps to keep the pitta dosh healthy by promoting metabolism and good digestion. Nutmeg facilitates the production of serotonin, a neurotransmitter, which induces sleep. It contains myristicin which helps to reduce the secretion of enzymes induced by stress. The potent anti-inflammatory components like monoterpenes, sabinene, terpineol, and pinene reduce swelling and soreness. Jaiphal powder contains essential volatile oils like myristicin, elemicin, eugenol, and safrole which have powerful anti-inflammatory properties that provide relief from pain, swelling of muscles and joints. The properties of Jaiphal stimulate the nerves in the brain and have been used since ages by many civilizations. Nutmeg with its adaptogen nature works both as a stimulant and a sedative. The distinct flavor and aroma of Jaiphal powder hold incredible medicinal properties and are effective in aiding digestive woes like indigestion, constipation, flatulence, and ulcers [14-17]. The exceptional fragrance of mace and Jaiphal powder relieves abdominal cramps, pain associated with gas and also treats diarrhea and nausea. It removes toxins from the liver and kidneys and cleanses the system and improves digestion. The powerful antibacterial properties in Jaiphal are effective against harmful bacteria that cause dental diseases. The essential eugenol oil provides relief from toothache. The impressive antimicrobial, anti-inflammatory properties, and cleansing properties of Jaiphal helps to fight off blackheads, treats acne, and unclog the pores. The compound mace lignan in Jaiphal powder slows down aging. The oils in Jaiphal have skin rejuvenating properties. Nutmeg acts as a natural aphrodisiac with the hormone serotonin, which is primarily responsible for increased libido and a relaxed body. It boosts immunity and plays a key role in maintaining good health by enhancing immune function. The presence of various minerals and vitamins in this spice is responsible for the potent anti-inflammatory and antioxidant action, which in turn improves your overall health. Induces a good menstrual flow, stimulates healthy blood circulation, provides relief from the pain of joints and muscles. [18-20]

Chemical Composition *M. fragrans* Fruit

Mace used as a tropical spice having a pleasant aromatic fragrance, for this property it has been used widely as flavoring agent in cakes, pudding, beverages, meat, and sausages. Besides this, it has a special ability to enhance the taste of food. Myristicin (5-allyl-1-methoxy-2, 3 (methylenedioxybenzene) constituent is responsible for flavoring property and also been known to produce important psychopharmacological responses. Most of the important chemicals of *M. fragrans* are from the seed which are volatile phenolics, terpenoids, proteins, starch, lignincompounds and multifunctional bioactive compounds including Trimyristine, Myristicin and Dihydrogualaretic acid. [21-23]. Aqueous extract of *M. fragrans* contain flavonoids, saponins, alkaloids, cardiacglycosides and anthraquinones. 10% of essential oils are contain in the fruit. In the essential oil, 60-90% contains camphene, sabinene, limonene, mycene, a-pinene and p-cymene. 5-15% contain terpene derivatives, 2-20% contain phenylpropanes including elemicin, myristicin and safrole. Myristicin and elemicin present in the seed cause for the intoxicating effects. 80% of alkenylbenzene derivatives consist of myristicinandelimicin. Myristic, palmitic, lauric, oleic, stearic and linoleic are the fixed oils present in the seed.

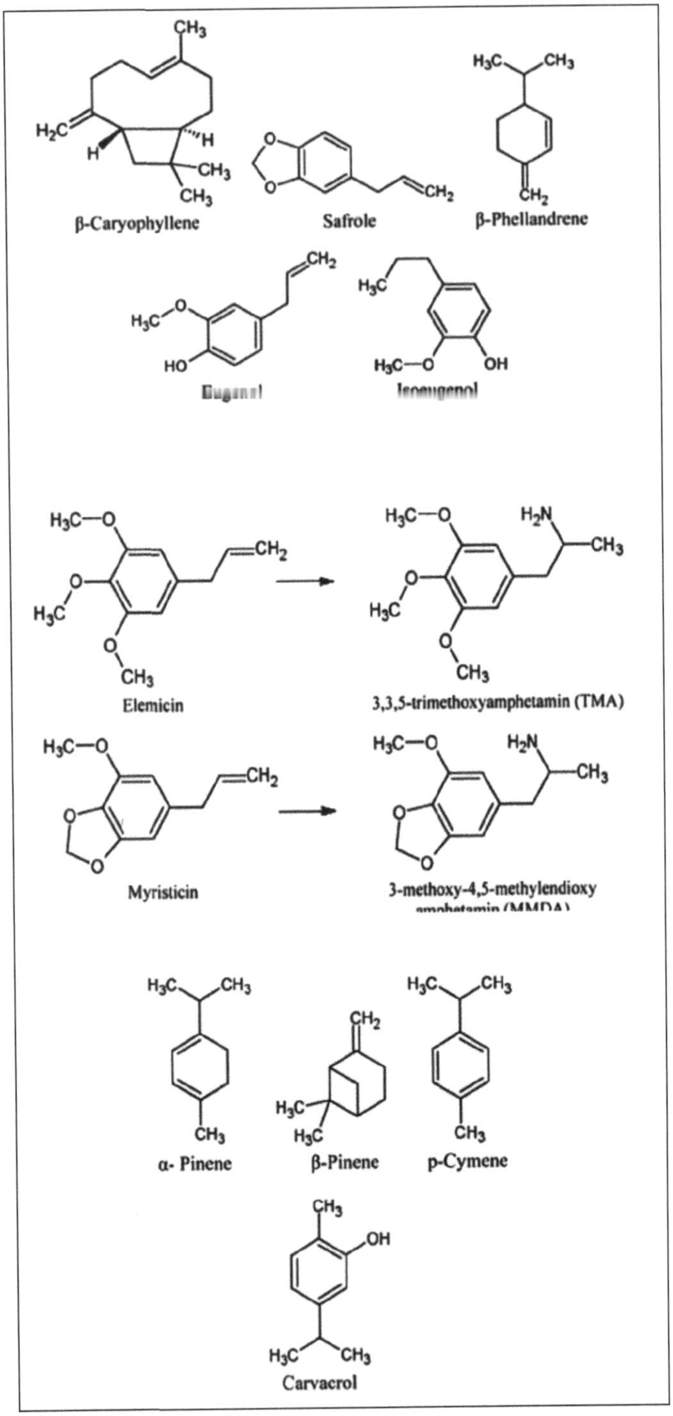

Major chemical constituents of Nutmeg seed and essential oil

Essential oil of nutmeg consists of β-pinene (7.3%), terpine-4-ol (5.8%), sabinene (41.7%), α-pinene (9.4%), limonene (3.7%), safrole (1.4%) and myristicin (2.7%). As major constituents in the *M. fragrans* leaves, α- pines (18.04%), sabinene (19.07%), β-pinene (7.92%), limonene (8.32%), 4-terpineol (11.83%) were identified. Lignin compounds such as meso-monomethyldihydroguaiaretic acid, (+) guaiacin, including (8R,8′S)-7′-(3′,4′-methyl enedioxyphenyl)-8,8′-dimethyl - 7-(3, 4 - dihydroxy - phenyl)-butane, 9-epoxylignan and many morelignins were isolated from *M. fragrans* seeds. Novel compounds (–)-1-(2, 6-dihydroxyphenyl)-9-[4-hydroxy-3-(p-menth-1-en-8-oxy) - phenyl]-1-nonanone and (7R, 8R)-7,8-dihydro-7-(3,4-dihydroxyphenyl)-32 -methoxy-8-methyl-12 -(E-propenyl)- benzofuran were characterized in the fruits of M. fragrans. Due to the presence of terpenes, Mace, dried seed covers of M. fragransare aromatic. Mace has same aromatic compounds as nutmeg but indifferent proportions. Mace has 30% fixed oils and 7-14% essential oils depending on their origin. Monoterpenes (87.5%), monoterpene alcohols (5.5%) and other aromatic compounds (7%) can be found in mace. Resorcinol malabaricone B and malabaricone C were also have been isolated from mace. [24-47]

Dihydroguaiaretic acid	Trimyristin
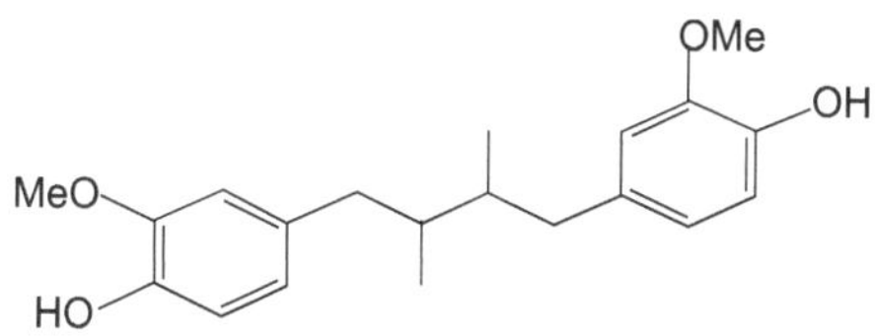	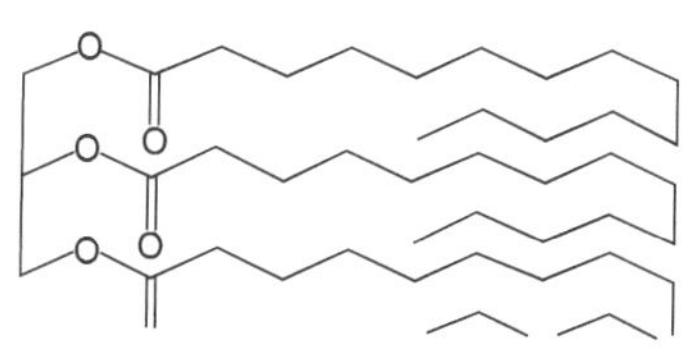

Elemental Contents of Nutmeg

The quantity of element in nutmeg is Mg (0.45%), Al (210 mg/kg), Si (167 mg/kg), P (0.17%), S (0.14%), Cl (402 mg/kg), K (0.63%), Ca (0.30%), Ti (13 mg/kg), Mn (124 mg/kg), Fe (151 mg/kg), Cu (73 mg/kg), Zn (44 mg/kg), Br (95 mg/kg), Rb (32 mg/kg), and Sr (11 mg/kg).[49] Current information shows furanocoumarins in nutmeg could be useful in the development of new drugs for the treatment of different diseases that suggest an opportunity that furanocoumarins can be further developed as a potential disease-curing remedy [30,33,36].

Preparation of Cosmetics and Culinary usage

A spice that is commonly used in the preparation of various dishes across various cuisines, nutmeg (jaiphal) is valued for its sweet aroma. Mace is the reddish, lacy aril or covering of the seed, which is known for its mild flavor and the orange tinge it imparts to the dishes it is used in. Besides being an exotic spice, nutmeg is grouped under the category of aphrodisiacs, and in cooking, only small quantities - such as a little grating or a pinch of the ground powder - are used to make soups, meat gravies, beef stew, steaks, roulades, and even desserts. In India, it is more commonly seen in Kerala, probably being brought in during the ancient spice trade. The locals use it to flavor meat curries and desserts, while the flesh of the fruit goes into the making of pickles, chutneys and other condiments. The spice is also a regular feature in Mughlai cuisine, being used as part of the various masala mixes for the meat preparations. Nutmeg, especially in the ground form, is used mainly in the food processing industry as a spice, cooking, or baking and also used as an ingredient in the pungent garam masalas (Spice) of North India. The oleoresin of nutmeg finds use in the preparation of vegetables, meat, and to flavor milk dishes, soft drink, punches, and canned food. Camphene presents in the oil of nutmeg is used in the manufacture of camphor and related compounds. Pinene one of the essential oils of nutmeg, is used to make camphor, plasticizers, solvents, perfume bases and synthetic pine oil. Myristic acid is used as a flavor ingredient in the food industry and also finds use in the preparation of soap, liquid detergents, shaving creams, shampoos, plastics, and perfumes, also used in compounding rubber, paints and greases, in the synthesis of esters for flavors and perfumes and as a part of good-grade additives. The constituents of nutmeg myristicin, elemicin, and isoelemicin when presented in aroma form, they act as stress relievers.

Conclusion

Myristica fragrans which is commonly known as nutmeg produces two spices called nutmeg and mace. From very ancient times *M. fragrans* fruit has been used as folk medicine. Apart from that due to the chemical composition of nutmeg and mace, it can be used in many other industries like microbial industry, bakery industry, beverage industry and cosmetic industry. Research works have done to elucidate antidiabetic, antibacterial, anti-fungal, memory enhancing, hypolipidaemic and hypocholesterolemic, anticonvulsant, anti-inflammatory and analgesic properties of the plant.ost of the important chemicals of *M. fragrans* are from the seed which are volatile phenolics, terpenoids, proteins, starch, lignin compounds and multifunctional bioactive compounds including Trimyristine, Myristicin and Dihydrogualaretic acid. Aqueous extract of *M. fragrans* contain flavonoids, saponins, alkaloids, cardiac glycosides and anthraquinones. Mace has same aromatic compounds as nutmeg but indifferent proportions.

REFERENCES

1. Sonavane GS, Palekar RC, Kasture VS, Kasture SB. Anticonvulsant and Behavioural Actions of *Myristica fragrans* Seeds. Ind JPharmacol. 2011; 33: 417-424.
2. Sonavane GS, Palekar RC, Kasture VS, Kasture SB (2002). Anticonvulsant and Behavioural Actions of *Myristica fragrans* seeds. Ind J Phamacol 34: 332-338.
3. Sonavane GS, Sarveiya VP, Kasture VS, Kasture SB. Anxiogenic Activity of *Myristica fragrans* Seeds. PharmacolBiochemBehav. 2002; 71: 247-252.

4. Orabi KY, Mossa JS, Feraly FS. Isolation and Characterization of Two Antimicrobial Agents from mace (*Myristica fragrans*). J Nat Prod. 1991; 54(3): 856-859.
5. Ozaki Y, Soedigdo S, Wattimena YR, Suganda AG. Antiinflammatory Effect of Mace, Aril of *Myristica fragrans* Houtt. and its Active Principles. Japan J Pharmacol.1989; 49(155): 63.32.
6. Pal M, Srivastava M, Soni DK, Kumar A, Tewari SK. Composition and Anti-microbial Activity of Essential Oil of *Myristica fragrans* from Andaman Nicobar Island. IntJ Pharm Life Sci. 2011; 2(10): 1115-1117.
7. Gomathi P, Aman K, Mebrahtom G, Gereziher G, Hassan GA. Nutmeg (*Myristica fragrans* Houtt.) Oils. In: Preedy, V.R. (Ed.), Essential Oils in Food Preservation, Flavorand Safety. Academic Press, San Diego, Chap. 2016; 69: 607-616.
8. Gopalakrishnan M. Chemical Composition of Nutmeg in the Spice Islands. J Spices Aroma Crops. 1992; 1: 49.54.
9. Weerakoon WMTDN, Perera WPRT, Rajapaksha RMH, 1J, A. Liyanage JA. A Review on Bioactive Compounds and Pharmacological Activities of *Myristica fragrans* as a Medical Plant. Int J Innov Scientif Res Rev. 2021; 3(06): 1316-1320.
10. Jaiswal P, Kumar P, Singh VK, Singh DK. Biological Effects of *Myristica fragrans*. 2009; 11: 21-29.
11. Narasimhan B, Dhake AS. Antibacterial Principles from *Myristica fragrans* Seeds. J Med Food. 2006; 9: 395-399.
12. Qiu Q, Zhang G, Sun X, Liu X. Study on Chemical Constituents of the Essential Oil from *Myristica fragrans* Houtt. by Supercritical Fluid Extraction and Steam Distillation. Zhong Yao Cai.2004; 27: 823-826.
13. Wang Y, Yang XW, Tao HY, Liu HX. GC-MS Analysis of Essential Oils from Seeds of *Myristica fragrans* in Chinese Market. ZhongguoZhong Yao ZaZhi2004; 29: 339-342.
14. Yang XW, Huang X, Ahmat M. New Neolignan from Seed of *Myristica fragrans*. Zhongguo Zhong Yao Za Zhi 2008; 33: 397-402.
15. Kalbhen DA. Nutmeg as a Narcotic. A Contribution to the Chemistry and Pharmacology of Nutmeg (Myristica Fragrans). Angew Chem Int Ed Engl. 1971; 10: 370-374.
16. Niyas Z, Variyar PS, Gholap AS, Sharma A. Effect of γ-irradiation on the Lipid Profile of Nutmeg (Myristica Fragrans Houtt.). J Agric Food Chem.2003; 51: 6502-6504.
17. Morsy NF. A Comparative Study of Nutmeg (Myristica fragrans Houtt.) Oleoresins Obtained by Conventional and Green Extraction Techniques. J Food Sci Technol. 2016; 53: 3770-3777.
18. Madhavan L, Gopalakrishnan M, Narayanan CS. Chemical Composition of Nutmeg Leaf and Flower Oils. Ind Perfumer. 1991; 35: 161-163.
19. Hada S, Hattori M, Tezuka Y, Kikuchi T, Namba T. New Neolignans and Lignans from the Aril of Myristica Fragrans. Phytochem. 1988; 27: 563-568.
20. Kasahara H, Miyazawa M, Kameoka H. Absoluteconfiguration of 8-O-4′-neolignans from Myristica Fragrans. Phytochem 1995; 40: 1515-1517.
21. Ananthakumar A, Variyar PS, Sharma A.Estimation of Aroma Glycosides of Nutmeg and their changes during Radiation Processing. J Chromatogr 2006; 1108: 252-257.
22. Jukic M, Politeo O, Miloš M. Chemical Composition and Antioxidant Effect of Free Volatile Aglycones from Nutmeg (Myristica Fragrans Houtt.) Compared to its Essential oil. CroaticaChemActa. 2006; 79: 209-14.
23. Asgarpanah J, Kazemivash N. Phytochemistry and Pharmacologic Properties of *Myristica fragrans* Hoyutt.: A review. Afr J Biotechnol 2012; 11(65): 12787-12793. doi:10.5897/AJB12.1043

24. Calliste CA, Kozlowski D, Duroux JL, Champavier Y, Chulia AJ, Trouillas P. A New Antioxidant from Wild Nutmeg. Food Chem. 2010; 118: 489-496.
25. Chatterjee S, Niaz , Gautam, S, Adhikari S, Variyar PS, Sharma A. Antioxidant Activity of Somephenolic Constituents from Green Pepper (Piper nigrum L.) and Fresh Nutmeg Mace (*Myristica fragrans*). FoodChem 2007; 101, 515-523.
26. Olajide OA, Ajayi FF, Ekhelar AL, Awe SO, Makinde JM, Alada ARA. Biological effect of Myristica Fragrans (Nutmeg) extract. Phytoth Res.1999; 13, 344-345.
27. Somani R, Karve S, Jain D, Jain K,Singhai AK.Phytochemical and Pharmacological Potential of Myristica fragrans Houtt: A Comprehensive Review. Pharmacog Rev. 2008; 2: 68-76.
28. Maya KM, John Zachariah T, Krishnamoorthy B.Chemical Composition of Essential Oil of Nutmeg (Myristica fragrans Houtt.) Accessions. J Spices Aroma Crops. 2004; 13: 135-139.
29. Gopalakrishnan M (1992) Chemical Composition of Nutmeg and Mace. J Spices Aroma Crops. 1992; 1: 49-54.
30. Mallavarapu GR, Ramesh S. Composition of Essential Oils of Nutmeg and Mace. J Med Aroma Plant Sci. 1998; 20: 746-748.
31. Jangid K, Jaykumar ND, Sheeja S, Varghese SS. Achievable Therapeutic effects of *Myristica fragrans* (Nutmeg) on Preodontitis: A Short Review. IntJ Pharm Pharm Sci. 2014; 6(5): 591-594.
32. Tan KP, Khoo HE, Azrina A. Comparison of Antioxidant Components and Antioxidant Capacity in different Parts of Nutmeg. Int Food Res J. 2013; 20: 1049-1052.
33. Thangaselvabai T, Sudha KR, Selvakumar T, Balakumbahan R. Nutmeg (*Myristica fragrans* Houtt.) The twin Spice – A Review. AgriRev. 2011; 32 (4): 283-293.
34. Jose H, Arya KR, Sindhu TJ, Syamjith P, Vinod KR, Sandhya SA. A Descriptive Review on *Myristica fragrans* Houtt. Hygeia J Drug Med. 2016; 35-43. doi:10.15254/H.J.D.Med.8.2016.155
35. Maeda A, Tanimoto S, Abe T, Kazama S, Tanizawa H, Nomura M. Chemical Constituents of *Myristica fragrans* Houttuyn Seed and their Physiological Activities. Yakugaku Zasshi. 2008; 128: 129-133.
36. Maya KM, Zachariah TJ, Krishnamoorthy B. Chemical Composition of Essential Oil of Nutmeg (*Myristica fragrans* Houtt.) Accessions. J Spices Aroma Crops. 2004; 13: 135-139.
37. Sonavane GS, Palekar RC, Kasture VS, Kasture SB. Anticonvulsant and Behavioural actions of *Myristica fragrans* Seeds. Indian J. Pharmacol. 2001; 33: 417. 424-427.
38. Ahmad ST, Latif A, Qasmi IA, Amin KM. An Experimental Study of Sexual Function Improving Effect of *Myristica fragrans* Houtt. (Nutmeg). BMC Complement Altern Med. 2005; 5: 16-18.
39. Varshney I P & Sharma SC. Saponins and Sapogenins. Part XXII. Chemical Investigation of Seeds of *Myristica fragrans* Houtt. Indian J. Chem. 1968; 6: 474.476.
40. Verghese J 2001 Nutmeg and Mace. IV. Essential Oils of *Myristica fragrans* Houtt. And of Myristicaargentea Warb. Spice India 2001; 14: 7.11.
41. Narasimhan B, Dhake AS. J Med Food. 2006; 9(3): 395-399.http://doi.org/10.1089/jmf.2006.9.395
42. Jangid K, Jayakumar, Va rghese SS. Achievable Therapeutic Effects of *Myristica fragrans* (nutmeg) on Periodontitis a short review. IntJ Pharm Pharmsci. 2014; 6(5): 591-594.
43. Jaiswal P, Kumar P, Singh VK, Singh DK, Biological Effects of *Myristica fragrans*. Annual Rev Bomed Sci. 2009; 11: 21-29.

44. Weerakoon WMTDN, Perera WPRT, Rajapaksha RMH, Liyanage JA. A Review on Bioactive Compounds and Pharmacological Activities of *Myristica fragrans* as a Medicinal Plant.Int J InnovScient Res Rev. 2021; 3(6): 1316-1320.
45. Ha MT, Vu NK, Tran TH, Kim JA, Woo MH, Min BS. Phytochemical and Pharmacological Properties of *Myristica fragrans* Houtt.: An Updated Review. 2020; 43(11): 1067-1092. doi: 10.1007/s12272-020-01285-4.
46. Kalbhen DA. Nutmeg as a Narcotic. A Contribution to the Chemistry and Pharmacology of Nutmeg (*Myristica fragrans*). Angew ChemInt Ed Engl. 1971; 10: 370-4.
47. Ali MA, Hamiduddin, Zaigham M, Ikram M. Phyto-pharmacological Potential of Jaiphal (*Myristica fragrans* Houtt): A Spice of Medicinal Importance and its Utilization in Unani Medicine. Int J Green Pharm. 2018; (Suppl)12 (1) | S26-S36.

CHAPTER
21

Versatile usage of Red Chilli (*Capsicum annuum* L.)

ABSTRACT

Capsicum annuum (Solanaceae), commonly known as chilli, is a medicinal spice used in various Indian traditional systems of medicine and it has been acknowledged to treat various health ailments. Therapeutic potential of chilli and capsaicin were well documented; however, they act as double-edged sword in many physiological circumstances. In traditional medicine, chilli has been used against various gastrointestinal complains such as dyspepsia, loss of appetite, gastroesophageal reflux disease, gastric ulcer and so on. Red Chilli contains a variety of carotenoids, including capsanthin, capsorubin, β-carotene, cryptoxanthin, lutein, phytofluene, and xanthophyll, and steroids, including capsicoside. Some of its active constituents play numerous beneficial roles in various gastrointestinal disorders such as stimulation of digestion and gastromucosal defense, reduction of gastroesophageal reflux disease (GERD) symptoms, inhibition of gastrointestinal pathogens, ulceration and cancers, regulation of gastrointestinal secretions and absorptions. However, further studies are warranted to determine the dose ceiling limit of chilli and its active constituents for their utilization as gastroprotective agents. This review summarizes the phytochemistry, various traditional uses and its various active constituents.

Keywords: GERD, Capsaicin, CAPS.

Introduction

Capsicum annuum L. belonging to Solanaceae family, popularly known as the nightshade family is a small herb that can grow up to 1 m tall. Leaves are oblong-ovate, ovate, obovate-lanceolate, 4-13 cm by 1.5-4 cm with entire margin. Flowers are small, white or tinged purple. Fruits are mostly red, but can be green, orange, yellow and cangrow up to 15 cm. Seeds are pale yellow, discoid obreniform and 3-5 mm. The fruits or berries of the Capsicum plant are varied in shape, color, size, and taste. The spicier versions are called chili peppers or chilis or just peppers in different parts of the world. The large mild green, yellow, or red bell peppers are called capsicum in India, Australia, New Zealand, and Singapore. Capsicum is a tropical and an important agricultural crop and one of the popular vegetables, not only because of its economic value, but also for the combination of color, taste and nutritional values of its fruit [1-5]. The interest in the consumption of capsicum is to a large extent due to its content of bioactive compounds and their importance as dietary antioxidants. One of the main constituents is capsaicin, which produces an intense burning sensation when it comes into contact with the skin, eyes, or mucous membranes and which gives peppers their burning taste. A hot shower or bath before topical application to the skin intensifies the burning sensation. Capsaicin is used internally for various conditions, including colic and for improving peripheral circulation, and externally for unbroken chilblains. Present review will highlight the chemical constituents and the pharmacological and therapeutic effects of *Capsicum annuum* [6-8].

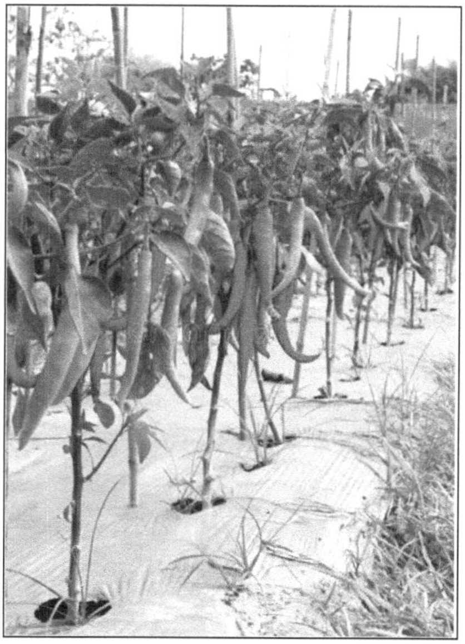

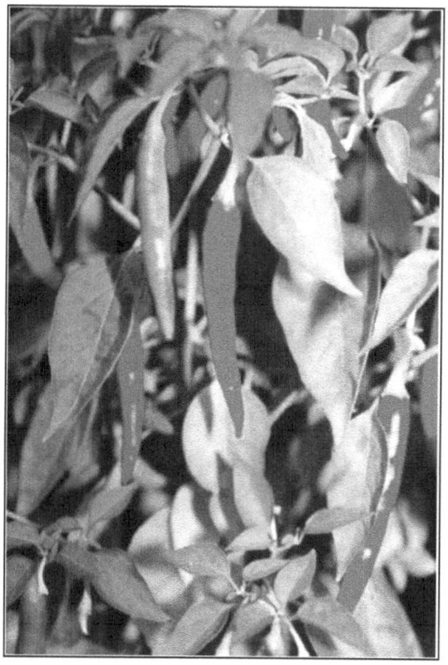

Chilli Plants

Health benefits of Capsicum

Capsicum comes in dried form, as a spice as chili pepper and paprika. The dried spice can be used in many sauces. The dried variety is available as whole dried peppers, as a single spice, or in dried spice blends. With chili's ready availability in many markets, it should be considered that though the dried spice is convenient and might be effective in its health benefits, eating it fresh may provide more benefits. Additionally, it might have been used in traditional medicine for the treatment of cough, toothache, sore throat, parasitic infections, and wound healing. The health benefits of capsicum may include relief from stomach issues, back pain, muscle spasms, headaches, skin aging, peptic ulcers, menopausal problems, lower risk of cardiovascular diseases, and diabetes management. It might have anti-inflammatory and analgesic properties, and may also provide relief from pain related to arthritis [9-12]. They can be an excellent source of vitamins A and C, among other nutrients. Capsicum is commonly applied to the skin for arthritis pain and other conditions. The fruit of the capsicum plant contains a chemical called capsaicin. Capsaicin is what seems to help reduce pain and swelling. A particular form of capsicum causes intense eye pain and other unpleasant effects when it comes in contact with the face. This form is used in self-defense pepper sprays. Capsicum is commonly used for nerve pain and other painful conditions. It is also used for many other purposes, including digestion problems, conditions of the heart and blood vessels and many others, but there is no good scientific evidence for many of these uses. Capsaicin, a water-insoluble derivative of homovanillic acid, and also the major active ingredient in capsicum is responsible for the hot and burning sensation to the tongue. With the varieties of chili peppers available, it is important to know that the capsaicin content of each type of chili pepper varies. This natural fruit may be used fresh or dried as a culinary spice, added to teas, or taken in capsules to reap its medicinal benefits [13-16].

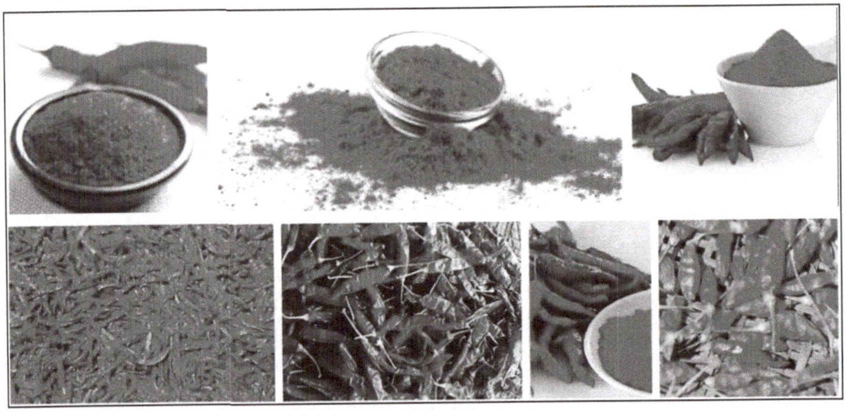

Dried chilies and powder

Peppers were used fresh, dried, fermented, or as an oleoresin extract. It has both nutritional and nutraceutical importance. Capsicum was used as a colorant, flavorant, and/or as a source of pungency. The main source of pungency in peppers is the chemical group of alkaloid compounds called capsaicinoids (CAPS), which are produced in the fruit. Capsaicin, trans-8-methyl-N-vanillyl-6-nonenamide, is the most abundant CAPS, followed by dihydrocapsaicin, with minor amounts of nordihydrocapsaicin, homocapsaicin, homodihydrocapsaicin, and others.

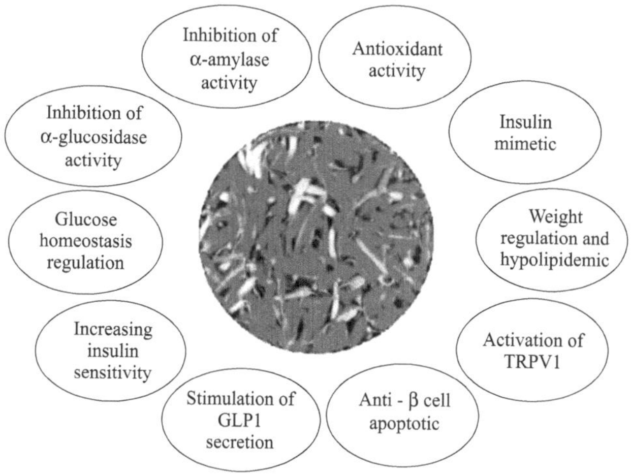

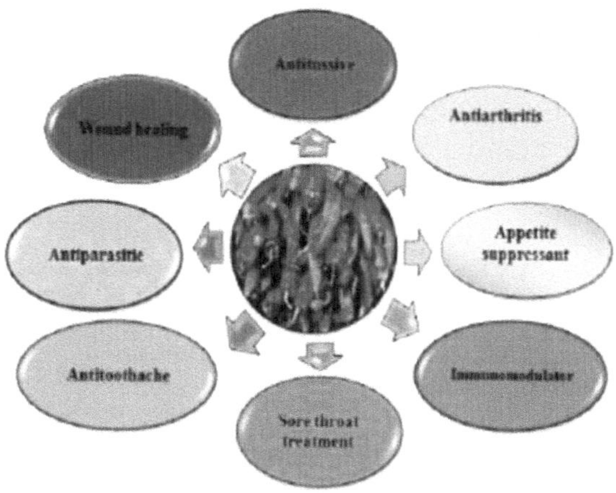

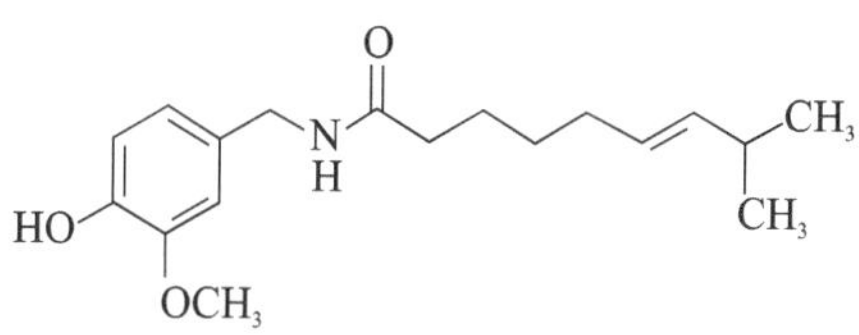

Capsaicin

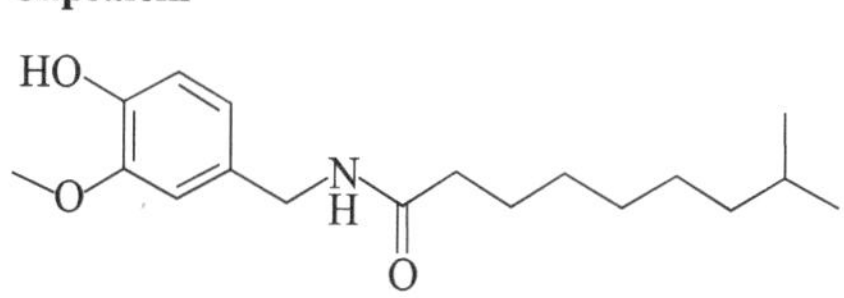

Dihydrocapsaicin

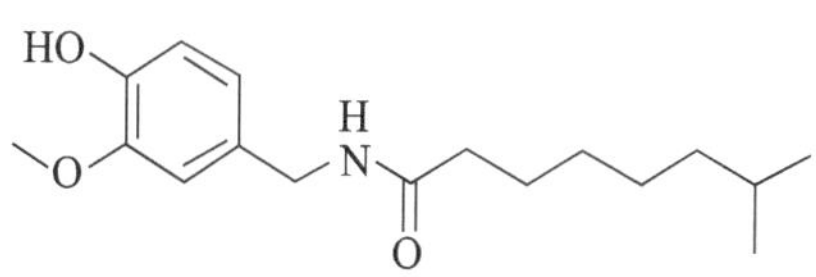

Capsaicin is a white crystalline, fat-soluble compound formed from homovanillic acid that is insoluble in water, odourless and tasteless. The red color of mature pepper fruits is due to several related carotenoid pigments, including capsanthin, capsorubin, cryptoxanthin, and zeaxanthin, which are present as fatty acid esters. The most important pigments are capsanthin and its isomer capsorubin, which make up to 30-60% and 6-18% respectively of the total carotenoids in the fruit. It is also important for its flavor in many products in addition to its color [17-19]. Dried chilli is also valued for its contribution to flavor in chilli sauces and chilli powders. The flavoring principle is associated with volatile aromatic compounds and color. As a general rule, when the color of paprika or chilli powder fades, the flavor also disappears. Both volatile and non-volatile substances contribute to its use as flavoring agent. *Capsicum annuum* was used traditionally to treat toothache. The fruits are used to stimulate gastric activities and increase blood circulation. It is also a stimulant, carminative, and used locally for neuralgia and for rheumatism. Uterine pain associated with childbirth istreated with soup containing the fruit. The Commission E approved *Capsicum annuum* for painful muscle spasms inareas of shoulder, arm and spines. Preparations are used to treat arthritis, neuralgia, lumbago and chilblains. The red color of capsicum is imparted by carotenoids with more than 50 identified structures. Carotenoids content in the reports varies from 0.1 to 3.2 g/100 g dry weight with marked difference in composition. The unique keto carotenoids capsanthin, capsorubin and cryptocapsin impart brilliant red color to ripen chilly pods, while the yellow orange color is from β-carotene, zeaxanthin, violaxanthin and β-cryptoxanthin [20-21]. Most of the xanthophylls in red pepper occur as esters with C12, C14 and C18 fatty acids whereas green pepper extracts comprised mostly of free carotenoids. The carotenoids such as capsanthin and capsorubin with ê-ring as end groups were previously reported to be characteristic of capsicum species. Capsanthin contributes 30-70% of carotenoids in most of the varieties and cultivars. The proportions of capsanthin and capsorubin increase in the advanced stages of ripening. Significant proportions of capsanthin-5,6-epoxide, capsanthin-3,6-epoxide, cucurbitaxanthin A, cucurbitaxanthin B, violaxanthin, antheraxanthin, capsanthone, neoxanthin, lutein etc. have also been reported in red pepper [19-23].

A small shrub like branched plant bearing green and red fruits is used as seasoning or enhancer. Chilies are an imperative ingredient in Indian, Thai and Mexican cuisines. More than 200 different species are discovered that contains capsaicin as an active ingredient and is helpful for respiration process, blood pressure and heart health. Chili belongs to the member of nightshade family, Solanaceae. Chili peppers are used in various cuisines to add heat to the dishes. Literally, chilies are originated in Mexico. Various cultivars spread across the word after Columbian exchange and used for both food purposes and as traditional medicine. The cultivars in Europe and North America are derived from *Capsicum annuum* and bears yellow, white, purple, red to black fruits. Unripe fruits are green and as it ripens turn to red color. Basically, it is a valuable source of minerals such as magnesium, iron, potassium, macronutrients and dietary fibers. This chilli is well-known for its intense pungent taste which is provided by the active constituent Capsaicin, a stimulant with no narcotic effect.

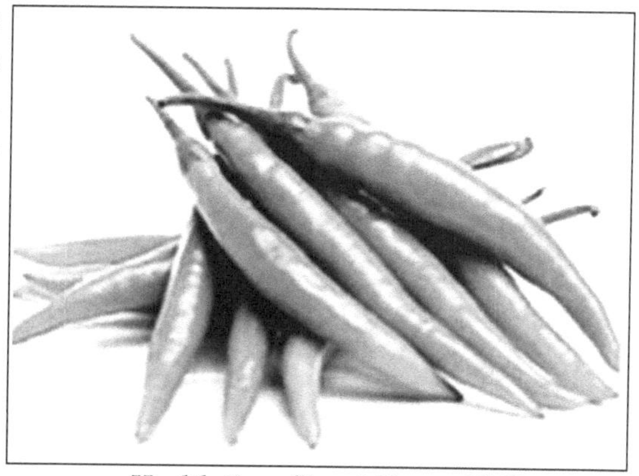

Health Benefits of Green Chill

It has a crucial role in boosting immunity and acts as anti-ulcer, anti-cancer, anti-inflammatory, analgesic, anti-hemorrhoidal and anti-epileptic agent. It also helps to manage burns, psoriasis, chronic migraine, diabetes and heart disorders. Green chilies are used raw, fried or added to curries. It has ample amounts of Vitamin C, A, B complex (B6 and B9). It reimburses the damaging effects of bacteria in the bodies and helpful to prevent blood clotting which is a major cause for cardiovascular problems such as cardiac arrest and heart stroke. It hinders the extent of cancer to colon, lungs and prostate. Green chilies provide relief from pain and swelling is associated with outraging bone ailments such as rheumatoid, osteoarthritis and arthritis. Chilies contain phytonutrients that relaxes respiratory passage and reduces the chances of lung cancer with prevention of problems related with lungs such as cough, asthma and cold. Green chilies have anti-bacterial properties that prevents from infections such as athlete's foot, colon infections and herpes zoster. It encompasses essential nutrients such as Vitamin C and B6 that enhance the immunity of the body to counteract diseases. Green chilies are packed with essential dietary fiber that cleanses colon and supports healthy bowel movements and also prevents the chances of constipation. Adequate amount of calcium in green chilies is must for keeping the bones and teeth healthy as well as strong. It also repairs tissues and helps in forming new blood cells. Green chilies contain Vitamin A, an essential nutrient required for improving vision and lower the chances of cataracts and macular degeneration that occurs as people ages. No calories are found in green chilies. Also, it promotes the body's metabolism and helps to burn excess fat from the body. Vitamin C facilitates the formation of collagen which maintains firmness as well as health of the skin. The phytonutrients found in it helps to cure rashes, acne, blemishes, pimples and wrinkles. Vitamin E forms natural oils which are beneficial for the skin. Capsaicin releases the good endorphins and acts as anti-depressant keeping the mood positive. Green chilies contain natural silicon that promotes blood circulation to the scalp and hair follicles. As a stimulator, it protects hair follicles. The chilies have Vitamin C that absorbs iron and provides oxygen to the hair by preventing of split ends and hair breakage. Use green chilies in breads, curries, stir fries and meat dishes. Especially, green chilies are used in pickles, chutney, sauces and spicy snacks.

Use chilies as a topping for burritos, egg dishes, enchiladas and fries. It is used in savory dishes such as dals, breads and appetizers. Green chilli helps to lower the appearance of scars and wrinkles. It is useful to treat malarial fevers, constipation, gout and hemorrhoids. It is used in tinctures and ointments for its anti-pruritic, astringent, analgesic and counter-irritant properties.

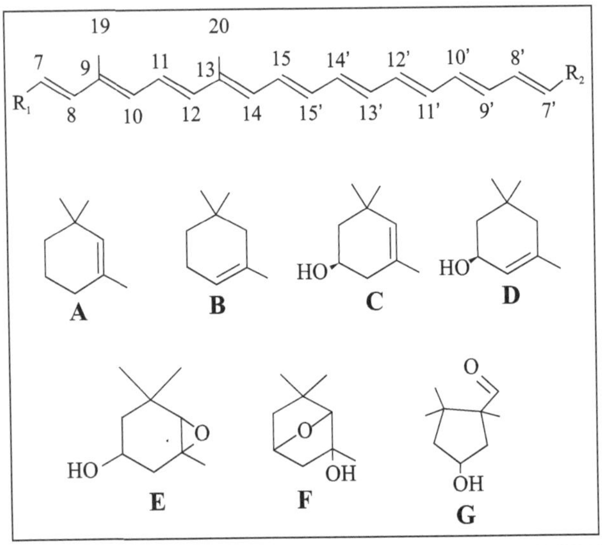

Major carotenoids in red pepper	R1	R2
β-carotene	A	A
α-carotene	A	B
Capsathin	C	G
Capsathin-5, 6-epoxide	E	G
Capsathin-3, 6-epoxide	F	G
α-cryptoxanthene	C	B
Capsorubin	G	G
Cryptpocapsin	A	G
β-cryptoxanthin	C	D
Lutein	C	D
Antheraxanthin	E	C
Violoxanthin	E	E
Zeaxanthin	C	C

Discussion and Conclusion

The uniqueness of pepper is the typical pungency due to the presence of capsaicinoids. Capsaicinoids are secondary metabolites and derivatives of phenylpropanoids produced in placental epidermis cells and accumulated in structures (blisters) located on the placenta surface. The hotness sensation when consumed is given by the interaction with vanilloid receptors, supposed to be a mechanism of defense against mammalian herbivory. Capsaicin and dihydro-capsaicin are the two predominant compounds, accounting for almost 90% of total capsaicinoids. Anti-inflammatory, anticancer and anti-obesity activities have been recognized within capsaicinoids. These properties are exerted by the release of substance P, a neuro-transmitter involved in pain transmission by nerve. Peppers are also an extremely good source of compounds exerting antioxidant properties and responsible for fruit pigmentation. Different colors are encountered in mature fruits as a result of accumulation of carotenoids in chromoplasts during ripening such as capsanthin and capsorubin (mainly in red fruits), violaxanthin and neoxanthin (mainly in yellow fruit), and lutein and b-carotene (mainly in orange fruit). High contents of other essential vitamins such vitamin A in the form of b-carotene and vitamins of group B (thiamine, riboflavin, and niacin) are recognized. All these compounds, of which content is determined by species, cultivar, environmental conditions, and maturation stage, exert their biological effects protecting cells against oxidative damage through the interaction with oxygen molecules and scavenging peroxyl radicals. Finally, antimicrobial and antivirulence properties, against Streptococcus pyogenes, a major human pathogen.

Fusarium infection, a polyphagous fungus affecting many vegetables, are reported. All these properties make pepper a good candidate against diseases. Other than food uses are recognized as active ingredient in cosmetics, pharmaceuticals, and pest management. The extractable colors from fruits due to the presence of compounds unique in pepper such as capsanthin, capsorubin, and cryptocapsin are extensively used in the food processing industry as natural colorant for a wide range of products such meats, cheeses, and other foods. Non-food uses include coloring and flavoring agents, from oleoresins (carotenoids) extracts or powder, as example, paprika powder can be used to inhibit lipid oxidation of pork meat while oleo-resin is used to enhance physical and sensory properties of food product.

REFERENCES

1. GarcíaGMR, AlejoON. Biochemistry and Molecular Biology of Carotenoid Biosynthesis inchili peppers (Capsicum spp). Int J Mol Sc. 2013; 14: 19025-19053.
2. Tewksbury JJ, Reagan KM, Machnicki NJ, Carlo TA, Haak DC, Penaloza ALC, Levey DJ. Evolutionary Ecology of Pungency in Wild Chilies. ProcNatlAcad Sci. 2008; 105: 11808-11811.

3. Baenas N, Beovíc M, Llic N, Moreno DA, García-Vi-guera C. Industrial use of Pepper (Capsicumannum L.) Derived Products: Technological Benefits and Biological Advantages. Food Chem. 2019; 274: 872-885.
4. Barceloux DG. Pepper and Capsaicin (Capsicum and Piper species) Dis Mon. 2009; 55: 380-390.
5. Singletary K. Red Pepper: Overview of Potential Health Benefits. *Nut Today.* 2011; 46: 33-47.
6. Pawar SS, Bharude NV, Sonone SS, Deshmukh RS, Raut AK, Umarkar AR. Chilles as Food, Spice and Medicine: A Perspective. Int J Pharm Biol Sci. 2011; 1: 311-318.
7. Maji AK, Banerji P. Phytochemistry and Gastrointestinal Benefits of the Medicinal Spice *Capsicum annuum* L.(Chilli): A Review. J Complement Integr Med. 2016; 13: 97-122.
8. Dog LT. A Reason to Season: The Therapeutic Benefits of Spices and Culinary Herbs. Explore (NY). 2006; 2: 446-449.
9. Kim WR, Kim EO, Kang K, Oidovsambuu S, Jung SH, Kim BS, *et al.* Antioxidant Activity of Phenolics in Leaves of Three Red Pepper (*Capsicum annuum*) Cultivars. J Agric Food Chem. 2014; 62: 850-859.
10. Papoiu AD, Yosipovitch G. Topical Capsaicin. The Fire of a 'Hot'Medicine is Reignited. *Expert OpinPharmacother.* 2010; 11: 1359-1371.
11. Hayman M, Kam PC. Capsaicin: A Review of its Pharmacology and Clinical Applications. CurrAnaesth Crit Care. 2008; 19: 338-343.
12. Srinivasan K. Spices as Influencers of Body Metabolism: An Overview of Three Decades of Research. Food Res Int. 2005; 38: 77-86.
13. Wesolowska A, Jadczak D, Grzeszczuk M. Chemical Composition of the Pepper Fruit Extracts of Hot Cultivars *Capsicum annuum* L. ActaSci Pol HortorumCultus. 2011; 10: 171-184.
14. D'Alonzo AJ, Grover GJ, Darbenzio RB, Hess TA, Sleph PG, Dzwonczyk S, *et al. In vitro* Effects of Capsaicin: Antiarrhythmic and Antiischemic Activity. Eur J Pharmacol. 1995; 272: 269-278.
15. Mason L, Moore RA, Derry S, Edwards JE, McQuay HJ. Systematic Review of Topical Capsaicin for the Treatment of Chronic Pain. BMJ. 2004; 328: 991.
16. Mueller M, Beck V, Jungbauer A. PPARalpha Activation by Culinary Herbs and Spices. Planta Med. 2011; 77: 497-504.
17. Arimboor R, Natarajan RB, Menon RK, Lekshmi P. Chandrasekhar LP, Moorkoth V. Red pepper (*Capsicum annuum*) Carotenoids as a Source of Natural Food Colors: Analysis and Stability—a Review J Food Sci Technol. 2015; 52(3): 1258-1271. doi: 10.1007/s13197-014-1260-7
18. Banergy P, Maji AK. Phytochemistry and Gastrointestinal Benefits of the Medicinal Spice, *Capsicum annuum* L. (Chilli): A Review. J Complement IntegrMed. 2016; 13(2): 97-122. doi: 10.1515/jcim-2015-0037.
19. RuizRM, Gordo GS, Cañas A, Campos, MJ, Paradela A, Corpas FJ, Palma JM. Sweet Pepper (*Capsicum annuum* L.) Fruits Contain an Atypical Peroxisomal Catalase That is Modulated by Reactive Oxygen and Nitrogen Species. *Antioxidants.* 2019, 8, 374. https://doi.org/10.3390/antiox8090374
20. Jha TB, Dafadar A, Ghorai A. (2012). New Genetic Resource in Capsicum L. from Eastern Himalayas. Plant Genet Resour Characteriz Utiliza. 2012; 10: 141-144.
21. Kehie M, Kumaria S, Tandon P, Ramchiary N. Biotechnological Advances on in vitro Capsaicinoids biosynthesis in Capsicum: A review. Phytochem Rev. 2014; doi: 10.1007/s11101-014-9344-6
22. Kim *et al.* Genome Sequence of the Hot Pepper provides insights into the Evolution of Pungency in Capsicum species. Nat Genet 2014; doi:10.1038/ng.287
23. Kumar RV, Sharma VK, Chattopadhyay B, Chakraborty S. An Improved Plantre Generation and Agrobacterium – Mediated Transformation of Red pepper (Capsicumannuum L.). Physiology and Molecular Biology of Plants 2012; doi: 10.1007/s12298-012-0132-8.

CHAPTER

22

Cinnamomum tamala
A Spice of Immense Culinary and Therapeutic Importance

ABSTRACT

C. tamala bark, fruits and leaves exhibits wider use of *C. tamala* in generation of chemopreventive anti-cancer, antiulcer, immunomodulatory, antilipidemic, antidiabetic and hepatoprotective drugs which might show broad-spectrum biological effectiveness. *C. tamala* essential leaves oil contains various components but majorly eugenol, sabinene, germacrene D, β-caryophyllene and curcumenol. This cinnamon oil consists of different class of sesquiterpenoids i.e. furanodienone, curzerenone, furanodiene and curzerene. The leaves have camphene, myrcene, limonene and alfapinene as its major constituents. Bark of *C. tamala* consist of cinnamaldehyde. Cinnamon oil is used as anti-flatulent, diuretic and carminative. Furanogermenone, β-caryophyllene, germacerene d, curcumenol, curzerenone, furanodiene, furanodienone, sesquiterpenoids compounds, and mainly contains some other phytochemical compounds cinnamaldehyde, eugenol, α- linalool, carophyllene oxide, geraniol, Benzaldehyde, 1,8-cineole, Salicylaldehyde, γ-terpinene, acetophenone, cis-sabinene hydrate, trans-sabinene hydrate, 3-phenyl propanala, Pinocarvone, borneol, 2-methylbenzofuran, tepinen4-ol, p-cymen-8-ol, α-terpineol, bornyl acetate, cinnamyl alcohol, hydrocinnamyl acetate, cinnamyl acetate, cinnamic acid, coumarin, cinnamyl acetate, α -humulene, nerolidol, spathulenol, Monoterpenoid Hydrocarbons, Oxygenated Monoterpenes, Sesquiterpens Hydrocarbons, Oxygenated Sesquiterpens, Phenylpropanoids and also includes in small quantity of α–humulene, α–muurolen. The present review explains therapeutic and pharmaceutical potential of *Cinnamomum tamala*, also emphasizes important uses of *C. tamala* constituents as spice.

Keywords: Cinnamaldehyde, β-caryophyllene, Immunomodulatory, Hepatoprotective, Antiulcer.

Introduction

Cinnamomum tamala Nees and Eberm (family-Lauraceae) is a multipurpose evergreen plant native of India commonly known as Tejpat or Bay leaf. This is an important traditional medicinal plant found in various parts of India, especially in Himalayan region. Plant contains aromatic leaves which are major source bioactive compounds of immense therapeutic, culinary and medicinal use. Plant has many synonyms and recognized by different names based on local area. In Bengali, it is called as tejpat, in Hindi tejpatta, in Marathi tamalpatra, in Telugu bagharakku, tamālapattram in Sanskrit, tejpata in Nepal and tsheringma herb that is used Bhutan in tea. Bay laurel leaves are shorter and light to medium green in color, with one large vein down the length of the leaf, while tejpat leaves are about twice as long and wider, usually olive green in color and with three veins down the length of the leaf. Dried leaves of *Cinnamomum tamala* spread are used to flavor a variety of food preparations. Plant bark and leaves are good source of aromatic essential oil which possess phenolic compounds which show multiple therapeutic effects against Alzheimer 's disease, diabetes, arthritis and arteriosclerosis. Plant emits clove-cinnamon like flavor. Essential oil is golden-yellow in color and possesses a very hot aromatic taste. Plant bark is rich source of cinnamaldehyde that provides a pungent taste and strong aroma that after exposure with oxygen, it become dark in color and forms resinous compounds [1-4]. Cinnamon essential oil contains more than 80 compounds including eugenol and cinnamaldehyde as major constituents. Plant leaves are used to generate special flavor to dishes, beverages and food items. In Ancient time, the plant also used as for its medicinal value and it contains an aromatic property. Due to the presence of this property, it is used in perfumery industry and used as mouth refreshing, useful for removal of bad odour from body, mouth and also used in pharmaceutical industries. The leaves of the plant possess flavoring agent property, it is used as a flavoring agent in food, curry, fast food, pickles and used as a spice. All parts of plant possess many major bioactive constituents due to the presence of major phytoconstituent like alkaloids, steroids, sugar, flavonoids, tannins, saponins, phenols, carbohydrate, etc. The different parts of this plants shows many pharmacological activities like immunosuppresive, antidiabetic, antibacterial, antiparasitic, antimicrobial, anti-HIV, antiulcer, antidiabetic, hyperlipidemic, anti-inflammatory, immunomodulatory, antitumour, antityrosinase, antioxidant, hepatoprotective, gastroprotective, cryptoprotective, mulluscidial, antifungal, antipyretic, antipathogenic, antigenotoxic, antidiarrheal and Alzheimer's prevention potential activities that are useful for the treatment of various diseases or disorders. *Cinnamomum tamala* leaves put strong effect on biological systems such as immune system, gastro-intestinal tract and liver. The bark is also sometimes used for cooking and flavoring the food [5-8]. Cinnamon bark, essential oils, bark powder showed multiple biological activity such as antioxidant, antidiabetic, anti-inflammatory, anticancer, and antimicrobial activity. Essential oil of *C. tamala* is found toxic to mosquito larvae and fire ants. It is also found therapeutically effective against Alzheimer's disease, diabetes, arthritis, and arteriosclerosis, cancer and inflammatory, cardioprotective and neurological disorders. Phytochemical analysis of *C. tamala* leaf extract revealed presence of important saponins, phytosterols, fatty acids, carbohydrates, monoterpene, sesquiterpene, geraniol, linolol, bornyl acetate, caryophylene oxide, p-coumaric acid and vanillic acid. Plant leaves also contain, procyanidin oligomers compounds, mainly cinnam, tannin B1, cinnamtannin D1 (CTD-1), parameritannin A1, procyanidin B2 and procyanidin C1 in bark. *C. tamala*, also contain cinnamtannin D-1 (CD1) as one of the main A-type procyanidin oligomers. Plant also contains steroids, terpenoids and tannins, polysaccharides, procyanidins cpd3, cpd4 and cpd6 and glycosides, cinnacassides F and G, with a rare geranylphenylacetate carbon skeleton [9-12].

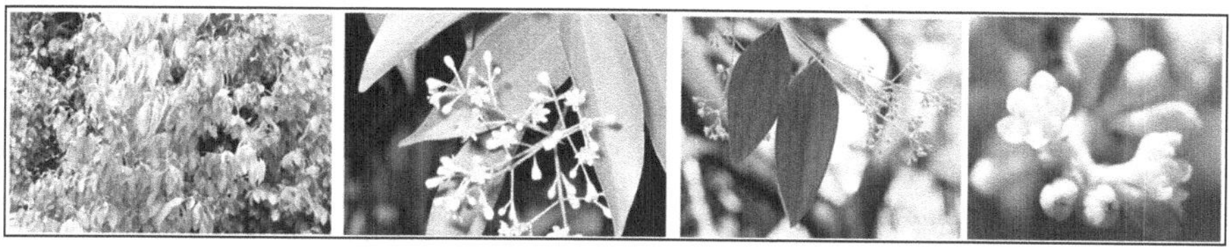

***C. tamala* Leaves, Flowers and seeds**

Phytochemical Constituents

Various chemicals of immense therapeutic applicability were isolated fron different parts of *C. tamala* viz. Cinnamaldehyde, trans-cinnamaldehyde, 3,4′, 5,7- tetrahyroxyflavone, 3, 3′, 4′, 5,7- pentahydroxyflavone (non-glycoside compounds), kaempferol-3- Oglycopyranoside (Astragalin), quercetin-3-Orutinoside, quercetin-3-O- sophoroside (flavonoid glycoside), kaempferol-3,7di-O-rhamnopyraoside, a-pinene, myrcene, camphene, p-cymene, limonene, eugenol (4-hydroxy-3- methoxyallylbenzene), methyl eugenol, methyl ether eugenol and eugenol acetate. In the evaluation of leaf oil of plant, the study found that plant leaf oil possess a major bioactive compound includes Furanogermenone, β- caryophyllene, germacerene d, curcumenol, curzerenone, furanodiene, furano dienone and contains a rich amount of sesquiterpenoids compounds, and mainly contains some other phytochemical compounds cinnamaldehyde, eugenol, α- linalool, carophyllene oxide, geraniol, Benzaldehyde, 1,8-cineole, Salicylaldehyde, γ-terpinene, acetophenone, cis-sabinene hydrate, trans- sabinene hydrate, 3-phenyl propanala, Pinocarvone, borneol, 2- methylbenzofuran, tepinen4-ol, p-cymen-8-ol, α-terpineol, bornyl acetate, cinnamyl alcohol, hydrocinnamyl acetate, cinnamyl acetate, cinnamic acid, coumarin, cinnamyl acetate, α -humulene, nerolidol, spathulenol, Monoterpenoid Hydrocarbons,

Oxygenated Monoterpenes, Sesquiterpens Hydrocarbons, Oxygenated Sesquiterpens, Phenylpropanoids and also includes in small quantity of α-humulene, α-muurolene. In a study, the chemical composition of the essential oils obtained from the fresh leaves of *Cinnamomum tamala* Neeset Eberm. determined by GC and GC-MS yielded the oil on a dry weight basis ranging from 1.2% to 3.9% (w/w). Phenyl propanoids constitute the major portion (88.9-95.0%) of the oils. Fifty-four compounds were identified from the oils. Eugenol (91.4-41.8%) was the main compound, followed by eugenyl acetate (0.0-47.1%) and α-phellandrene (0.6-2.5%) in the analyzed oils [13-16]. The extract of this plant reduces the oxidative damage and it is protective against renal toxicity induced by gentamicin. It is useful in the treatment of different diseases including anal and rectal disease, protective against flatulence, cancer, coryza (inflammation in mucous membrane), anorexia, liver and spleen diseases, prevent bleeding (used as a coagulating agent), cardio vascular diseases and used for induce blood circulation. Plant bark is a good source of essential oils and its phenolic compounds which show multiple beneficial effects against Alzheimer's disease, cardiac mainly arteriosclerosis. Plant also shows therapeutic effects against cancer and inflammation, cardiac, and neurological disorders. Leaves and bark have aromatic, astringent, stimulant and carminative qualities and used in rheumatism, colic, diarrhea, nausea and vomiting. The essential oil of the leaves called tejpat oil is medicinally used as carminative, anti-flatulent, diuretic and in cardiac disorders. It is also used in pharmaceutical preparations because of its hypoglycemic, stimulant and carminative properties. This plant shows moderate level of pharmacological activities such as immunosuppressive activity, antidiabetic activity, antibacterial activity, antimicrobial activity, anti-HIV activity, anti-inflammatory activity, antitumour activity, antityrosinase activity, anti-oxidant activity, antifungal activity, antidiarrheal activity and Alzheimer's prevention potential activity, etc. Bark and dried leaves powder are used for reducing fever, anaemia (lack of blood), unpleasant body odour, bad mouth odour and the plant seed powder are combined with honey prescribed for children in purpose of diarrhoea, cough problem. The plant possesses aromatic property due to the presence of its property, it is useful in perfumery industry and also useful in preparation of soaps, detergents, cosmetics, toothpaste etc. and also useful in food industry as a spice. *C. Tamala* plant parts are useful for preparation of some ayurvedic formulation like Sudarshanchurna, Chandraprabhavati etc. Leaves extract of plant used as a clarifier in dyeing method with emblicmyrobalans. *C. tamala* plant is also used as a food, fodder, medicine etc. Numerous studies shown that the plant leaves are also used for its green dyeing property [17-19].

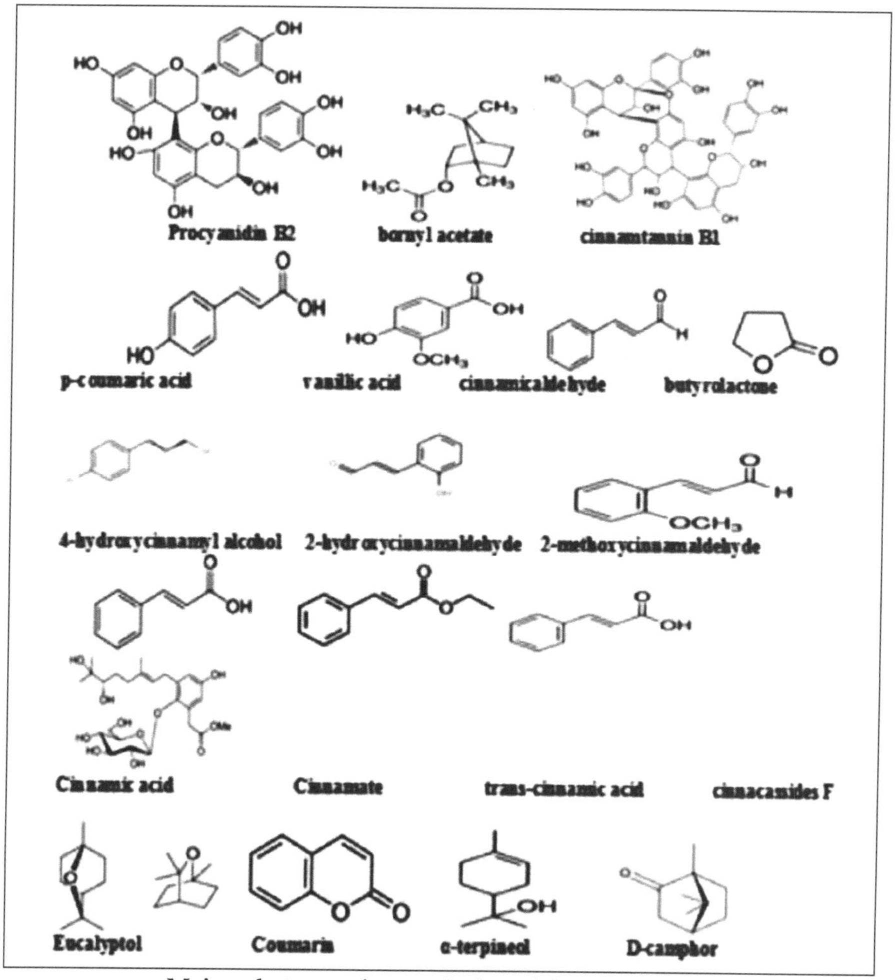

Major phytoconstituents isolate d from *C. tamala*

Traditional and Ethnopharmacological Relevance

The plant is used in many years ago in Indian system, ayurvedic system and also traditionally system for its medicinal property, aromatic property and used as a flavoring agent in food. Traditionally, tejpatta is used in food, beverages, fast food, pickle used as a flavoring agent or as a spices and also useful for its aromatic property. The presence of flavoring agent, mouth refreshening property, the plant is also used in chewing gums and also beneficial for breath problems. Tejpatta powder is used for some dental problems like reducing tooth pain. Traditionally, the plant is useful for the treatment of many diseases and disorders includes colon cancer, Diabetes, cardiac disease, CNS disorders, bleeding disorder (useful for increase blood circulation in uterus) and it is also useful in appetite problem, mouth problems like dryness of mouth, unpleasant/poor breath problem, rheumatism, etc.

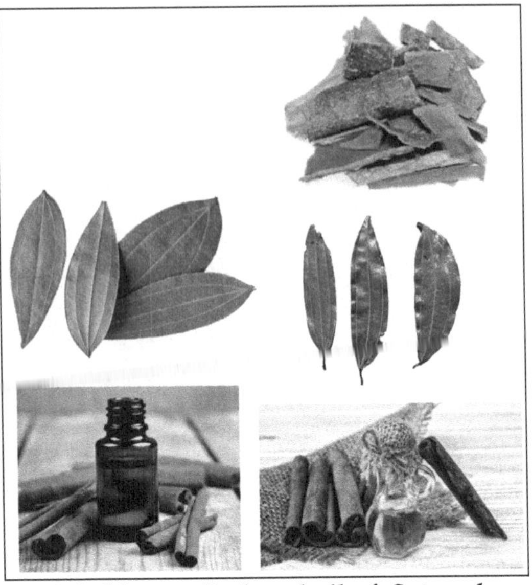
Dried leaves, Bark and oil of *C. tamala*

Tejpatta leaves and bark also exhibits astringent, antiemetic, antidiarrheal, anti-inflammatory includes wound healing property, carminative property (relieving flatulence) [20-22]. *C. tamala* and its associating species are rich source of economically important bio-organic products which can be largely used for preparation of flavored foods, pharmaceuticals and pesticides. Both leaves and plant bark of this plant is widely used in folk medicine. *C. verum* bark is used as Dalchini, a specific spice. Its leaves are used to provide a specific aroma to vegetable curries. Its bio-organic ingredients can kill drug resistant pathogens. *Cinnamomum* species contains alkaloids, triterpenes, cinnamaldehyde which showed antioxidant, anti-inflammatory, antidiabetic, anti-inflammatory, immunomodulatory, immunosuppressive antimicrobial, anticancer effects and anti-food spoilage/ antipathogenic activity. Essential oils obtained from this plant possess various active ingredients which can be used to control insects and nematodes and drug resistant bacteria and fungi. These can be processed to obtain pharmaceutical agents mainly against gastric, diabetic, high blood pressure and neurological problems. *Cinnamomum* species contain major group of biologically active chemicals that can be used to make highly efficacious broad spectrum pharmaceutical products. The different parts of plant like stem, bark, leaves and also the whole plants shows many activities. The different phytochemical of these plants has been taken out from several extract from various part of these plants which contain so many chemicals such as alkaloids, steroids, sugar, flavonoids, tannins, saponins, amino acids and phenolic compounds carbohydrates, glycosides, phytosterols, proteins, oils and fats that are used as medicinal purpose. Also, the leaves of *Cinnamomum tamala* are widely used as spice throughout the world since ancient times. It is used in Indian system of traditional medicines in various ayurvedic formulations [20-24].

Culinary usages

Tejpatta leaves is commonly used in foods, beverages, pickles, meats, fast foods, chewing gums as a flavouring agent, it also exhibits a mouth freshening property. It is a natural food preservative agent used in some juices like pineapple juice. Oil of *Cinnamomum* is used in baked goods and to flavor various alcoholic beverages. Cinnamon is mixed during distillation process to prepare cinnamon liqueur or brandy. It is also added to flavor white wine mainly maiwein and vodka in Europe. Cinnamon bark is used as spice to flavor food. It is used in cookery as a condiment and flavoring material. It is also used to produce flavored chocolates in Mexico. Cinnamon is used in preparing buns, apple pie and dough nuts and in other desert recipes. Cinnamon mixed with sugar is used to flavored, sweet and savoury dishes, cereals, breads, toasts. It is also rubbed on fruits to provide a specific aroma. Cinnamon is used in important spices, pickling, soups, drinks and sweets [7,9,11-13].

Conclusion

The major component of Cinnamon oil is eugenol (4-hydroxy-3-methoxy- allylbenzene), (β caryophyllene, sabinene, germacrene D and curcumenol. The leaf oil was characterized by a high content of sesquiterpenoids, dominated mainly by furanosesquiterpenoids. The main constituent of *C. tamala* leaves are camphene, myrcene, limonene, methyl ether of eugenol and alfapinene. Barks of cinnamon also having medicinal value it possesses cinnamaldehyde which is responsible for its aroma. Medicinally tejpatta oil used as anti-flatulent, diuretic and carminative also it has anti-oxidative potentiality. *Cinnamomum tamala* shows moderate level of activities such as immunosuppressive activity, antidiabetic activity, antibacterial activity, antiparasitic activity, antimicrobial activity, anti-HIV activity, antiulcer activity, antidiabetic activity, hyperlipidemic activity, anti-inflammatory activity, immunomodulatory activity, antitumour activity, antityrosinase activity, anti-oxidant activity, hepatoprotective activity, gastroprotective activity, cryptoprotective activity, mulluscidial activity, antifungal activity, antipyretic activity, antipathogenic activity, antigenotoxic activity, antidiarrheal activity and Alzheimer's prevention potential activity. The phytochemical analysis of the methanolic extract of *Cinnamomum tamala* leaves confirmed the presence of various secondary metabolites including alkaloids, flavonoids, terpenoids and tannins. Alkaloids show anthelminthic, antidiarrheal and antimicrobial activities. Numerous researchers study shown that the tejpatta possess a various pharmacological activity such as anti-hyperlipidemic activity, anti-diabetic activity, gastro protective activity, anti-helminthic/antiprotozoal activity, anti-inflammatory property, antiemetic activity, anti-diarrheal, antifungal activity, it has shown potent antibacterial property against various micro-organism (*Escherichia coli, Bacillus subtilis, Saccharomyces cerevisiae*), anti-oxidant property, free radical scavenging activity, also exhibit CNS protective activity like anticonvulsant and hypothermic activity. The extract of plant reduces the oxidative damage and useful for the protective against renal toxicity induced by gentamicin etc. and useful for treat various diseases includes anal and rectal disease, protective against flatulence, cancer, coryza (inflammation in mucous membrane), anorexia, liver and spleen diseases, prevent bleeding (used as a coagulating agent), cardio vascular diseases and used for induce blood circulation. Leaves oil is useful for dermatophytic infection.

REFERENCES

1. Upadhyay RK. Therapeutic and Pharmaceutical Potential of Cinnamomum Tamala. Res Rev: Pharm Pharmaceut Sci. 2017; 6 (3): 18-28.
2. Sharma V and Rao LJ. An Overview on Chemical Composition, Bioactivity and Processing of Leaves of Cinnamomumtamala. Crit Rev Food SciNutr. 2014; 54(4): 433-448.
3. Satyal P, *et al*. Bioactivities and Compositional Analyses of Cinnamomum Essential Oils from Nepal. C. camphora, *C. tamala*, and C. glaucescens. Nat Prod Commun. 2013; 8(12): 1777-1784.
4. Taha AM, Eldahshan OA. Chemical Characteristics, Antimicrobial, and Cytotoxic Activities of the Essential Oil of Egyptian Cinnamomum glanduliferum Bark. Chem Biodivers. 2017; 14(5).
5. Shahwar D, *et al*. Anticancer Activity of Cinnamon tamala Leaf Constituents towards Human Ovarian Cancer Cells. Pak J Pharm Sci. 2015; 28(3): 969-972.
6. Ahmed A, *et al*. Essential Oil Constituents of the Spice *Cinnamomum tamala* (Ham.) Nees and Eberm. FlavFragra J 2000; 15(6): 388-390.
7. Pandey AK, Mishra AK. Antifungal and Antioxidative Potential of Oil and Extracts derived from Leaves of Indian Spice Plant Cinnamomumtamala. Cell Mol Biol. 2012; 58(1): 142-144.
8. Wang J, Su B, Jiang H, Cui N, Yu Z, Yang Y, Sun Y. Traditional uses, Phytochemistry and Pharmacological activities of Thegenus Cinnamomum (Lauraceae): A Review. Fitoterapia. 2020; 146: 104675.
9. Sankaran V, Chakraborty A, Jeyaprakash K, Ramar M, Chellappan DR. Chemical Analysis of Leaf Essential Oil of *Cinnamomum tamala* from Arunachal Pradesh, India. J Pharm Sci. 2015; 8: 246-248.
10. Tiwari S, Talreja S. Importance of Cinnamomum Tamala in the Treatment of Various Diseases. Pharmacog J. 2020, 12: 1792-1796.doi:10.5530/pj.2020.12.241
11. Sharma G *et al*, Cinnamomumtamala: A valuable Tree from Himalayas, Int. J. Med. Arom. Plants, 2011, Vol. 1(1): 1-4.
12. Sharma V, Rao LJM. An Overview on Chemical Composition, Bioactivity and Processing of Leaves of Cinnamomum tamala Crit Rev Food SciNutr. 2014; 54(4): 433-48. doi: 10.1080/10408398.2011.587615
13. Rana VS, Langoljam RD, Verdeguer M, Blázquez MA. Chemical Variability in the Essential Oil of Cinnamomum tamala L. leaves from India. Nat Prod Res. 2012; 26(14): 1355-7. doi: 10.1080/14786419.2011.599806
14. Jeyasree P, Dasarathan P. Screening of Phytochemicals and Immuneomodulatory Potential of Amedicinal Plant, Cinnamomumtamala. Int J PharmaSci Res. 2012; 3: 1049-1052.
15. Kumar S, Kumari R. Cinnamomum: Review Article of Essential Oil Compounds, Ethnobotany, Antifungal and Antibacterial effects. Open Access J Sci, 2019; 3(1): 3-16.
16. Kumar S, Kumari R. Cinnamomum: Review Article of Essential Oil Compounds, Ethnobotany, Antifungal and Antibacterial effects. J Sci. 2019; 3, 13-16.
17. Mehta, S, Purohit VK, Andola, HC. Pharmacological Activities of Cinnamomum tamala Nees & Eberm. and Medical Implication: A Review. Med Aroma Plants. 2014; 2(4): 12-13.

18. Shah M, Panchal M. (2010). Ethnopharmacological Properties of Cinnamomum tamala—A review. International Journal of Pharmaceutical Sciences Review and Research, 5(3): 141-144.
19. Gill S, Panthari P, Kharkwal H. Phytochemical Investigation of High Altitude Medicinal Plants Cinnamomum tamala (Buch-ham) Nees and Eberm and Rhododendron Arboreum Smith. Am J PhytomedClinTher. 2015; 3(6): 512-528.
20. Hassan W, Kazmi SNZ, Noreen H, Riaz A, Zaman B. Antimicrobial Activity of Cinnamomum tamala Leaves. J Nutr Disorders Ther. 2916; 6: 190-195.doi:10.4172/2161-0509.1000190
21. Gulati BC, Agarwal S, Thappa RK, Dhar KL. Essential Oil of Tejpat (Kumaon) from Cinnamomum tamala. Indian Perfum. 21.1(1977): 15-20.
22. Sood RP, Padha CD, Talwar IP, Jamwal RK, Chopra MM, Rao PR. Essential Oils from the Leaves of Cinnamomum tamala Nees and Ebern. Growing in Himachal Pradesh, Indian Perfumer, 23(1979): 75-78.
23. Simic A, Sokovic MD, Ristic M, *et al.* The Chemical Composition of some Lauraceae Essential Oils and their Antifungal activities. Phytother Res. 18(2004): 713-770.
24. Kapoor PS, Singh B, Singh F, Isidorov C, Szczepaniak L. Chemistry, Antimicrobial and Antioxidant Potentials of Cinnamomum tamala Nees & Eberm. (Tejpat) Essential Oil and Oleoresins. Nat Prod Radiance. Nat Prod Radiance. 2009; 8(2): 106-116.
25. Mal D, Gharde SK, Chatterjee R. Chemical Constituent of Cinnamomum tamala: An Important Tree Spices. Int J CurrMicrobiol App Sci. 2018; 7(4): 648-651. doi: https://doi.org/10.20546/ijcmas. 2018.704.073

CHAPTER
23

An appraisal on Nutritional, Phytochemical and traditions aspects of Tamarind (*Tamarindus indica* Linn.)

ABSTRACT

Tamarind, a podded fruit constitutes pulp, seeds, shell and fibers. The various constituents of the pulp include tartaric acid, reducing sugars, pectin, protein, fiber and cellulosic materials. The pulp is widely used for domestic and industrial purposes, and also claims some medical uses. It is found in all medicinal system for a number of diseases, these includes its usefulness in jaundice, in liver, complains, as an acid refrigerant, as a gentle laxative, in yellow fever, as a blood tonic, and as a skin cleanser. It contains, citric acid, oleic acid, linoleic acid, volatile oils (geraniol, limonene), pipecolic acid, lupeol, orientin, vitamin B_3, vitamin C, vitexin, phenylalanine, leucine, potassium, Campesterol, β-amyrin, β-sitosterol, Tannins, saponins, glycosides. It has various pharmacological activities like hypolipidemic, weight reducing, antimicrobial, hepatoprotective, anthelmintic, antioxidant, analgesic and anti-inflammatory etc. Tamarind kernel powder is an important sizing material in textile, paper and jute industries. This paper reports the brief information of tamarind fruit, composition of tamarind pulp and its uses.

Keywords: Tamarind seed, Tannin, Proanthocyanidin, Xyloglucan, Chrysanthemin Ascorbic acid, Fluorosis.

Introduction

Tamarind, an arboreal fruit of *Tamarindus indica* L. which belongs to family Leguminosae or Caesalpiniaceae, is a tropical evergreen tree native to Africa and Southern Asia. Tamarind grows naturally all over Asia up to an altitude of about 500 m that is from Burma to Afghanistan. In the In Indian subcontinent, it is distributed continuously in Southern and Central regions. It also occurs in sparse patches up in northern India. In Africa, *T. indica* is commonly found in woodlands and is well adapted to the arid and semi-arid zones. Its various parts such as seeds, root, leaves, bark and fruits have been extremely used in traditional Indian and African medication. Flowers are in bunches, yellow in color and boat-shaped; seeds are reddish brown, thick, bark of the trunk is scaly; leaves are paripinnate and 15 cm in length [1-3]. Tamarind can be eaten fresh (ripe or unripe) and it can be consumed processed into different products. One of the most known health benefits of tamarind is its use as medicine since the ancient times. It has been known to be useful for treating constipation and liver problems among others. For years, tamarind has proven to be particularly useful for treating liver and gall disorders and has severally on the role it plays in treating bile problems. Tamarind is particularly useful for managing pain and inflammation on joints. It has been seen that crushed leaves and pulp applied on swollen joints provides great relief and reduces inflammation. Tamarind used for treating sore throat. It is either gargled or drunk as tamarind juice to help relief pain and discomfort of sore throats. In Northern Nigeria, the fresh stem bark and leaves are used as decoction variegated with potash for the treatment of stomach disorder, general body pain, jaundice, yellow fever and as a blood tonic and skin cleanser. The phytochemical study in the human system due to their therapeutic properties cures many ailments which cannot be cured by the modern drugs. Tamarind mostly used as two different varieties i.e. they are sweet and sour. Sweet tamarind is harvested ripe and directly consumed. On the other side, sour tamarind is processed into a range of value-added product [4-6]. *Tamarindus indica* is a plant that can be used traditionally in wound healing, snake bite, abdominal pain, colds, inflammations, diarrhea, helminthic infections and fever. It may also play a role as antimicrobial, antidiabetic, anti-inflammatory and effects on the control of satiety, playing a potential role in the treatment or prevention of obesity and other chronic diseases. These effects are probably due to the presence of polyphenols. *T. indicus* includes a variety of bioactive compounds in the leaves, seeds, bark, pulp and flowers with beneficial effects to human health and the possibility of application in the pharmaceutical industry. This review gives broad information about the bioactive constituents and ethnopharmacology along with the scientifically claimed medicinal uses. The tree grows wild, though cultivated to limited extent. It is almost found throughout the tropics and subtropics of the world and has become naturalized at many places particularly in India, South East Asia, tropical America, the Pacific Islands and the Caribbean. In India, the tree is particularly abundant in states of Madhya Pradesh, Bihar, Andhra Pradesh, Chhattisgarh, Karnataka, Tamilnadu and West Bengal [7-9].

Tamarind trees have a variety of use from the pulp that is used in sauce and chutney to the leaves and barks that has important medicinal applications. Tamarind bark is processed into wood and can be used in making furniture and wood flooring. The pods and flowers are usually pickled and used as side dish. They are most often used as ornamental plants to provide shades along roadside [10-11].

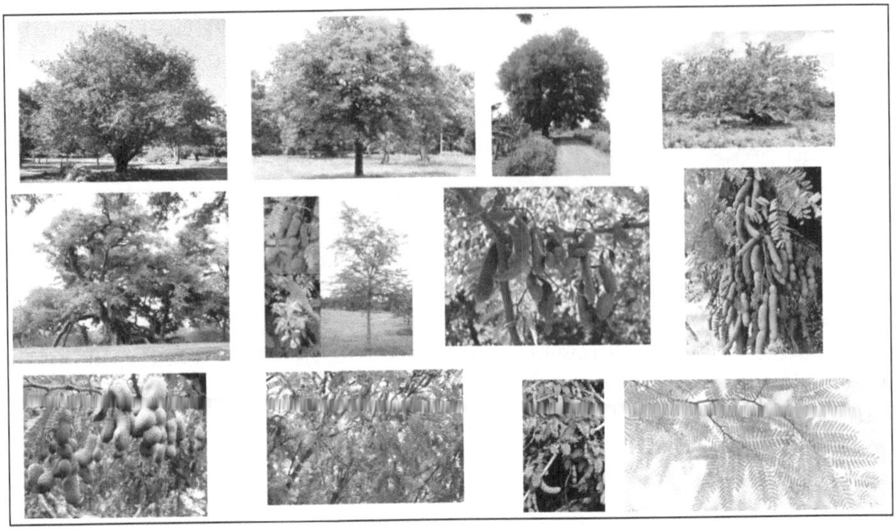

Tamarind trees, Leaves and pods

Tamarind pods contain 3-12 seeds, which are irregularly shaped, flattened or rhomboid. Seeds are very hard, shiny, reddish or purplish brown, enveloped by a tough leathery membrane, the so called endocarp. Outside the endocarp is the light brownish-red, sweetish, acidic edible pulp traversed by tough ligneous fibers. A typical fruit/pod contains about 55% pulp, 34% seeds, and 11% shell and fibers. Mainly there are two varieties of tamarind found in India, including red and common brown variety. The pulp of the red variety of tamarind is less acidic in taste while the pulp of brown variety has more acidic or sour taste. The pulp of brown variety contains high proportion of free acids as compared to red variety. The anthocyanin pigment, chrysanthemin is responsible for the color of the pulp in case of red variety of tamarind and the brown color of pulp of brown variety is due to leucocyanidin.

Tamarind Fruit Pulp and its Composition

Tamarind tree is a multipurpose tree, of which almost every part finds at least some use, either nutritional or medicinal. The most valuable and commonly used part is the fruit which yields acidic pulp.

Uses of Tamarind Pulp

Due to its pleasant acidic taste and rich aroma, the pulp is widely used for domestic and industrial purposes. The pulp is used for seasoning, to flavor confections, curries and sauces and is used as a substitute for chemical acidulants in the preparation of certain beverages. Tamarind pulp can be processed into number of products including tamarind juice, concentrate, powder, pickles and paste. Tamarind pulp also claims some medical uses and is regarded as a digestive, carminative, laxative, expectorant and blood tonic. The pulp has been found to possess hypolipidemic activity. Tamarind intake helps in delaying the progression of fluorosis in humans by enhancing the urinary excretion of fluorine. In traditional practice, he pulp is applied on inflammations and is also used in a gargle for sore throat. The pulp is said to aid the restoration of sensation in cases of paralysis [12-14].

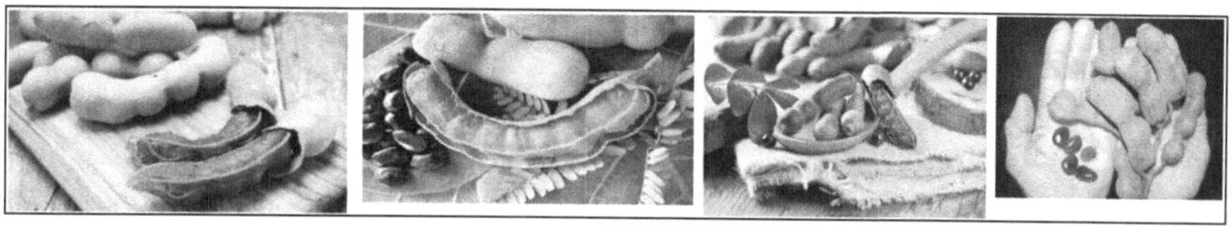

Tamarind pods and seeds

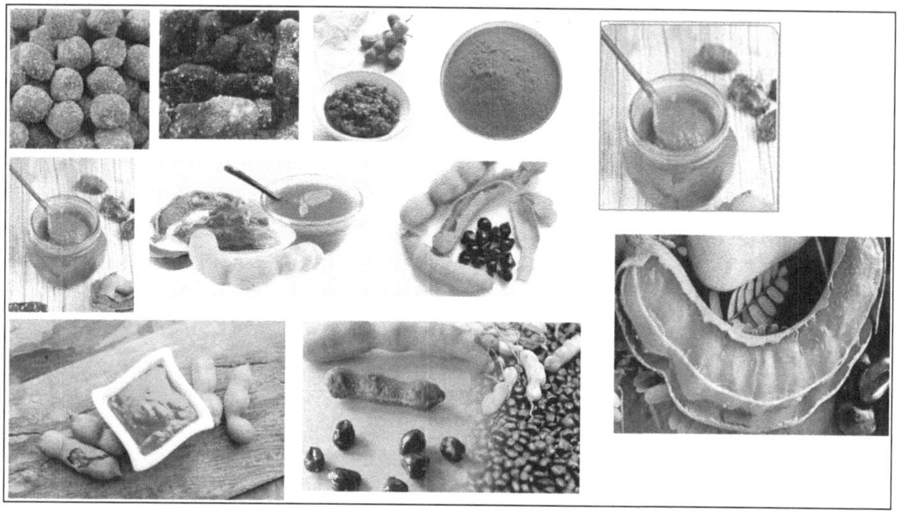

Tamarind seeds, seed extract, candies, chutney, powder

Phytochemical Attributes

Phytochemicals from different plant genera are reported to be biologically active, endowed with antimicrobial, allelopathic and antioxidant properties. Tamarind contains a compound known as hydroxycitric acid (HCA), which inhibits an enzyme that prompts your body to store fat. Tamarind seed husk mainly contains polyphenols which can be classified as flavonoids and polymeric proanthocyanidins known as condensed tannin. Tamarind seed contains polysaccharide including xyloglucan. The leaves have a proven hepatoprotective activity associated with the presence of poly-hydroxylated compounds, with many of them flavonolic in nature.

Various parts have been expansively studied in terms of the pharmacological activity potent antibacterial, antifungal, hypoglycaemic, cholesterolemic, hypolipidemic, antioxidant, antihepatotoxicant antiinflammatory and antidiabetic properties. Tamarind leaves are a fair source of vitamin C and α-carotene; mineral content is high, particularly P, K, Ca and Mg. Vitamin B content is quite high; carotene and vitamin C contents are low. Presence of tannins and other dyeing matters in the seed testa make the whole seed unsuitable for consumption, but they become edible after soaking and boiling in water. Seeds are gaining importance as an alternative source of proteins, and are besides rich in some essential minerals. Seed pectin can form gels over a wide pH range. Chemically tamarind kernel powder is highly branched carbohydrate polymer. The pulp of the fruit contains tartaric acid, reducing sugars, pectin, protein, fiber and cellulosic materials. The percentage of the constituents varies from sample to sample with tartaric acid ranging from 8-18%, 25-45% reducing sugars, 2-3.5% pectin and 2-3% protein. Besides being a rich source of sugars, tamarind pulp is an excellent source of B-vitamins and exhibit high antioxidant capacity that appear to be associated with a high phenolic content. The fruit pulp is a good source of minerals especially potassium, calcium, phosphorous magnesium and sodium. Nevertheless, the proximate composition of the tamarind pulp depends on locality. The major volatile constituents of tamarind pulp include furan derivatives (44.4%) and carboxylic acids (38.2%), the components of which are furfural (38.2%), palmitic acid (14.8%), oleic acid (8.1%) and phenyl acetaldehyde (7.5%). Most abundant volatile constituent of tamarind is 2-acetyl-furan, coupled with traces of furfural and 5-methylfurfural, which form the total aroma of tamarind pulp. Tartaric acid is the major acid present in tamarind pulp which gives the pulp acidic taste. Tamarind pulp also contains malic, succcinic, citric and quinic acid. Tamarind fruit is an ideal source of all essential amino acids except tryptophan [12-19].

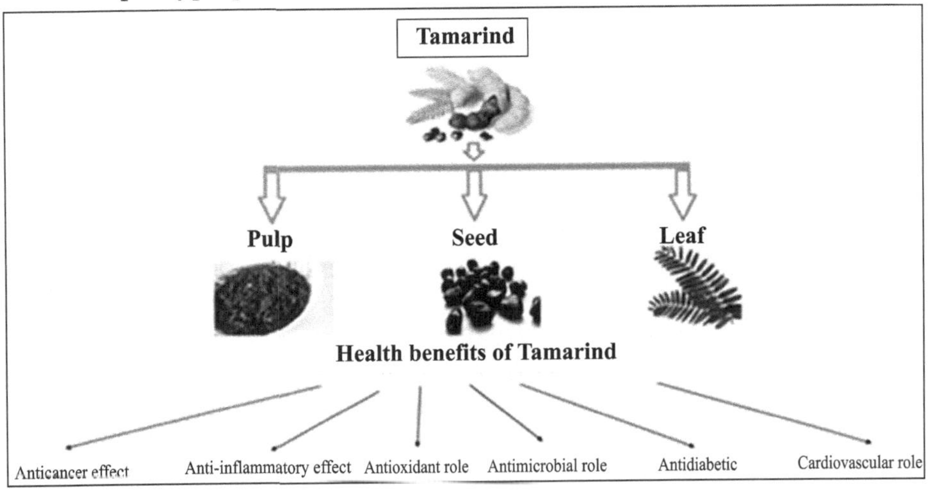

Phytopharmacological Assets and Specific Therapeutic Uses of Various parts of Tamarind

Tamarind is used in wound healing, abdominal pain, diarrhea, dysentery, parasitic infestation, fever, malaria and respiratory problems. It is also commonly used in tropical countries because of its laxative and aphrodisiac properties. *T. indica* fruit is used as a laxative in traditional medicine because of its high malic acid, tartaric acid and potassium content. There are various reasons of abdominal pain. Mostly encountered reasons are diarrhea and constipation. For diarrhea, *T. indica* leaves; for constipation, *T. indica* fruit; for abdominal pain, soft parts of bark and root can be used. It has been shown that *T. indica* seed extract has dose dependent protective effect on ulcer models induced by ibuprofen, alcohol and pylorus ligation. The protective effect of *T. indica* seed comes from its polyphenolic compounds, mainly procyanidin, epicatechin and polymeric tannins. These compounds have antioxidant effect and protective role against free radicals. Tannins also prevent the ulcer development via causing protein accumulation and vasoconstriction. Tamarind fruit content cause smooth muscle relaxation via calcium channel blockage. It also explains the usage of *T. indica* in diarrhea treatment [20-22]. Fluoride, especially found in drinking water, can be harmful in a dose dependent manner. According to World Health Organization report, optimum fluoride level of drinking water is between 0.5-1.0 mg/L. Above this limit it causes fluoride toxicity. Fluoride toxicity is an important global health problem in India and approximately 66.62 million people are affected. Fluoride may also be found in foods but it is especially found in drinking water. Excess fluoride intake alters gene expression, cell cycle, cell proliferation, cell migration, and has negative effect on respiration, metabolism, ion exchange, changes in cellular level (i.e. secretion, endocytosis, apoptosis and necrosis). Oxidative stress, loss of antioxidant capacity may also cause metabolic problems. Extract obtained from *T. indica* leaves ameliorates fluoride toxicity effects via its antiperoxidant and antioxidant properties. Extract obtained from *T. indica* fruit decreases plasma fluoride concentration and ameliorates fluoride induced liver and kidney damage. And also it has been shown that after some procedures *T. indica* fruit can be used in effective drinking water cleaning from fluoride, nickel and lead [23-25].

It is used as a mild laxative to treat digestive system disorder and thus it is able to promote bowel movement and relieve digestive ailments. It is used in the treatment of bronchial disorders. It is used in relieving the sore throat. It is used as an antiseptic in eye hoths and the treatment of ulcers. Because of tamarind acidic nature it is able to excites bile and digestive juices and as such serve as a remedy in relieving biliousness in the body. It is rumored to destroy worms in the intestine of children. It is useful in the treatment of jaundice. Tamarind is high in vitamin C content and as such is used in the treatment and subsequent cure of scurvy and also as an antiscorbutic agent. Tamarind is also used as a blood purifier. Tamarind is used in body cleansing. Because of its refrigerant properties, tamarind is used as a remedy for fever. In the Philippines, tamarind is used to treat and reduce malaria fever. It is used in folk medicine as remedy for pains and swellings. It is effective in the treatment of burn and healing of skin by preventing oedema. Oedema is same as edema and is built of excess of fluid around skin tissues, which is a characteristic in many burn victims [22-27]. Oil from tamarind helps promote moisture and healthy skin and also restricts the entry of harmful germs. Tamarind is used to treat dysentery. Dysentery is a disease of the lower intestine caused by many parasites especially protozoan that often leads to pain, persistent severe diarrhea, inflammation and the passage of blood and mucus. Tamarind pulp because of its fibrous nature is useful in relieving constipation. Tamarind has also been rumored to lower cholesterol levels due to their fibrous nature they are able to bind to bile salts restricting its reabsorption in the colon. Tamarind with other remedial ingredients in the form of soup helps to alleviates and helps to clear nasal blockage. Tamarind is used for diarrhea. The ingredients in tamarind helps promote healthy heart by indirectly lowering blood cholesterol. It is used as a treatment for leucorrhea, which is a white discharge. Tamarind comprises of tartaric acid that provides and serves as a powerful antioxidant for the body. The fiber binds also to toxin chemicals that often binds to mucus and expels them from the body. These toxin chemicals are often the precursor for many cancer especially colon cancer. The tamarind is a source of many minerals such as potassium, calcium, copper, selenium, zinc, magnesium and especially copper where iron facilitates the production of red blood cells and as a co-factor for cytochrome oxidase enzymes [25-28]. The tamarind is also used for the treatment of gall bladder problems and hemorrhoid. Polysaccharide in tamarind aids in the relieve of dry eye syndrome. Presence of antioxidant in tamarind helps to boost the body's immune system. Tamarind helps delay the progress of fluorosis caused by excess fluorides. Tamarind is used in cases of gingivitis and eye inflammation. Pulp is used for the treatment of Scurvy, fever, biliousness, flatulence, indigestion, constipation, loss appetite, bile disorder. It used for the inclination of food intake and reduces the probability of colon cancer. Pulp is smeared on skin for skin-itching and used for common cold. It is also used as a mild laxative, to alleviate alcohol intoxication and datura poisoning. Leaves are used as poultice for cuts and burn, treatment of fever and rheumatism (stiffness in joints and muscles). Herbal tea from tamarind leaves is used to treat eye infections and is usually taken internal for the treatment of diabetes and common cold and flu [28-29], help to prevent edema, used for liver disorders such as jaundice, worms and liquid drawn is used as a wash for sore eyes. Crushed leaves are usually applied to joints of skin as pain reliever. Bark is useful in asthmatic attack and aids in the removal of freckles. Bark is prepared into an astringent and tonic for chest disorders. Poultice extracted from the bark are used on open sores and caterpillar rashes. Roots aids in the removal of freckles, improves appetite, treat urinary problems, constipation, diarrhea, asthma, skin irritations and infections caused by mite and tick bites such as scabies.

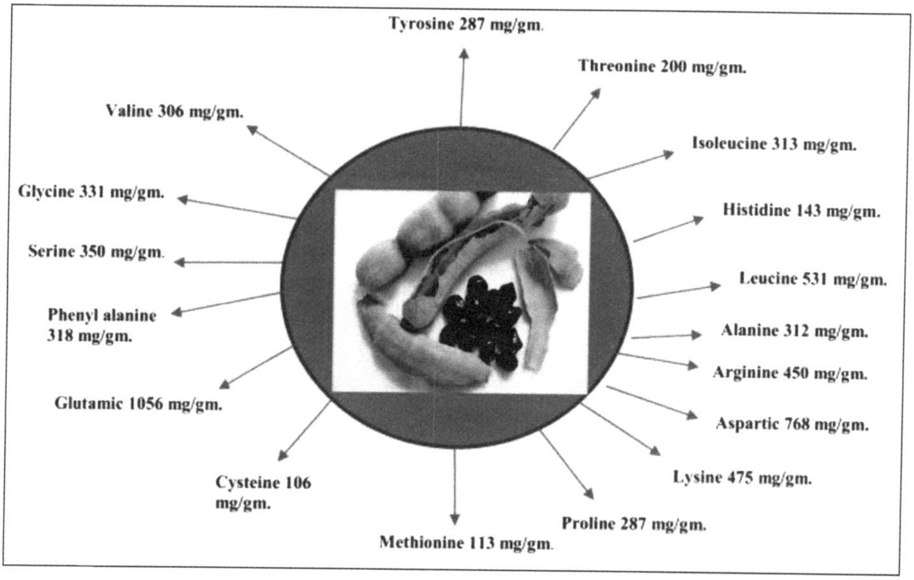

Also used as a remedy for chest complaints and used as an ingredient in the prescription for leprosy. Powdered tamarind seed is used in chronic diarrhea, digestive disorder such as dysentery. Seed coat also has astringent properties and is used in the treatment of the latter also. Tamarind kernel is an ingredient in various medicines and is effective in curing fever, treating intestinal diseases and diarrhea. The seed powder is applied locally to the vagina for contraction of the vaginal passage. Shell used for treating running stomach. Flowers are used for digestive disorders, popularly used by natives [26-30]. Boiled or dried flower is useful for pains, swelling and boils. Juice extracted from flowers is useful for treating bleeding piles. Tamarind leaves has a myriad of benefits chief of them being providing relief from malaria. Its medical benefit though is not confined to just that as it can also cure jaundice and diabetes, helps cure scurvy, treats ulcer, inhibits genital infections, protects the whole body from infections and provides relief from hyper tension. It has anti-inflammatory properties and can also be used to provide relief from menstrual cramps. Tamarind has been used in Indian cuisines since centuries to give that classic sour taste but not just the fruit, the leaves too have featured in cuisines and Ayurveda since ages ago. Tamarind leaves are green in colour and is longitudinal in shape. In cuisines, it is used both in fresh and dried form. The benefits of tamarind leaves are versatile. They contribute as much to medicine as they do to cuisines. Its cathartic, astringent and antiseptic properties make it an important element in Ayurveda while the light tart flavor that its leaves impart, makes it a viable ingredient in Indian cuisines. Tamarind has high ascorbic level acid content that mitigate scurvy. Tamarind leaves are useful in healing wounds thanks to the antiseptic properties present in it. When the juice of tamarind leaves are applied on the wound, it tends to heal faster. Not only that, the juice also serves to prevent infections and parasitic growth which are common in wounds. The quality of breast milk is improved when a lactating mother consumes tamarind leaves extracts. Genital infections are common if proper hygiene is not maintained. Tamarind leaf extracts does not only stop genital infections but also provide relief from its symptoms. Menstrual cramps are terrible and make menstruation a very uncomfortable experience but what is worse is that it is recurring phenomena. Tamarind leaf extracts can dampen the cramps as they are analgesic. Efficiency of the leaves can be increased if they are mixed with papaya leaves, salt and water but care should be taken that too much salt is not added to the mixture. Joint inflammations are painful and can restrict movement heavily. It is also a source of massive discomfort that prevents you from going about your day to day life smoothly. Tamarind leaves have anti-inflammatory properties that help cure joint pain and other inflammations. Maintaining oral hygiene is very important. Two of the most common oral problems faced by people are bad breath and tooth ache. Tamarind leaves are an ideal treatment for both these oral problems [27-30].

Traditional and Culinary uses

Tamarind fruit pulp has a sweet acidic taste due to a combination of high contents of tartaric acid and reducing sugars. The pulp is used for seasoning, in prepared foods, to flavor confections, curries and sauces, and as a major ingredient in juices and other beverages. Commercial tamarind-based drinks are available from many countries. Tamarind is used in Indian spices as a souring agent to provide the desired acidity in the various food recipes. In this era of increased concern on safety of chemical food additives, natural methods of preservation and natural preservatives are receiving increased attention. The tamarind tree produces edible, pod- like fruits which are used extensively in cuisines around the world. Tamarind seeds are traditionally used to treat diabetes, fevers and intestinal infections [26-29]. They are also used in the treatment of diarrhoea and as a laxative. Leaves and flowers can be eaten as vegetables, and are prepared in a variety of dishes. They are used to make curries, salads, stews and soups. Tamarind fruit pulp is used for seasoning, as a food component, to flavor confections, curries and sauces and is a main component in juices and certain beverages. Tamarind fruit pulp is eaten fresh and often made into a juice, infusion or brine and can also be processed into jam and sweets. The refreshing drinks arc popular in many countries around the world, though there are many different recipes. In some African countries, the juice obtained from the fruit pulp is mixed with wood ash to neutralize the sour taste of the tartaric acid. However, the most common method is to add sugar to make a pleasantly acid drink. In Ghana, the pulp is mixed with sugar and honey to make a sweet drink. Most of the producing countries manufacture drinks commercially. Sometimes pulp is fermented into an alcoholic beverage. Tamarind seeds or Kernel is a byproduct of Tamarind pulp industry. Tamarind gum is obtained from endosperm of seeds of the tamarind tree, which is a seed gum with potential industrial applications. Tamarind gum is having applications in paper, food and textile industry etc. In Recent years, research has been initiated on the use of tamarind gum in pharmaceutical and cosmetic applications. Tamarind leaves are powdered and used in various dishes. Tender tamarind leaves are used in coconut chutney. It is also used in the preparation of dal [30-34].

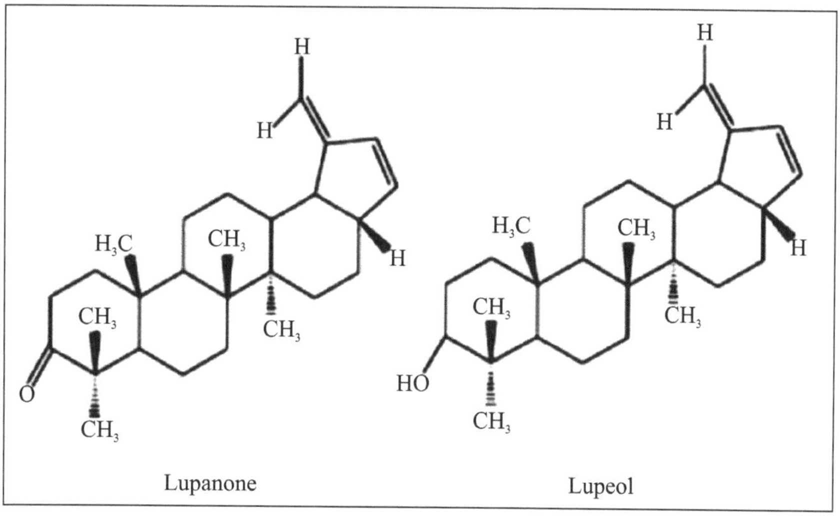

Phytochemical occurring in leaves, pulp and sedds of tamarind

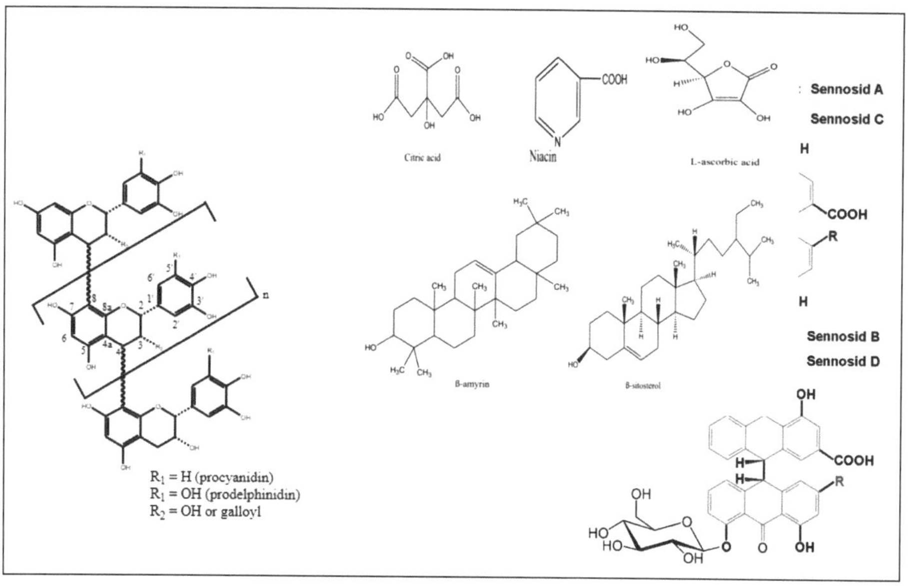

Conclusion

Every part of *T. indica* plant (root, body, fruit and leaves) not only has rich nutritional value and broad usage area in medicine but also has industrial and economic importance. Tamarind is a rich source of most of the essential amino acids and phytochemicals and hence the plant is reported to possess antidiabetic, antimicrobial, antivenomic, antioxidant, antimalarial, cardioprotective, hepatoprotective, antiasthmatic, laxative and anti-hyperlipidemic activity. *T. indica* has ameliorative effects on many diseases.

Tamarind is highly valued for its pulp. Tamarind fruit pulp has a sweet acidic taste due to a combination of high contents of tartaric acid and reducing sugars. The pulp is used for seasoning, in prepared foods, to flavor confections, curries and sauces, and as a major ingredient in juices and other beverages. Commercial tamarind-based drinks are available from many countries. Vitamin B content is quite high, carotene and vitamin C contents are low. Presence of tannins and other dyeing matters in the seed testa make the whole seed unsuitable for consumption, but they become edible after soaking and boiling in water. Tamarind kernel powder is an important sizing material in textile, paper and jute industries. Seeds are gaining importance as an alternative source of proteins and are besides rich in some essential minerals. Seed pectin can form gels over a wide pH range. Leaves and flowers can be eaten as vegetables and are prepared in a variety of dishes. They are used to make curries, salads, stews and soups. Tamarind leaves are a fair source of vitamin C and α-carotene, mineral content is high, particularly, P, K, Ca and Mg. Anti-oxidant, anti-inflammatory, anti-microbial and anti-fungal activity has been documented from several plant parts. The traditional uses, its phytochemistry and pharmacognostic reviewed to provide with a particular orientation to its value.

REFERENCES

1. Doughari JH. Antimicrobial Activity of *Tamarindus indica* Linn. Trop J Pharmaceut Res.2006; 5: 597-603.
2. Arranz JCE, Roses, RP, Laffita, IU, Pozo, MIC, Amado, JR, Licea-Jiminez IL. Antimicrobial Activity of Extracts from *Tamarindus indica* L. leaves. Pharmacog Mag. 2010; 6: 242-247.
3. Lefebvre JC. Tamarind – A Review. Fruits. 1971; 26: 687-695.
4. Lewis YS, Neelakantan S. The Chemistry, Biochemistry, and Technology of Tamarind. J Sci Ind Res. 1964; 23: 204-206.
5. Hasan SK, Ijaz S. Tamarind – A Review. Sci Indus Pak. 1972; 9: 131-137.
6. Shankaracharya NB. Tamarind – Chemistry, Technology and uses: A Critical Appraisal. J Food Sci Technol. 1998; 35: 193-208.
7. Tsuda T, Ohshima K, Yamamoto A, Kawakishi S, Osawa T. Antioxidative Components Isolated from the Seed of Tamarind (*Tamarindus indica* L.). J Agric Food Chem. 1994; 42(12): 2671-2674

8. Sudjaroen Y, Haubner R, Wartele G, Hull WE, Erben G, Spiegelhalder B, Changbumrung S, Bartsch H, Bartsch HW. Isolation and Structure Elucidation of Phenolic Antioxidants from Tamarind (*Tamarindus indica* L.) Seeds and Pericarp. Food ChemToxicol. 2005; 43(11): 1673-1682.
9. Sinchaiyakit P, Ezure Y, Sriprang S, Pongbangpho S, Povichit N, Suttajit M. Tannins of Tamarind Seed Husk: Preparation, Structural Characterization and Antioxidant Activity. Nat Prod Commun. 2011; 6(6): 829-834.
10. Savur GR. Constitution of Tamarind Seed Polysaccharides, and the Structure of Xylan. J Chem Soc. 1956; 2600-2603.
11. Srivastava HC, Krishnamurthy TN. Tamarind Kernel Polysaccharides. II. Fraction and Examination of Minor Component Polysaccharide. Staerke. 1972; 24(11): 369-73.
12. Taylor IEP, Atkins EDT. X-ray diffraction Studies on the Xyloglucan from Tamarind (*Tamarindus indica*) Seeds. FEBS Lett. 1985; 181(2): 300-302.
13. Heq QN, Nabi MN, Kiamuddin M. Oil from Tamarind seed (*Tamarindus indica*). Bangladesh J SciInd Res 1973; 8(1-4): 42-46.
14. Pitke PM, Singh PP, Srivastava HC. Fatty Acid Composition of Tamarind Kernel Oil. J Am Oil ChemSoc 1977; 54(12): 592-595.
15. Doughari JH. Antimicrobial Activity of *Tamarindus indica* Linn. Trop J Pharmaceut Res. 2006; 5 (2): 597-603.
16. Komakech R, Y Kim Y, Matsabisa GM Kang Y. Anti-inflammatory and Analgesic Potential of *Tamarindus indica* Linn. (Fabaceae): A Narrative Review Integrat Med Res.2019; 8 (3): 181-186.
17. Zohrameena S, Mujahid M, Bagga P, Khalid M, Noorul H, Nesar A, Saba P. Medicinal uses & Pharmacological activity of *Tamarindus indica* World J Pharm Sci. 2017; 5(2): 121-133.
18. Khanzada SK, Shaikh W, Sofia W, Kazi T, Usmanghani K, Kabir A, Sheerazi TH. Chemical Constituents of *Tamarindus indica* , Medicinal Plant in Sindh. Pak J Bot. 2008; 40(6): 2553-2559.
19. Dhasade VV, Nirmal SA, Patil RY. Pharmacognostic and Phytochemical Evaluation of *Tamarindus indica* Linn. Leaves. Curr Pharm Res. 2016; 8(2): 66-73.
20. Kalpesh P, Harisha CR, Shukla VJ. Phytochemical Evaluation of Fruit Pulp of Tamarindusindica Linn. JAyurMed 5(1): 37-42.
21. Pramila G, Jirekar D (2021) *Tamarindus Indica*: An Important Medicinal Plants.Int J Innov Res Technol. 2014; 8(4): 321-325.
22. Tsuda T, Watanable M, Ohshima K, Yamanato A, Kawakishi S, Osawa T: Antioxidative Components Isolated from the Seed of Tamarind (*Tamarindus indica* L.). J Agri Food Chem. 1994; 42: 2671-1674.
23. Rimbau V, Cerdan C, Vila R, Iglesia J. Antiinflammatory Activity of some Extracts from Plants used in Traditional Medicines of North African Countries (II). Phytother Res. 1999; 13: 128-132.
24. APP, Trevisan SCC, Sandra Maria Barbalho SM, Guiguer E. *Tamarindus indica* L.: A Plant with Multiple Medicinal Purposes, Journal of Pharmacog Phytochem. 5(3): 50-54.
25. Siddhuraju P. Antioxidant Activity of Polyphenolic Compounds extracted from Defatted Raw and Dry Heated *Tamarindus indica* Seed Coat. LWT Food Sci Tech. 2007; 40: 982-90.
26. Osawa T, Tsuda T, Watanabe M, Ohshima K, Yamamoto A. Antioxidative Components Isolated from the Seeds of Tamarind (*Tamarindus indica* L) J Agric Food Chem.; 1994; 42: 2671-2674.

27. Luengthanaphol S, Mongkholkhajornsilp D, Douglas S, Douglas PL, Pengsopa L, Pongamphai S. Extraction of Antioxidants from Sweet Thai Tamarind Seed Coat: Preliminary Experiments. J Food Eng. 2004; 63: 247-52.
28. Gupta C, Prakash D, Gupta S. Studies on the Antimicrobial Activity of Tamarind (*Tamarindus indica*) and its Potential as Food Bio-preservative. Int Food Res J. 2015; 21(6): 2437-2441.
29. Komakech R, Kim YG, Matsabisa GM, Kang Y. Anti-inflammatory and Analgesic Potential of *Tamarindus indica* Linn. (Fabaceae): A Narrative review. Integra Med Res. 2019; 8(3): 181-186.
30. Emmy De Caluwé, Katerina Halamová, Patrick Van Damme. Tamarind (*Tamarindus indica* L.): A Review of Traditional Uses, Phytochem Pharmacol. ACS Symposium Series 2010; 23(1) 1010-105.doi: 10.1021/bk-2009-1021.ch005
31. Jyothirmayi T, Rao GN, Rao DG. Studies on Instant Raw Tamarind Chutney Powder. J Food Service. 2006; 17(3): 119-123.
32. Muzaffar K, Kumar P. Tamarind-a mini Review. OJ Food Process Technol. 2017; 5(3): 296 297.
33. Kuru P. *Tamarindus indica* and its Health related Effects. Asian Pac J Trop Biomed. 2014; 4(9): 676-681.
34. Vasant RA, Narasimhacharya AV. Ameliorative effect of tamarind leaf on Fluoride-induced Metabolic Alterations. Environ Health Prev Med. 2012; 17(6): 484-487.
35. Arranz JCE, Rosés RP, Amado JR, Quevedo HJM, Mwasi LB, Sotomayor OC, García RM, Lórez OF, Castillo AA, Zapata EP. Antioxidant and Toxicological Evaluation of a *Tamarindus indica* L. leaf Fluid extract. Natural Product Research. 2016; 30(4): 456-459. doi:10.1080/14786419.2015.1019350
36. Leng LY, binti Nadzri N, bin Shaari AR, Yee KC. Antioxidant Capacity and Total Phenolic Content of Fresh, Oven-dried and Stirfried Tamarind Leaves. Curr Res Nut Food Sci J. 2017: 5(3): 282-287.

CHAPTER
24

A particular Orientation to multifaceted Turmeric worth

ABSTRACT

Curcuma longa L. or turmeric is highly regarded as a universal panacea in the herbal medicine with a widespectrum of pharmacological activities. Curcumin (diferuloylmethane), the main yellow bioactive component of turmeric has been shown to have a wide spectrum of biological actions. These include its antiinflammatory, antioxidant, anticarcinogenic, antimutagenic, anticoagulant, antifertility, antidiabetic, antibacterial, antifungal, antiprotozoal, antiviral, antifibrotic, antivenom, antiulcer, hypotensive and hypocholesteremic activities. For traditional Ayurvedics, turmeric plant was an excellent natural antiseptic, disinfectant, antiinflammatory and analgesic, while at the same time the plant has been often used to aid digestion, to improve intestinal flora and to treat skin irritations. It is the purpose of this review to provide a brief overview of the plethora of research regarding the potential health benefits of curcumin.

Keywords: Curcumin, Antiinflammatory, Anticarcinogenic, Sesquiterpenes.

Introduction

Turmeric is a plant distributed throughout tropical and subtropical regions of the world. It is widely cultivated in Asian countries, mainly in China and India. Turmeric is an herbaceous evergreen plant in the Zingiberaceae (ginger) family. Turmeric (*Curcuma longa*) is extensively used as a spice, food preservative and colouring material in India, China and South East Asia. Turmeric powder is best known as one of the main ingredients used to make the curry spice; it also gives ballpark mustard its bright yellow colour. Turmeric is an essential spice all over the world with a distinguished human use particularly among the Eastern people. Apart from the uses as spice, it is used as traditional medicine in Asian countries such as India, Bangladesh and Pakistan because of its beneficial properties [1-3]. It is called turmeric and has been in continuous use for its flavoring, and medicinal properties. Turmeric is a sterile plant and does not produce any seeds. The plant grows up to 3-5 ft tall and dull yellow flowers. The rhizome is an underground stem that is thick and fleshy ringed with the bases of old leaves is part of turmeric which possess a potential medicinal property. Rhizomes are boiled and then dried and ground to make the distinctive bright yellow spice. The purpose of this review to focuses on the medicinal and pharmacological properties of turmeric as anti-inflammatory, antioxidant, hepatoprotective, anticarcinogenic, antidiabetic, antimicrobial and antidepressant in addition to its use in cardiovascular disease, gastrointestinal and neurological disorder. Due to these biological activities turmeric widely used as medicinal plant [4-6].

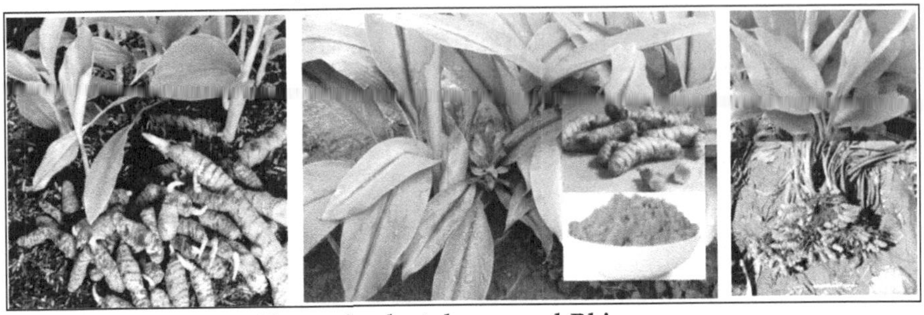

Turmeric plant, leaves and Rhizome

Recent and Traditional Assets

Fresh, woody with spicy notes - turmeric, the bright yellowish-orange root, a staple spice in Indian and Asian cooking, literally means 'sacred earth' in Latin - and rightly so. Brimming with powerful phytochemicals this amazing "superfood" is packed with incredible health-promoting benefits! The activities of turmeric include antibacterial, antiviral, anti-inflammatory, antitumor, antioxidant, antiseptic, cardioprotective, hepatoprotective, nephroprotective, radioprotective and digestive. Used in the Indian sub-continent and parts of Asia for thousands of years, turmeric hails from the Zingiberaceae plant family (the same family as ginger) and has both been used as a spice to flavor and color food and also as a medicinal herb. Studies conducted by modern science today have backed what people in India and Asia have known for centuries - that turmeric does in fact contain active compounds making it one of the most powerful healing herbs on the planet. One of the major active compounds in turmeric is curcumin, a super-powerful antioxidant and anti-inflammatory. Curcumin has been used extensively in ayurvedic medicine for centuries, as it is nontoxic and has a variety of therapeutic properties including antioxidant, analgesic, anti-inflammatory, antiseptic activity and anticarcinogenic activity.

Apart from its culinary uses, turmeric has been used widely in the traditional medicine all over the world. Current traditional medicine claims its powder against gastrointestinal diseases, especially for biliary and hepatic disorder, diabetic wounds, rheumatism, inflammation sinusitis, anorexia, coryza and cough. The coloring principle of turmeric is called curcumin, which has yellow color and is the essential component of this plant. The plant has also shown to possess anti HIV activity to combat AIDS. These medicinal properties of turmeric caused it to be considered as a spice with multifunctional medicinal properties. Besides flavoring food, to purify the blood and skin conditions remedy is probably the most common use of Turmeric in Ayurveda. The main organs that turmeric treats are the skin, heart, liver and lungs. Turmeric is used for epilepsy and bleeding disorders, skin diseases, to purify the body-mind, and to help the lungs expel Kapha. Activities of Turmeric include: Alterative, analgesic, antibacterial, anti-inflammatory, anti-tumor, anti-allergic, antioxidant, antiseptic, antispasmodic, appetizer, astringent, cardiovascular, carminative, cholagogue, digestive, diuretic, stimulant, and vulnerary. Therapeutic uses of Turmeric: Anemia, cancer, diabetes, digestion, food poisoning, gallstones, indigestion, IBS, parasites, poor circulation, staph infections, and wounds. Turmeric helps to regulate the female reproductive system and purifies the uterus and breast milk, and in men it purifies and builds semen, which is counterintuitive for a pungent bitter. Turmeric reduces fevers, diarrhea, urinary disorders, insanity, poisoning, cough and lactation problems in general. Turmeric is used to treat external ulcers that respond to nothing else. Turmeric decreases Kapha and so is used to remove mucus in the throat, watery discharges like leucorrhea, and any pus in the eyes, ears, or in wounds, etc. In Ayurvedic cooking, turmeric is everywhere, this multifaceted wonder spice helps to detoxify the liver, balance cholesterol levels [4-8]

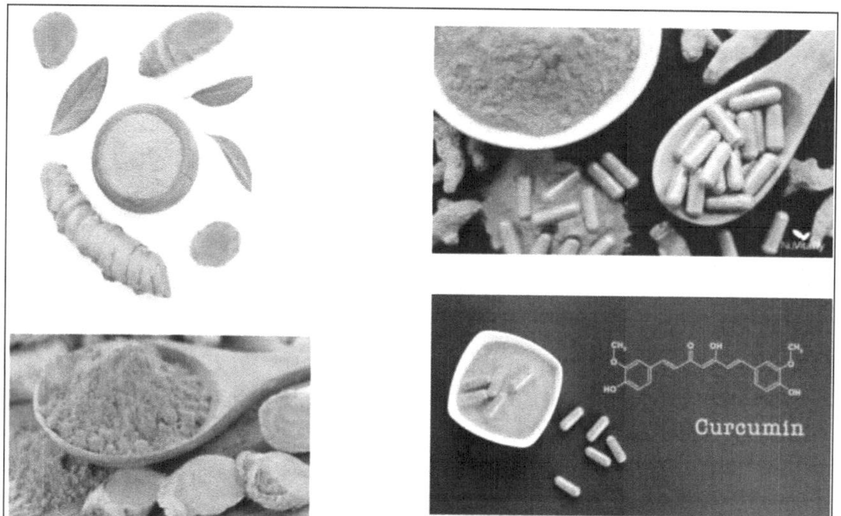

Turmeric (Haldi), its powder and Capsules

Fight allergies, stimulate digestion, boost immunity, enhance the complexion. It is also an antioxidant Ayurveda recognizes turmeric as a heating spice, contributing bitter, pungent and astringent tastes. Since ancient time turmeric has been used in ayurvedic medicine with various biological application. Now a day's researcher found enthusiasm in treating various diseases with natural product. Although some work has been done on the possible medicine application but not much study had done for drug development carried out yet. *Curcumin* is a nontoxic, highly promising natural antioxidant compound having a wide spectrum of biological functions. Curcumin is now available in pure form, which shows a wide spectrum of biological activities, it would be easier to develop new drugs from this compound after extensive studies on its mechanism of action and pharmacological effects. It is expected that *Curcumin* may find application as a novel drug in the near future to control various disease, disorders and oxidative stress. Recent studies have authenticated the use of turmeric for various diseases especially oxidative stress induced ones such as cancer, diabetes mellitus and inflammatory disorders. It also is used as hepatoprotective, nephroprotective, anticoagulant and anti-HIV to combat AIDS. *Curcumin*, as a spice, exhibits great promise as a therapeutic agent. It has very low toxicity, too. As the global scenario is now changing towards the use of non-toxic plant products having traditional medicinal use, development of modern drugs from turmeric should be emphasized for the control of various diseases. Further evaluation needs to be carried out on turmeric in order to explore the concealed areas and their practical clinical applications, which can be used for the welfare of mankind [9-12]

Benefits of Turmeric Oil, Milk and Water

Extracted from the roots, also called rhizomes, via the process of steam distillation, turmeric essential oil is a lot more concentrated than the powdered form. The aroma of turmeric oil is also very much like the fresh cut root - woody and earthy with a touch of spice. And just like the powder, the oil is also packed with antibacterial, antifungal, antiviral, anti-worm, anti-allergic, and anti-parasitic healing properties. At times the words 'turmeric' and 'curcumin' are used interchangeably, but *Curcumin* is only one of the many active ingredients found in the turmeric plant. The many other phytochemicals (biologically active compounds) found in turmeric oil are actually quite complex. In fact turmeric oil is known to contain over 300 phenolic compounds! The major compounds, ar-turmerone, alpha-turmerone, beta-turmerone and curcumin are sesquiterpenes, molecules that have to ability to pass through the blood brain barrier promoting oxygen in the brain. Sesquiterpenes also have excellent antiseptic and anti-inflammatory properties and can bring hormonal balance, promote liver health, soothe inflamed tissues and stimulate the glands. In South Asia and Ayurvedic medicine, turmeric has been used for centuries as a natural remedy to treat skin conditions including curbing acne, reducing blemishes and scars and discouraging facial hair growth in women. Applying turmeric essential oil topically can help treat skin conditions, improve skin elasticity, reduce wrinkles and treat sunburn. Being a powerful antimicrobial turmeric essential oil makes an excellent acne fighter [7-12]. The oil helps to naturally dry out pimples and prevent future breakouts. Turmeric is often a key ingredient used in anti-blemish and anti-scar skin creams. Curcuma longa extract, or turmeric essential oil used in skin creams, can protect against the harmful effects of the sun. Brimming with antioxidants, turmeric oil can keep facial skin soft and supple, reduce fine lines and give your skin a healthy glow. Turmeric essential oil is rich in antioxidants making it excellent for stimulating new cells to grow, promoting healthy hair follicles and preventing hair loss. The anti-inflammatory properties of the oil contribute to reducing scalp inflammation and improving hair growth. The powerful anti-inflammatory properties of turmeric oil help to keep dandruff at bay and soothe an irritated scalp. Turmeric oil's antiseptic and anti-inflammatory qualities can relieve your scalp symptoms and stop an infection in its tracks. *Curcumin* can "act as a chemopreventive agent in cancers of colon, stomach and skin," and can actually work on the molecular level to potentially prevent and even treat cancer. There's promising research to show that curcumin combined with turmerones (the essential oil component of turmeric) inhibits colon cancer in lab mice, and that this combination, may become a powerful method for prevention of inflammation-associated colon carcinogenesis [8-15].

Curcumin is a strong candidate for use in the prevention or treatment of major disabling age-related neurodegenerative diseases like Alzheimer's, Parkinson's, and stroke. Inhaling turmeric essential oil is highly effective for boosting memory, cognitive function, and improving concentration. *Curcumin* is a powerful anti-inflammatory and can actually fight inflammation at the molecular level. *Curcumin* blocks the molecule NF-kB responsible for activating genes in cells nuclei that trigger inflammation. In fact studies have described its potency to be as effective as anti-inflammatory drugs - without the unpleasant side effects. High quality therapeutic-grade turmeric oil contains over 60% alpha-curcumene, a sesquiterpene hydrocarbon that gives turmeric its incredible anti-inflammatory healing properties. This compound allows turmeric oil to alleviate inflammation associated with chronic disease, joint pain, muscle aches, gout, inflammation of the digestive tract and more. Turmeric has been used holistically to maintain liver health and studies show that turmeric is "hepatoprotective," meaning it protects the liver, mainly due to it being a powerful anti-inflammatory. When it comes to building immunity turmeric essential oil contains powerful active ingredients that offer solid support to your body's innate natural defenses. Turmeric's immune-boosting benefits can actually support the body's response in dealing with allergens. *Curcumin* activates the release of bilirubin, an important antioxidant responsible for strengthening immune response [16-18].

The combination of biologically active compounds in the oil offer everything from being antibacterial and antifungal to antiseptic and anti-inflammatory. This helps to ward off invaders, build immunity and keep inflammation in control. Turmeric essential oil contains powerful healing properties to combat the symptoms of cold, cough and flu. It can help everything from congestion and cough to relieving bronchial infections. Being a potent anti-inflammatory there is strong research to suggest that *Curcumin* could potentially help support arthritis pain. In fact in ancient Ayurvedic medicine and traditional Chinese medicine turmeric has long been used to relieve joint and arthritic pain and swelling. Turmeric essential oil's active compounds block inflammatory enzymes and chemicals that can trigger joints to swell. Additionally, the highly concentrated antioxidants present in the oil quash free radicals that tear down cartilage. *Curcumin* soothes inflammation, speeds blister healing and support immunity which keeps the infection at bay and controls it from flaring up further. Curcumin is by far one of the best natural remedies to promote cardiovascular health and lower cholesterol. More importantly, *Curcumin* improves the lining of blood vessels or the endothelium. Its powerful antioxidants prevent free radicals from destroying blood vessels and restrict plaque from adhering to blood vessel walls. Damaged and plaque-lined blood vessels impede blood flow causing the two biggest killers - heart attack and stroke. By protecting the endothelium, along with its anti-inflammatory and antioxidant benefits, curcumin helps to lower blood pressure, promote the growth of fresh red blood cells and protect against fatigue, anemia, high blood pressure, heart disease and stroke. Being a potent anti-microbial and anti-inflammatory it's no surprise that turmeric can help reduce inflammation related to teeth, gum and oral health problems. A study documented that "turmeric is definitely a good adjunct to mechanical plaque control" when compared to medicated mouthwash, and that it could actually be a better low-cost alternative.

Another study reported that at a 100% concentration, turmeric oil possesses antimicrobial activity against *P. gingivalis* and can help in the prevention and treatment of periodontitis, which is the inflammation of the tissues supporting the teeth. Turmeric has been used traditionally to help with digestion issues and is known to reduce bloating and cramping, encourage the elimination of gas from the system and support the digestive system. Zingeriberene and 6-gingerol are the key components of turmeric essential oil, known to have a strong impact on the digestive/gastrointestinal system. Turmeric oil stimulates the production of gastric juices and helps to alleviate the symptoms of irritable bowel syndrome, ulcers and other digestive ailments. Being an all-natural antiseptic and antimicrobial, turmeric oil can be used as a disinfectant for minor scrapes, cuts and burns. As a potent anti-inflammatory turmeric oil helps to reduce inflammation and also the antioxidant properties help to accelerate healing and decrease the formation of scars [19-22].

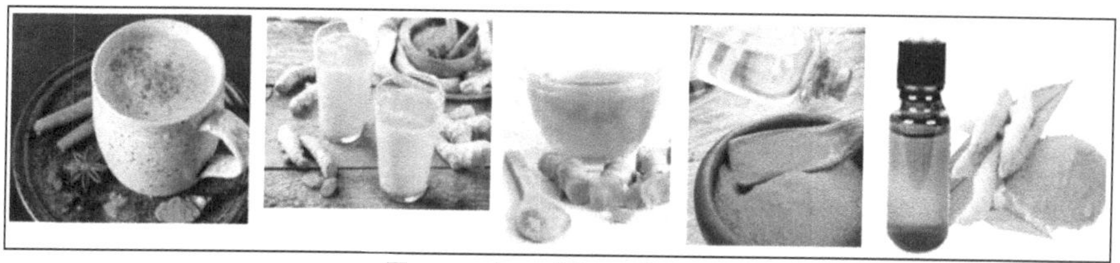

Turmeric milk and water

Turmeric Milk, or Haldi Doodh (as we call it in India), is an ancient recipe. It is used to treat several diseases. Turmeric milk can help reduce joint pain, control blood sugar, improve memory & brain function and help recover wounds. In addition, it can relieve cough and cold and help give you better sleep. Since milk contains calcium and vitamin D, it also helps strengthen bones. It is a straightforward homemade recipe and has many natural qualities. Another easy way of adding turmeric to your diet is turmeric water or Haldi Wala Paani (as we call it in India). There are many benefits of drinking turmeric water. First, it is perfect for your heart as it reduces cholesterol levels. In addition, it prevents atherosclerosis. Turmeric water also protects against blood clots and plaque build-up in the arteries.

Phytocomponents of Turmeric

Turmeric contains 69.4% carbohydrates, 6.3% protein, 5.1% fat, 3.5% minerals, and 13.1% moisture. The essential oil (5.8%) obtained by steam distillation possesses Sesquiterpenes (53%), zingiberene (25%), a-phellandrene (1%), sabinene (0.6%), cineol (1%), and borneol (0.5%). Curcumin (3-4%) is responsible for the yellow colour and comprises curcumin I (94%), curcumin II (6%) andcurcumin III (0.3%). Demethoxy and bisdemethoxy derivatives of curcumin have also been isolated from turmeric. Presence of tumerone a, tumerone b, curzerenone, curdione, mono- and di-demethoxycurcumin have been reported in the rhizomes. The essential oils of leaves of *C. longa* have been analyzed by GLC and reported to contain linalool, caryophyllene, geraniol, α-pinene, β-pinene, sabinene, myrcene, α-phellandrene, 1,8-cineole, p-cymene, C8-aldehyde, and methyl heptanone. A novel sesquiterpene, (6S)-2-methyl-6-(4- hydroxyphe-nyl-3-methyl)-2-hepten-4-one, two new bisabolaneses-quiterpenes, (6S)-2-methyl-6- (4-hydroxyphenyl)-2-hep-ten-4-one, (6S)-2- methyl-6- (4-formylphenyl)-2-hepten-4-one, and two calebin derivatives, 4''-(4'''-hydroxyphenyl-3'''-methoxy)- 2''-oxo-3''-butenyl-3-(4'-hydroxyphenyl)-propenoate and 4''-(4'''-hydroxyphenyl)- 2''-oxo-3''-butenyl-3-(4'-hydroxyphenyl- 3'-methoxy)-propenoate were isolated along with five known bisabolane sesquiterpenes from turmeric [13-22].

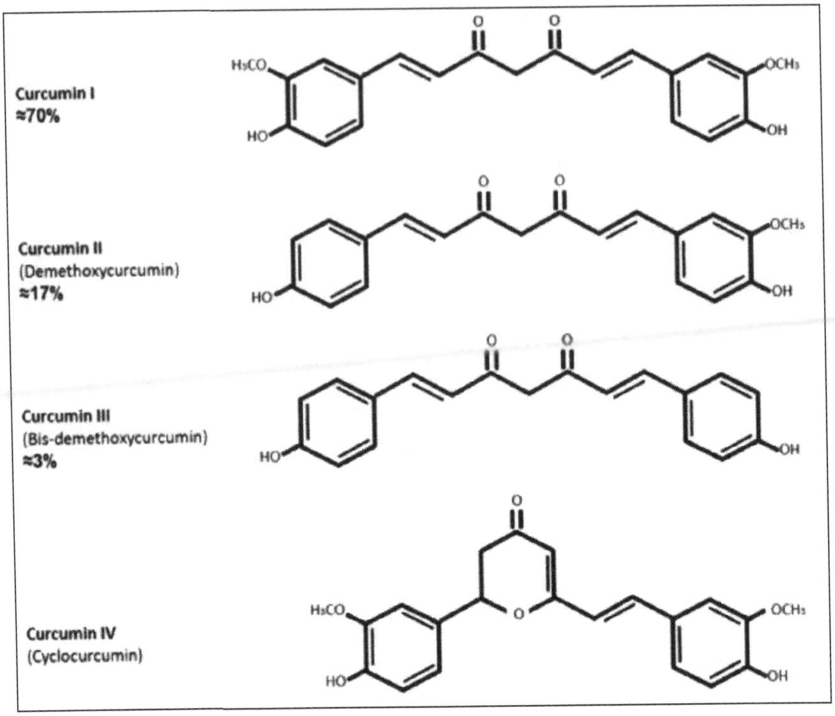

Curriculum	**3.1-3.4%**
Anthocyanins	18.9-37.0 g/g
Phenols	0.15-0.62%
Tannins	0.32-0.76%
Protein content	3.6-6.8%
Sugars	20.5-43.4%
Oil	3.7-5.3%
Ash	6.9-9.8%
Moisture	90.2-91.3%

Biochemical contents of dried turmeric rhizome (12)

Methyleurcumin	Anti protozoan
Demethoxycurcumin and Bisdemethoxycurcumin	Antioxidant
Volatile oil	Anti-inflammatory, Antibacterial, Antifungal
Curcumin	Antibacterial, Anti protozoan, Antiviral Antitumor and Antioxidant

Pharmacological activities of Turmeric chemical constitutions

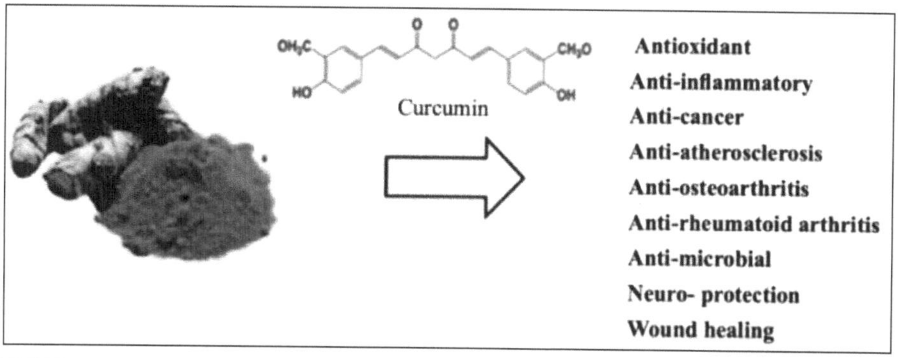

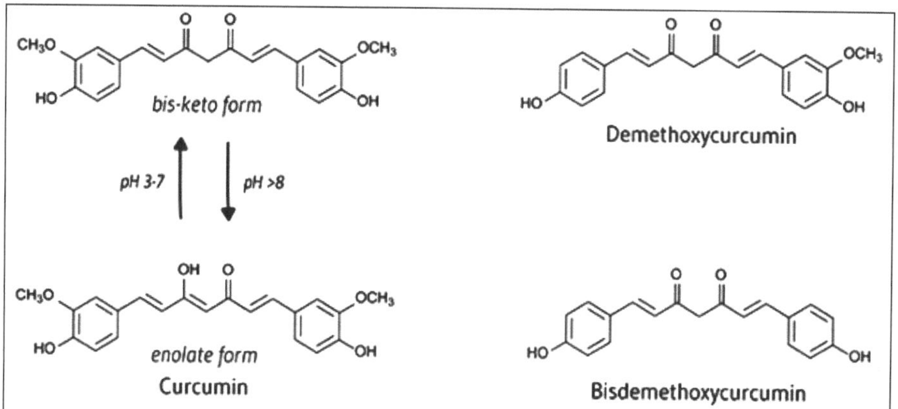

Curcuminoids in turmeric roots are a mixture of three main compounds: curcumin (~77%), demethoxycurcumin (~17%), and bisdemethoxycurcumin (~3%). Curcumin exists in two molecular configurations (known as tautomers): the bis-keto form is predominantly found in neutral and acidic conditions and in a solid phase, while the enolate form is

Conclusion

Curcuma longa (Turmeric) is one of the most useful herbal medicinal plants. Extensive researches have proven that most of the turmeric activities of the turmeric are due to curcumin. *Curcumin* has received worldwide attention for its multiple health benefits, which appear to act primarily through its anti-oxidant and anti-inflammatory mechanisms. These benefits are best achieved when Curcumin is combined with agents such as piperine, which increase its bioavailability significantly. Research suggests that curcumin can help in the management of oxidative and inflammatory conditions, metabolic syndrome, arthritis, anxiety, and hyperlipidemia. It also has antifungal, antimicrobial, renal and hepatoprotective activities. Therefore, it has the potential against various cancer, diabetes, allergies, arthritis, Alzheimer's disease and other chronic and hard curable diseases.

REFERENCES

1. Verma RK, Kumari P, Maurya RK, Kumar V, Verma RB, Singh RK. Medicinal Properties of Turmeric (Curcuma longa L.): A Review. Int J Chem Stud. 2018; 6(4): 1354-1357.
2. Apisariyakul A, Vanittanakomm N, Buddhasukh D. Antifungal Activity of Turmeric Oil Extracted from Curcuma longa (Zingiberaceae). J Ethnopharmacol. 1995; 49: 163-169.
3. Chandra D, Gupta SS. Antiinflammatory and Antiarthritic Activity of Volatile Oil of Curcuma longa (Haldi). Ind J Med Res. 1972; 60: 138-142.
4. Chattopadhyay I, Biswas K, Bandyopadhyay U, Banerjee RK. Turmeric and Curcumin: Biological actions and Medicinal Applications. CurrSci Ind. 2004; 87: 44-53.
5. Gujral ML, Chowdhury NK, Saxena PN. The Effect of Certain Indigenous Remedies on the Healing of Wounds and Ulcers. J Ind State Med Assoc., 1953; 22: 273-276.
6. Murugananthi D, Selvam S, Raveendaran N, Meena ST. A Study on the Direction of Trade in the Indian Turmeric Exports: Markov Chain Approach. IUP J Agr Econ. 2008; 4: 20-25.
7. Nasri H, Sahinfard N, Rafieian M, Rafieian S, Rafieian M, Shirzad. Turmeric: A Spice with Multifunctional Medicinal Properties. J HerbMed Pharmacol. 2014; 3(1): 5-8.
8. Naz S. Antibacterial Activity of Curcuma longa Varieties against Strains of Bacteria. Pak J Bot. 2010; 42: 455-462.
9. Negi PS. Antibacterial Activity of Turmeric Oil: A byproduct from Curcumin manufacture. J Agri Food Chem. 1999; 47: 4297-4300.
10. Sarangthem K, Haokip MJ. Bioactive Component in Curcuma caesiaRoxb. Grown in Manipur. The Bioscan. 2010; 5: 113-115.
11. Sinha M, Mukherjee BP, Mukherjee B, Sikdar S, Dasgupta SR. Study of the Mechanism of action of Curcumin; an Antiulcer Agent. Ind J Pharmacol. 1975; 7: 98-102.
12. Niranjan A, Dhan P, Tewari SK, Pandey A, Pushpangadan P, Prakash D. Chemistry of Curcuma spp. Cultivated on Sodic soil. J. Medicinal and Aromatic Plants Sciences. 2003; 25: 69-75.
13. Ruby AJ, Kuttan G, Dinesh Babu K, Rajasekharan KN, Kuttan R. Antitumor and Antioxidant Activity of Natural Curcuminoids. Cancer Lett. 1995; 94: 79-83.
14. Nasri H, Sahinfard N, Rafieian M, Rafieian S, Shirzad M, Turmeric: A Spice with Multifunctional Medicinal Properties. J Herb Med Pharmacol. 2014; 3(1): 5-8.
15. Ravindran PN, Nirmal Babu K, Sivaraman K. Turmeric. The Golden Spice of Life. In: Turmeric. The Genus Curcuma. Boca Raton, FL, USA: CRC Press; 2007. p. 1-14.
16. Chattopadhyay I, Biswas K, Bandyopadhyay U, Banerjee RK. Turmeric and Curcumin: Biologicalactions and Medicinal Applications. CurrSci Ind. 2004; 87: 44-53.
17. Ammon HP, Wahl MA. Pharmacology of *Curcuma longa*. Planta Med 1991; 57: 1-7.
18. Bernard GT, Esteban P, Christopher JS. Turmerones: Isolation from Turmeric and their Structure Determination. Chem Commun. 1982; 6: 363.
19. Priyadarsini KI. The Chemistry of Curcumin: From Extraction to Therapeutic Agent. *Molecules*. 2014; 19: 20091-20112. doi: 10.3390/molecules191220091.
20. Gupta SC. Patchva S, Aggarwal BB. Therapeutic Roles of Curcumin: Lessons Learned from Clinical Trials. *AAPS J*. 2013; 15: 195-218. doi: 10.1208/s12248-012-9432-8.
21. Aggarwal BB, Kumar A, Bharti AC. Anticancer Potential of Curcumin: Preclinical and Clinical Studies. *Anticancer Res*. 2003; 23: 363-398.
22. Hewlings SJ, Kalman DS. Curcumin: A Review of its' Effects on Human Health. Foods. 2017; 6(10): 92. doi: 10.3390/foods6100092

Index

❐ ❐ ❐ ❐ ❐